SCHIZOPHRENIA AND PSYCHOTIC SPECTRUM DISORDERS

Primer on Series

Anxiety Disorders
Kerry J. Ressler, Daniel S. Pine, Barbara Olasov Rothbaum

Autism Spectrum Disorder
Christopher J. McDougle

SCHIZOPHRENIA AND PSYCHOTIC SPECTRUM DISORDERS

Edited by

S. Charles Schulz, MD

Professor Emeritus
Department of Psychiatry
University of Minnesota Medical School

Michael F. Green, PhD

Professor-in-Residence
Department of Psychiatry and Biobehavioral Sciences
Semel Institute for Neuroscience and Human Behavior
Geffen School of Medicine at University of California Los Angeles

Katharine J. Nelson, MD

Assistant Professor
Vice Chair for Education, Department of Psychiatry
Program Director, Psychiatry Residency
University of Minnesota Medical School

OXFORD
UNIVERSITY PRESS

OXFORD
UNIVERSITY PRESS

Oxford University Press is a department of the University of Oxford. It furthers the University's objective of excellence in research, scholarship, and education by publishing worldwide. Oxford is a registered trade mark of Oxford University Press in the UK and certain other countries.

Published in the United States of America by Oxford University Press
198 Madison Avenue, New York, NY 10016, United States of America.

Library of Congress Cataloging-in-Publication Data
Schizophrenia and Psychotic Spectrum Disorders / edited by S. Charles Schulz, Michael F. Green, Katharine J. Nelson.
p.; cm. — (Primer on series)
Includes bibliographical references.
ISBN 978–0–19–937806–7 (alk. paper)
I. Schulz, S. Charles, editor. II. Green, Michael Foster, editor. III. Nelson, Katharine J., editor.
IV. Series: Primer on.
[DNLM: 1. Schizophrenia. WM 203]
RC514
616.89′8—dc23
2015035271

9 8 7 6 5 4 3 2 1
Printed by Webcom, Canada

CONTENTS

FOREWORD

People with mental illnesses have long been marginalized or misunderstood. The primary focus of this volume is to explore essential aspects of schizophrenia and other disorders on the psychosis spectrum based on the scientific literature describing the pathophysiology, symptoms, approach to accurate diagnosis, and treatment. Multiple disciplines engage in care of people with schizophrenia and related disorders. Learning about these disorders and the impact on people and our communities can lead to better outcomes and comfort for people with mental illnesses and their families.

It is through the continued understanding of the pathophysiology, phenomenology, intervention, and shaping of community and societal attitudes that we can advance the quality of life and reduce the suffering for those impacted by schizophrenia.

CONTRIBUTORS

Sue Abderholden, MPH
Executive Director, NAMI Minnesota (National Alliance on Mental Illness)
Saint Paul, MN, USA

Afshan Anjum, MD
Department of Psychiatry
University of Minnesota
Minneapolis, MN, USA

Wanlop Atsariyasing, MD
Department of Psychiatry
Faculty of Medicine Siriraj Hospital, Mahidol University
Bangkok, Thailand

Krista Baker, LCPC
Clinical Supervisor
Early Psychosis Intervention Clinic and Adult Schizophrenia Clinic
Johns Hopkins Bayview
Baltimore, MD, USA

Donald W. Black, MD
Department of Psychiatry
University of Iowa Roy J. and Lucille A. Carver College of Medicine
Iowa City, IA, USA

Morris D. Bell, PhD
Department of Psychiatry
Yale University School of Medicine
New Haven, CT, USA
Rehabilitation Research and Development, Department of Veterans Affairs
VA Connecticut Healthcare System
West Haven, CT, USA

Tyrone D. Cannon, PhD
Department of Psychology
Department of Psychiatry Yale University
New Haven, CT, USA

Ryan Coon, MD
Department of Psychiatry
University of Minnesota
Minneapolis, MN, USA

Eric A. Epping, MD, PhD
Department of Psychiatry
University of Iowa Carver College of Medicine
Iowa City, IA, USA

S. Hossein Fatemi, MD, PhD
Departments of Psychiatry and Neuroscience
University of Minnesota Medical School
Minneapolis, MN, USA

Robert Findling, MD, MBA
Leonard and Helen R. Stulman Professor in Child and Adolescent Psychiatry
Kennedy Krieger Institute
The Johns Hopkins Hospital
Baltimore, MD, USA

Timothy D. Folsom, MS
Departments of Psychiatry and Neuroscience
University of Minnesota Medical School
Minneapolis, MN, USA

Rebecca Fortgang, PhD
Department of Psychology
Yale University
New Haven, CT, USA

Oliver Freudenreich, MD, FAPM
Associate Professor of Psychiatry
Medical Director, Massachusetts General Hospital Schizophrenia Program
Erich Lindemann Mental Health Center
Harvard Medical School
Boston, MA, USA

Kathryn M. Gill, PhD
Department of Neuroscience
University of Pittsburgh
Pittsburgh, PA, USA

Morris Goldman, MD
Department of Psychiatry
Feinberg School of Medicine
Northwestern University
Chicago, IL, USA

Sherilyn Goldstone, PhD
Orygen, the National Centre of Excellence in Youth Mental Health
Parkville, Australia

Anthony A. Grace, PhD
Department of Neuroscience
University of Pittsburgh
Pittsburgh, PA, USA

Michael F. Green, PhD
Department of Psychiatry and Biobehavioral Sciences
Semel Institute for Neuroscience and Human Behavior
Geffen School of Medicine at University of California Los Angeles
Los Angeles, CA, USA

Robert Haight, PharmD, BCPP
University of Minnesota Medical Center
Minneapolis, MN, USA

Jonathan Homans, MD
Department of Psychiatry
University of Minnesota
Minneapolis, MN, USA

Carolyn Howell, MD
Division of Child and Adolescent Psychiatry
Department of Psychiatry
Johns Hopkins University Hospital
Baltimore, MD, USA

Kumail Hussain, MD
Rush University Medical Center
Chicago, IL, USA

Philip G. Janicak, MD
Psychiatric Clinical Research Center
Rush University Medical Center
Chicago, IL, USA

Suzanne Jasberg, MD
Department of Psychiatry
University of Minnesota
Minneapolis, MN, USA

Alex Kopelowicz, MD
Department of Psychiatry and Biobehavioral Sciences
David Geffen School of Medicine at University of California Los Angeles
Los Angeles, CA, USA

Matthew Kruse, MD
Department of Psychiatry
University of Minnesota
Minneapolis, MN, USA

Kelvin O. Lim, MD
Department of Psychiatry
University of Minnesota Medical School
Minneapolis, MN, USA

Angus W. MacDonald III, PhD
Department of Psychology
Department of Psychiatry
University of Minnesota
Minneapolis, MN, USA

Patrick D. McGorry, AO MD PhD FRCP FRANZCP
Orygen, the National Centre of Excellence in Youth Mental Health
Parkville, Australia

Stephen Miller, MD
University of Minnesota Medical Center
Minneapolis, MN, USA

Katharine J. Nelson, MD
Department of Psychiatry
University of Minnesota Medical School
Minneapolis, MN, USA

Tasha M. Nienow, PhD
Minneapolis Veterans Affairs Health Care System
Department of Psychiatry
University of Minnesota
Minneapolis, MN, USA

Laura Pientka, DO
Department of Psychiatry
University of Minnesota
Minneapolis, MN, USA

Ian S. Ramsay, PhD
Department of Psychology
University of Minnesota
Minneapolis, MN, USA

S. Charles Schulz, MD
Department of Psychiatry
University of Minnesota Medical School
Minneapolis, MN, USA

Naomi T. Tabak, PhD
Department of Psychology
University of California, Los Angeles
VA Greater Los Angeles Health care System
Los Angeles, CA, USA

Dawn I. Velligan, PhD
Department of Psychiatry
Division of Schizophrenia and Related Disorders
University of Texas Health Science Center
San Antonio, TX, USA

Amanda B. Zheutlin, PhD
Department of Psychology
Yale University
New Haven, CT, USA

PART I

BACKGROUND AND PHENOMENOLOGY

/// 1 /// OVERVIEW OF SCHIZOPHRENIA AND TREATMENT APPROACHES

MATTHEW KRUSE and S. CHARLES SCHULZ

INTRODUCTION

Schizophrenia is frequently cited as the most severe and disabling mental illness. With a lifetime risk of approximately 1 percent (McGrath, Saha, Chant, & Welham, 2008) and a chronic course associated with significant medical comorbidity, decreased life expectancy, and significant societal and economic costs, it ranks among the top causes of disability worldwide (Whiteford et al., 2013).

Schizophrenia is classified as a psychotic disorder, defined by the presence of at least two of the five following domains of symptoms:

1. Delusions: Fixed, false beliefs that do not respond to contrary evidence. Delusions may be further classified as *nonbizarre* or *bizarre*. A bizarre delusion describes a belief that is not considered plausible by a patient's culture or society. For example, a patient's avoidance of standing near windows for fear of being shot by a spaceship would be considered a bizarre delusion.
2. Hallucinations: The perception of an external stimulus without a stimulus actually being present. Hallucinations may occur via any of the five senses. Auditory hallucinations, the perception of an external voice distinct from internal thoughts, are commonly documented in schizophrenia.
3. Disorganized thought: Abnormality in logic or progression of ideas, often detected on interview through the patient's communication.

4. Disorganized behavior: Abnormal or excessive behaviors. Disorganized behavior may include symptoms of *catatonia,* a reduced or inappropriate reactivity that may include purposeless movement, prolonged posturing, or complete absence of speech and movement.
5. Negative symptoms: This domain broadly refers to the lack of features typical of healthy individuals. Negative symptoms may include blunting of affect, social withdrawal, and reduced speech.

The five symptom domains of psychotic disorders provide the current diagnostic basis of schizophrenia. The time course of symptoms, level of severity, and presence or absence of mood disturbance allow clinicians to distinguish schizophrenia from the other psychotic disorders, including schizoaffective disorder, substance-induced psychotic disorder, bipolar disorder with psychosis, and psychotic depression. The *Diagnostic and Statistical Manual of Mental Disorders,* 5th ed. (*DSM-5*) outlines specific criteria required for the diagnosis of schizophrenia (American Psychiatric Association, 2013).

Although diagnostic criteria for schizophrenia can be succinctly described, schizophrenia remains a mysterious illness that has puzzled researchers and physicians for hundreds of years. A brief historical summary is now presented to describe our evolution in understanding of schizophrenia and to highlight the questions that, to this day, remain unanswered. Chapter 2 contains more information and a case discussion regarding the diagnosis of schizophrenia and related disorders.

HISTORICAL PERSPECTIVES

Vague descriptions of "madness" that likely represent psychotic illness can be found among some of the earliest medical literature. Imprecise phenomenology, however, has created an ongoing debate about whether schizophrenia was common before the nineteenth century. Medical historians often cite case studies by John Haslam (1764–1844) and Philippe Pinel (1745–1826), both published in 1809, as the first reliable accounts of schizophrenia (Heinrichs, 2003).

Haslam described the case of James Tilly Matthews, a British tea merchant committed to the asylum in Bethlem Hospital. In response to Matthews' families assertions that he was sane, Haslam, the hospital apothecary, chronicled Matthews' delusions and hallucinations, which closely mimic the current diagnostic criteria of paranoid schizophrenia (Howard, 2001).

Throughout much of the nineteenth century, few physicians drew a distinction between psychotic disorders. The variations in presentation of psychosis were thought to reflect the different stages of a single disease process. The *unitary psychosis* model remained prevalent until Emil Kraepelin (1856–1926), a German psychiatrist, proposed a new classification for psychotic disorders (Angst, 2002). Kraepelin argued that, although definitive diagnostic tests remained elusive, the natural course and ultimate outcomes of a psychotic illness could help distinguish distinct disorders. His work in the late 1800s introduced the *Kraepelinian dichotomy,* which distinguished *dementia praecox* ("premature dementia"), a chronic disease of progressive functional deterioration beginning in adolescence or young adulthood, and *manic-depressive insanity,* a relapsing and remitting psychosis analogous to the current diagnosis of bipolar disorder (Jablensky, 1999).

Eugen Bleuler (1857–1939) felt that Kraepelin's description of *dementia praecox* was problematic. He noted that some patients meeting criteria for this diagnosis had more mild courses of the illness. These patients often had later onset of illness and exhibited a less progressive course than was suggested by the term *dementia.* In 1908, Bleuler introduced the term *schizophrenia,* derived from Greek meaning "splitting of the mind." Bleuler's terminology reflected his theory of the illness as disconnected or even competing psychological processes, including thoughts and emotions. The frequent mischaracterization of schizophrenia as "multiple personality disorder," which still persists today, likely evolved from interpretations of Bleuler's theories (Moskowitz & Heim, 2011). Throughout his work, Bleuler often used the plural term "*the schizophrenias*" to suggest a family of distinct but related disorders, a concept that maintains relevance today (Jablensky, 2010).

Bleuler's conceptualization of schizophrenia identified several fundamental signs and symptoms that he considered unique to the illness. His fundamental symptoms of schizophrenia are often summarized as the 4 A's: flat or inappropriate *affect,* loosening of *associations, autism* (social withdrawal and preoccupation with one's own thoughts), and *ambivalence.* Although Bleuler classified the 4 A's as fundamental to schizophrenia, he believed the central pathology of schizophrenia was the splitting of psychological functions described earlier. Meanwhile, he considered psychotic symptoms, including delusions and hallucinations, to be secondary symptoms resulting from the splitting process, and less important for conception and diagnosis of the illness (Moskowitz & Heim, 2011).

Kurt Schneider (1887–1967) developed his own diagnostic criteria for schizophrenia. Based on his own observations of patients, he described a list of easily identifiable symptoms that would allow clinicians to diagnose schizophrenia. He referred to these symptoms as *first rank,* highlighting their importance in schizophrenia diagnosis. First-rank symptoms included auditory hallucinations, thought broadcasting (the delusion that others can hear an individual's thoughts), thought withdrawal (the delusion that thoughts have been taken out of an individual's mind). In contrast to Bleuler, Schneider's first-rank symptoms placed heavy emphasis on psychotic symptoms for diagnosis (Trimble, 1990).

DSM-I AND *DSM-II*

Despite advances in medical documentation and more reliable descriptions of schizophrenia, differing diagnostic methods prevailed worldwide throughout much of the twentieth century. Variability in diagnosis of schizophrenia among American psychiatrists became especially apparent and problematic when World War II forced collaboration between practitioners across the country. At that time, there was no standardized classification system for disease. It was unclear whether two clinicians describing schizophrenia were truly referring to the same illness (Andreasen, 1989).

In order for psychiatrists to communicate reliably, the Veterans Administration sought to establish a national standardized psychiatric nomenclature. The nomenclature standards implemented by the Armed Forces were ultimately amended by the American Psychiatric Association (APA) and published in 1952 as the *Diagnostic and Statistical Manual* of the American Psychiatric Association (*DSM-I*; Andreasen, 1989).

Despite efforts to standardize classification of schizophrenia, diagnosis of schizophrenia in the 1950s and 1960s, continued to be imprecise, particularly in the United States. The *DSM-I,* and later, the *DSM-II,* were strongly influenced by psychodynamic theory that dominated American psychiatry at the time. American psychiatrists believed that schizophrenia was a result of psychological conflict and disordered personality. They put little emphasis on psychotic symptoms for diagnosis, and instead based the diagnosis of schizophrenia on interpretation of psychodynamic conflict. Such diagnostic criteria could theoretically include nonpsychotic or even healthy individuals, raising the risk of overinclusive and unreliable diagnosis of schizophrenia (Andreasen, 1989; Mayes & Horwitz, 2005).

British psychiatrists, meanwhile, relied heavily on the presence of psychotic symptoms to diagnose schizophrenia. As might be expected, studies during the *DSM-I* and *DSM-II* eras suggested that American psychiatrists were much more likely to diagnose a patient with schizophrenia than a British colleague (Kendell et al., 1971).

DSM-III AND BEYOND

The wide variation in rates of schizophrenia diagnoses in the 1950s and 1960s was suspected to be due to unreliable and nonstandardized diagnostic criteria. In the early 1970s, the International Pilot Study of Schizophrenia (IPSS) examined the reliability of diagnostic signs and symptoms across nine separate countries to further standardize diagnostic criteria of schizophrenia. The findings of the IPSS recommended emphasis on the presence of psychotic symptoms for reliable schizophrenia diagnosis, reminiscent of Schneider's first-rank symptoms. The findings of the IPSS heavily influenced the *DSM-III*, published in 1980, which served as a stark departure from the *DSM-I* and *DSM-II*. In contrast to its predecessors, the *DSM-III* placed emphasis on objective psychotic features that could clearly distinguish schizophrenia from nonpsychotic disorders (Andreasen, 1989; Nordgaard, Arnfred, Handest, & Parnas, 2008).

The paradigm shift of the *DSM-III* has persisted through multiple revisions of the DSM to present day. Although a clear etiology or definitive diagnostic test for schizophrenia remains elusive, the *DSM-5* bases diagnosis on the time course and history of clearly identifiable symptoms, as described earlier in this introduction (APA, 2013).

EPIDEMIOLOGY

The epidemiology of schizophrenia has been of particular interest to investigators since the end of the nineteenth century for several reasons. First, a careful census of schizophrenia across regions and cultures might provide valuable clues for the heritable and environmental factors leading to illness. Second, such studies would reveal whether symptoms, course, and outcomes of schizophrenia were consistent across cultures, providing evidence for schizophrenia as valid diagnosis. Third, some scholars hypothesized that schizophrenia might be an illness unique to Western culture, a product of a developed industrial society. Epidemiological studies were the key to addressing these important issues, and to further understand this puzzling illness (Jablensky, 1997). Before reviewing the epidemiology of an illness, it is often best to start with a review of common epidemiological terms.

Common Epidemiological Terms:

Incidence: The risk of developing a disease within a given period.

Point Prevalence: The proportion of a population with a given disease at a specific time point.

Lifetime Prevalence: The proportion of a population with a given disease at any point in their lifetime at time of assessment.

Lifetime Morbid Risk: The proportion of a population that might become afflicted with a given disease at any point in their lifetime.

A review of the literature suggests schizophrenia has a median annual incidence of onset of approximately 0.15 per 1,000. Of note, there is a considerable range in incidence depending on the study and the methodology used. Meanwhile, point prevalence of schizophrenia has been estimated to be 4.6 per 1,000, period prevalence of 3.3 per 1,000, lifetime prevalence of 4.0 per 1,000, and lifetime morbid risk of 7.2 per 1,000 (McGrath et al., 2008).

Whether discussing incidence, prevalence, or lifetime morbid risk, the epidemiological studies of schizophrenia have demonstrated a striking range of values. Variation in findings may be due to several factors. As noted, the diagnostic criteria of schizophrenia has been a subject of ongoing debate long after the identification of the illness, and comparisons of diagnostic rates of schizophrenia in the 1960s demonstrated much higher rates of diagnosis among American psychiatrists than their European counterparts (Kendell et al., 1971).

The figures for incidence, prevalence, and morbid risk are compiled from many studies over time and across populations. As noted, however, the differences in rates of illness between settings and populations are an important concern. Although some hypothesized that schizophrenia may be a disease specific to industrialized societies, decades of population-specific study has been unable to identify any geographic regions with zero incidence of schizophrenia. In fact, incidence has been found to be relatively consistent worldwide, with variation commonly attributed to study methodology (Hafner & Heiden, 1997).

Prevalence, however, does seem to be lower in less industrialized and developing settings, and highest in urban settings. This pattern is not completely understood, but evidence suggests that less industrialized settings correlate with greater social support, particularly from closer-knit communities and closer ties with extended family. Greater levels of social support and smaller observable decline in function may promote a less severe course of illness with improved recovery, reducing the number meeting criteria for illness at any given time, and subsequently reducing prevalence (Padma, 2014). A broader discussion of epidemiology is found in Chapter 3.

COURSE OF ILLNESS

Kraepelin was one of the first investigators to emphasize the importance of understanding the natural course and outcome of schizophrenia. His term *dementia praecox* suggested an invariable course of cognitive decline. He furthermore believed that until specific etiology or a definitive marker for the disease could be elucidated, studying the course and outcome of the illness could help validate the diagnosis and separate it from similar illnesses, as he did when differentiating it from manic psychosis (Jablensky, 1999).

In contrast to Kraepelin's conception of *dementia praecox* as conferring a uniformly dire prognosis, decades of studies, both before and after widespread use of antipsychotic medication, have suggested that the course and outcome of schizophrenia can vary significantly, with a significant portion of patients achieving relatively robust reduction in symptoms and a greater recovery in function (van Os & Kapur, 2009). Milder courses of illness and more optimal outcomes are seen in both industrialized and developing countries, likely due to different factors. Industrialized countries may have greater access to antipsychotic medication and other evidence-based interventions known to improve the symptoms and course of schizophrenia. Developing and rural communities, meanwhile, may face fewer environmental stressors and greater social supports, factors shown to improve function and outcomes in schizophrenia (Padma, 2014).

INCREASED MORTALITY

Despite a milder course of illness in a substantial portion of patients with schizophrenia, it is important to note that the disease burden and outcome of schizophrenia is not limited to the psychotic and cognitive symptoms of the illness. Patients diagnosed with schizophrenia are expected to live 15 years less than individuals without serious mental illness. A portion of this average reduction in life expectancy can certainly be linked to increased rate of suicide. The risk of suicide in patients with schizophrenia is up to 12-fold higher than in the general population. Chapter 17 explores this relationship and an approach to clinical management in greater detail. Despite the high risk of suicide, patients with schizophrenia are noted to have decreased life expectancy even when correcting for suicide (Saha, Chant, & McGrath, 2007; Chesney, Goodwin, & Fazel, 2014).

Though incompletely understood, much of the increased mortality can be linked to comorbid medical problems, including diabetes, heart disease, and cancer, often related to poor self-care and lifestyle. Antipsychotic medications have additionally been linked to metabolic syndrome and diabetes, introducing some treatment-related causes for increased morbidity and mortality in schizophrenia. Accordingly, attention to medical comorbidities should be a regular component of management of schizophrenia (Saha et al., 2007; Chesney et al., 2014).

GENDER DIFFERENCES

Although available evidence suggests that morbid risk between males and females is equivalent at approximately 1 percent, some gender-specific patterns have been identified. The onset of schizophrenia in men has been shown to be somewhat bimodal, with a particularly high risk of onset between ages 20 and 25, and a second, smaller peak between 30 and 35 years. After age 35, the risk of new-onset schizophrenia diminishes gradually. Women, however, have average new-onset of illness five years later than men, with a second, smaller peak in incidence in the late 40s, correlating with menopause. In addition to a later onset of illness, evidence suggests that women, on average, may have a milder course of illness and better response to treatment. Current theories for this discrepancy have suggested a role for estrogen in regulation of dopamine (an important neurotransmitter implicated in the pathogenesis of psychotic disorders), but investigations are ongoing.

GENETICS

Schizophrenia is currently believed to result from a complex interaction of genetic and environmental factors. Whereas some disorders, such as cystic fibrosis, arise due to a variant in a single gene, schizophrenia is considered a complex genetic disorder, with susceptibility resulting from hundreds—if not more—genetic variants, each conferring a small risk of ultimately developing the illness. Jenny Koller's pioneering 1895 family aggregation study of psychiatric illness suggested that the heritability of psychotic disorders was particularly high. For the next several decades, however, there was significant concern that this heritability might arise from shared environment, including being raised among individuals with schizophrenia. Adoption studies, however, suggested that increased susceptibility persists even if raised in a home away from affected relatives, lending strong support for a genetic contribution to schizophrenia (Kety, Rosenthal, Wender, & Schulsinger, 1976). The genetic contribution to schizophrenia is further exemplified by rates of lifetime morbid risk of schizophrenia. In the general population, the risk is approximately 1 percent. Among individuals with a first-degree relative with schizophrenia, the lifetime risk rises to 6.5 percent, and individuals with an affected monozygotic twin have a risk to 40 percent.

Significant efforts have been made to identify genes that may confer a risk for development of schizophrenia. The search for candidate genes employs several strategies. One strategy, whole genome association studies (WGAS), examines millions of variants across the genome, and identifies which variants associate with higher frequency with an illness. Whole gene association studies are beneficial in identifying which regions of the genome (and associated genes) may confer a risk for developing an illness. Whole gene association studies for schizophrenia have identified many regions of the genome suspected to confer a risk for development of schizophrenia. Rarely, however, has any such region been consistently replicated.

A second strategy in the genetic study of schizophrenia relies on our knowledge of the etiology of schizophrenia to identify candidate genes a priori that may have an impact on systems implicated in its pathogenesis. Catechol-O-methyl transferase (COMT) continues to be one of the most studied of such genes. Catechol-O-methyl transferase is responsible for the degradation and inactivation of several neurotransmitters, including dopamine. Alteration in dopamine signaling has been implicated in the pathogenesis of schizophrenia, and indeed several studies have associated genetic variants in COMT with risk of schizophrenia.

Outside of common variants, rare genetic variants have additionally been associated with schizophrenia. These rare variants often involve either a duplication or deletion of some portion of the genome. Most individuals carry at least several rare duplications or deletions, but few ever become clinically relevant, as many are located in the large regions of the genome that do not contain any coded genes. When a duplication or deletion involves a coding gene, the phenotypic result may be quite large. One such deletion, occurring on chromosome 22, deletes one copy of the COMT gene. This deletion has been associated with velocardiofacial syndrome, a genetic syndrome associated with multiple features including cleft palate, heart defects, and an increased risk of schizophrenia. Rare insertions and deletions in the genome have additionally been associated with other psychiatric disorders, including autism and bipolar disorder.

The inconsistency of genetic findings combined with cases of rare duplication or deletion syndromes paint schizophrenia as a phenotypically similar but biologically heterogeneous illness, recalling Bleuler's use of the term "the schizophrenias." A full discussion of the role of genetics in schizophrenia is located in Chapter 8.

NEUROPATHOLOGY AND BRAIN IMAGING

Though the diagnosis of schizophrenia has been revised extensively over the past 100 years, diagnosis still continues to be based on a patient's signs and symptoms. Former theories that schizophrenia was a product of psychological conflict have fallen out of favor among the medical community, and it is accepted that schizophrenia is an organic illness with a neuropathological etiology.

The hypothesis that schizophrenia is an organic brain disease has been present since the 1800s. Ewald Hecker noted an increased ventricle size in psychotic patients in 1871. Kraepelin was aware of the findings of Paul Broca and Carl Wernicke, consistently correlating specific brain lesions with specific cognitive or neurological deficits. Kraepelin believed that such a defining lesion might be associated with *dementia praecox*. During his career, Kraepelin reported several anatomical variants in post-mortem brain studies of patients with *dementia praecox*. Unfortunately, none of the early neuropathological findings from the early twentieth century have been consistently replicated (Weinberger, Wagner, & Wyatt, 1983).

In 1919, neurosurgeon Walter Dandy introduced pneumoencephalography (PEG), an imaging technique that replaces the cerebrospinal fluid (CSF) with a gas to enhance the clarity of brain structures on X-ray. After its introduction, PEG studies in patients with schizophrenia identified several findings, including a replication of Hecker's findings of increased ventricular size (Knable & Weinberger, 1995).

These initial findings of the PEG studies were later replicated by computed tomography (CT), the majority of which did show increased ventricular size in patients with schizophrenia. Attempts were made to correlate the degree of ventricular enlargement to clinical phenotype. Though some studies found a correlation of ventricular size with cognitive impairment, poor response to treatment, and more negative symptoms, the true clinical or etiological significance of enlarged ventricles remains elusive.

The next major leap in neuroimaging studies in schizophrenia came with the introduction of magnetic resonance imaging (MRI). Whereas PEG and CT primarily distinguish tissue of varied density (e.g., bone versus soft tissue), MRI introduced the ability to distinguish soft tissues, greatly increasing the information obtainable on imaging studies. MRI studies in schizophrenia have unveiled a great number of structural brain changes correlated with schizophrenia. Whereas MRI studies allowed for the distinction between soft tissues, diffusion tensor imaging (DTI) allows for brain imaging in even greater detail. Diffusion tensor imaging measures the flow of water within brain cells, allowing for the imaging of distinct tracts of neurons within the brain.

An important takeaway from decades of imaging studies is that although early investigators such as Kraepelin and Bleuler believed a large, characteristic lesion would eventually be identified and associated with schizophrenia, it is now accepted that the anatomical and structural differences in the brains of those with schizophrenia are widespread, varied, and subtle, explaining the inconclusive and conflicting findings of the early neuropathology studies. Nevertheless, the advancement in imaging technology allows researchers more powerful tools to detect the subtle structural and connectivity variants characteristic of schizophrenia.

FUNCTIONAL IMAGING

Although the imaging modalities described demonstrate an ever-growing ability to image brain structures and connections in greater detail, functional imaging additionally plays a key role in elucidating neuropathology of schizophrenia and psychotic disorders. As opposed to demonstrating static information about brain structures, functional imaging allows for the visualization of activity of brain structures in real time. Important functional imaging technologies include positron emission tomography

(PET), single photon emission computed tomography (SPECT), and functional magnetic resonance imaging (fMRI).

Early functional imaging demonstrated decreased frontal lobe activity in patients with schizophrenia as compared to controls. The consistency of this finding increased when patients with schizophrenia were further stratified into subgroups: for instance, reduced frontal lobe activity was more frequently found in individuals further into the course of illness than individuals at onset of illness. Other functional studies correlated decreased frontal lobe action with poorer performance on tasks that require executive function, including the Wisconsin Card Sorting Test (WISC), a task on which individuals with schizophrenia typically perform poorly.

Additional subgroups of schizophrenia have additionally yielded distinct patterns in brain function. The domains of hallucinations and delusions, disorganized thought, and negative symptoms have all been linked to specific regional alterations in brain activity, lending support for Bleuler's description of "the schizophrenias" as a related but heterogeneous group of disorders. Chapter 9 provides greater details regarding advances neuroimaging.

NEUROTRANSMITTERS

Although brain architecture, connectivity, and activity have all been implicated in the pathogenesis of schizophrenia, abnormalities in neurotransmitter systems have additionally been studied in the search for understanding the illness.

The first neurotransmitter hypothesis of schizophrenia can be traced back to the 1940s. In 1947, chlorpromazine was developed as a new antihistamine for use in sedation for surgery. Early trials with the drug showed that in addition to expected sedation and indifference, rats who were administered chlorpromazine reacted less to aversive stimuli. It was hypothesized that a sedating drug might be helpful in controlling the agitation frequently observed in psychotic patients in asylums. Unexpectedly, the first trials of chlorpromazine in asylums in the 1950s produced a reduction in psychotic symptoms, including hallucinations and delusions. Until that time, no useful intervention had been identified to manage psychotic symptoms, and treatment had been focused merely on control of agitation. For the first time, treatment of psychotic symptoms was possible.

Chlorpromazine was not without side effects. Most commonly, it induced symptoms resembling Parkinson's disease, including dystonia and decreased movement. Animal studies eventually demonstrated that antipsychotic activity and Parkinsonism were both linked to the antidopaminergic activity of chlorpromazine and related compounds. This insight led to the dopamine hypothesis of schizophrenia: excessive dopamine activity produces psychosis. The dopamine hypothesis was further supported by observations that dopaminergic drugs, including cocaine and amphetamine, worsened psychotic symptom.

The original dopamine hypothesis of schizophrenia suggested that excess dopamine signaling was responsible for schizophrenia. Although dopamine is still implicated in schizophrenia's pathogenesis, its role is now considered far more nuanced and complex due to several observations. Not all patients treated with dopamine blockers experience resolution of psychotic symptoms. Among those that do respond to antipsychotic medications, many have enduring negative symptoms, which may even worsen with treatment with dopamine blockers. New insights into the dopamine system also note significant heterogeneity in dopamine receptors: at least five have been identified, each with distinct distribution and function in the brain.

Though dopamine continues to be the focus of much of the neurotransmitter research in schizophrenia, other neurotransmitters have been suspected to play a role in schizophrenia. Many serotonergic hallucinogens manage to produce psychotomimetic effects via activation of serotonin 2A receptors. Indeed, many current antipsychotic medications have antagonistic effects at these very receptors. Notably, serotonin transmission has regulatory effects on other neurotransmitter systems, including dopamine, glutamate, norepinephrine, and GABA.

Glutamate has additionally been implicated in the pathogenesis of schizophrenia. Similar to serotonergic hallucinogens, glutamate antagonists, including phencyclidine and ketamine, are additionally capable of producing psychosis-like states.

In conclusion, the story of neurotransmitters in schizophrenia continues to evolve. Although dopamine continues to be of primary focus in much of the literature, the symptoms of schizophrenia are likely impacted by the complex interaction of multiple, if not all, neurotransmitter systems. Chapters 10 and 11 provide an in-depth discussion of neurotransmitters and neuropeptides.

ENVIRONMENTAL FACTORS

If genetic susceptibility alone does not predict who will develop schizophrenia, as evidenced by monozygotic twin concordance far from 100 percent, the question lingers about which environmental factors might impact the development of schizophrenia. Studies have found several environmental associations, including marijuana use, exposure to urban environments, in utero insults, and psychosocial stressors. Few, if any, identified environmental factors have established themselves as causal links. Instead, the development of schizophrenia is likely the result of a complex interaction between environmental factors and an individual's genes (both predisposing and protective).

One such gene/environment interaction was demonstrated by Caspi et al. (2005), which showed that adolescents carrying at least one Val allele of the COMT gene who additionally used marijuana before the age 15 had an increased risk of psychosis later in life. This increased risk of psychosis disappeared if adolescents had no exposure to marijuana before age 15, or even if they were exposed to marijuana, but not until later in life.

Additional environmental factors have been associated with risk of schizophrenia, including urban environments, childhood trauma, and maternal viral infection during pregnancy. Although the debate of whether specific environmental factors represent correlation or causation for schizophrenia is ongoing, evidence is strong that schizophrenia represents a complex and subtle interplay between the environment and innate susceptibility that may never be completely understood.

NEUROCOGNITION

The field of neurocognition describes how specific pathways of the brain process data and allow for the broad range of tasks required for day-to-day functioning, including attention, learning, memory, and reasoning. A neurocognitive deficit is impairment in any of these functions, often occurring after an insult such as neurologic illness, brain injury, or mental illness.

Primary diagnostic symptoms of schizophrenia include delusions, hallucinations, disorganization, and negative symptoms. Neurocognitive deficits, meanwhile, are important factors contributing to the impaired functioning of individuals with schizophrenia, such as an average reduction in educational and vocational achievement. Even when the primary psychotic symptoms are managed with antipsychotic medication, neurocognitive deficits persist.

The neurocognitive deficits noted in schizophrenia are broad (virtually all areas of neurocognitive tasks have been shown to be impaired in schizophrenia) and are relatively stable over the entire course of illness with little correlation with psychotic symptom severity. In some patients, neurocognitive deficits are measurable before the first onset of psychosis, even in childhood, and worsen during the onset of the illness. In other patients, deficits only manifest at the onset of psychosis or during the prodromal phase. Virtually all domains of cognitive performance are affected, including processing speed, attention, memory, social cognition, and executive function. Across the population of those with schizophrenia, approximately a quarter will not register as impaired on neurocognitive assessment. Those individuals, however, still score lower on a neurocognitive battery than would be predicted based on their premorbid levels of functioning and functional levels of their parents.

The hypothesis that the distracting presence of psychotic symptoms, such as hallucinations, is responsible for the deficits in memory, attention, and executive function has been largely dismissed. Instead, such symptoms are likely a product of the neurologic and biochemical abnormalities present in schizophrenia. Hence, understanding the neurocognitive deficits in schizophrenia may allow for newer insights into the pathogenesis of the illness. In addition, as the neurocognitive deficits in schizophrenia have a considerable impact on the functional outcomes of patients with schizophrenia (Green, 1996), interventions to improve cognitive function may provide a new treatment modality that improves function and, ultimately, quality of life. Such issues and remedial therapies will be discussed further in Chapters 7 and 15.

INTRODUCTORY INFORMATION ON TREATMENT

The introduction of chlorpromazine, the first antipsychotic medication, served as an important paradigm shift in the treatment of schizophrenia. Prior to antipsychotic medication, treatment of schizophrenia focused on management of agitation, with heavy use of sedating medications, prolonged hospitalization, and risky experimental treatments including insulin-induced coma and prefrontal lobotomy. None of these treatments ever gained a strong evidence basis for their usefulness, and were abandoned quickly after chlorpromazine's antipsychotic effects were discovered. Not long after the introduction of chlorpromazine, additional antipsychotic medications were developed, including haloperidol and fluphenazine, known as first-generation antipsychotics (FGAs).

Although effective in managing psychotic symptoms, these medications were associated with significant side effects, notably extrapyramidal symptoms (EPS). Extrapyramidal sympotms may include akathisia (an uncomfortable and at times unbearable sensation of restlessness compelling an individual to continually move), dystonia, or Parkinsonism (including tremor and rigidity). Extrapyramidal symptoms can occur at any time, including immediately after starting an antipsychotic medication.

In addition to EPS, antipsychotic medications may produce tardive dyskinesia (TD), a side effect of abnormal and involuntary movements. The term "tardive" reflects that, unlike EPS, it typically has a slow or delayed onset after initiation of medication, and "dyskinesia" refers to abnormal, involuntary body movements. The most common manifestation of TD is oral and facial, including tongue protrusion, lip puckering, or grimacing. In severe cases, TD can affect the trunk and limbs, significantly reducing quality of life and functionality. Unlike EPS, which tend to resolve when the inciting medication is discontinued, TD was typically noted to persist indefinitely, even after cessation of antipsychotic treatment. Over time, individuals treated with an FGA have a 20 to 30 percent chance of developing TD, with 5 percent of young patients treated with FGAs developing TD each year. Patients with organic brain injury and advanced age are at higher risk for developing TD.

Clozapine is an antipsychotic medication introduced and studied in the 1960s. Unlike the FGAs in use at the time, clozapine did not have the typical association with EPS. Since the link between antipsychotic medication and EPS was so high, some worried that clozapine's lack of EPS indicated a lack of antipsychotic efficacy. Surprisingly, trials indicated that clozapine not only had antipsychotic activity but was even effective in treatment-resistant patients. After investigation and introduction in Europe, clozapine was noted in the 1970s to carry a risk for producing agranulocytosis, a potentially lethal reduction in white blood cells that led to the deaths of several patients. This side effect delayed its approval in the United States until 1990, and was indicated only for treatment-resistant patients. Approximately 0.3 percent of patients taking clozapine will develop agranulocytosis within the first year, and clozapine therapy still requires regular blood draws to monitor white blood cell counts.

Aside from agranulocytosis, additional side effects of clozapine may include seizures, myocarditis, and weight gain. Nevertheless, its efficacy in managing psychotic symptoms remains unparalleled, and continues to be a mainstay in treatment-refractory patients.

Options for antipsychotic medication did not change much until the 1990s when newer antipsychotic medications were introduced, including risperidone, olanzapine, quetiapine, aripiprazole, and others. These newer medications were labeled atypical antipsychotics, or second-generation antipsychotics (SGAs).

Though SGAs are similar to FGAs in efficacy in treating psychotic symptoms, SGAs differ from FGAs in their side-effect profile. Both generations of medications bind to D2 dopamine receptors, but SGAs tend to bind less tightly and dissociate from these receptors more quickly, allowing for a greater level of normal dopamine transmission via these receptors. As D2 blockade is responsible for mediating the EPS and Parkinsonian symptoms associated with antipsychotic medications, SGAs are associated with lower rates (but not absence) of these side effects. SGAs are additionally associated with a lower rate of TD.

Although producing fewer movement side effects, SGAs, particularly olanzapine and quetiapine, are associated with metabolic side effects, including risk for weight gain, diabetes, and dyslipidemia. Chapter 13 contains a broad discussion on medication treatment strategies.

Prevention of relapse of psychotic symptoms is an important indicator for the prognostic outcome in schizophrenia. Accordingly, much time has been invested in identifying strategies to improve consistent engagement in care. Unfortunately, medication nonadherence is high in people with schizophrenia, significantly raising the risk of relapse of psychotic symptoms. One method for improving medication adherence has been the introduction of long-acting injectable antipsychotics (LAIs). As opposed to oral medications, which require once- or twice-daily administration, LAIs require a shot only once every two or four weeks. Multiple FGAs and SGAs, including haloperidol, fluphenazine, and risperidone, are available in LAI form. Though many patients prefer oral medications because of the pain associated with an injection or the inconvenience of traveling to a clinic to receive an injection, LAIs remain an option that should be considered, particularly if the risk of medication nonadherence is high (Kishimoto et al., 2014). Chapter 14 discusses various approaches to improving treatment adherence in schizophrenia.

COMPREHENSIVE TREATMENT

Antipsychotic medications are effective in managing positive psychotic symptoms of schizophrenia. Medications alone, however, are not sufficient for optimizing the clinical course of schizophrenia for multiple reasons, including:

1. Patients with schizophrenia often discontinue taking antipsychotic medication against medical advice, increasing the risk of symptom exacerbation and repeat hospitalizations.
2. Even with stable antipsychotic treatment, negative symptoms and neurocognitive deficits persist regardless of antipsychotic treatment, limiting the educational and vocational potential of affected individuals (Green, 1996).
3. Among populations with schizophrenia, lack of insurance or prohibitive out-of-pocket costs frequently prevent regular access to mental health services and medical care.
4. Longer periods of untreated psychosis and irregular contact with providers have been associated with poorer clinical and functional outcomes (Polari et al., 2011).
5. Patients in developing countries often have better outcomes than in industrialized settings, even with less access to antipsychotic medications, suggesting strong social support may improve prognosis.

These insights have led investigators to seek proactive, multifaceted interventions to improve the outcome in serious mental illness. The 1984 Buckingham study was one of the first programs to examine the benefits of early, comprehensive intervention in psychosis. It employed several key strategies including case management, supportive psychotherapy, education for patients and families, and cognitive-behavioral therapy. In the decades since, programs adopting similar strategies, often referred to as first episode of psychosis (FEP) programs, have been established. First episode of psychosis programs are specialized multidisciplinary programs that seek optimization of long-term outcomes in schizophrenia by promoting early recognition of new-onset psychosis, initiating prompt treatment, and employing multifaceted strategies to improve functioning and treatment adherence. The specific resources and structure of FEP programs varies by site, but several modalities are frequently used.

Assertive community treatment (ACT) teams are collaborations among multiple providers, including psychiatrists and social workers, and provide proactive, comprehensive community care to patients. Though pharmacotherapy is provided, the ACT model places additional emphasis on strengthening a patient's support network, coordination of social services, and maintenance of regular contact with providers. Though the ACT model does employ a higher level of outpatient care, it is intended primarily for patients at risk for disengagement from treatment and multiple hospitalizations. The hypothesis that ACT teams can improve medication adherence, reduce emergency department visits, and shorten hospital stays has been supported in the literature.

Even with appropriate antipsychotic medications, many with schizophrenia experience a reduction, but not elimination, of psychotic symptoms. Cognitive behavioral therapy (CBT) provides a thorough evaluation of a patient's residual symptoms and helps a patient develop coping strategies to manage them. In addition to symptom management, CBT may also be employed to improve social skills. Though evidence has been inconsistent, there is compelling evidence that a 4–9 month course of individual or group CBT may reduce severity of both positive and negative symptoms (Wykes, Steel, Everitt, & Tarrier, 2008).

The symptoms and disability associated with schizophrenia can be distressing not only for patients, but also for his or her family members, and may even put a strain on familial relationships. In addition, a strong support network may improve the course and outcomes of schizophrenia. For these reasons, interventions including education, therapy, and training have been recommended for family members and significant others of people with schizophrenia. The length of these interventions may vary and the services provided may be tailored to the family's specific needs. Family-based services have been shown to be beneficial for patients, with improved treatment adherence and vocational outcomes. Families additionally benefit from this modality, noting reduced distress and improved relationships. Chapter 16 explores family therapy and its role in schizophrenia treatment.

Even when an antipsychotic medication produces substantial symptomatic benefit, the virtually universal neurocognitive deficits remain, contributing substantially to the reduced educational and vocational function in schizophrenia. Cognitive rehabilitation seeks to limit the impact of cognitive deficits through nonpharmacological interventions. Some approaches are compensatory, and improve function by assessing a patient's specific deficit, and altering the patient's home or work environment to minimize the sources of difficulty he or she may encounter. Remediation, meanwhile, uses specialized tasks and exercises (often computerized) to improve cognitive abilities. Variations in the specific rehabilitation programs likely contribute to the mixed evidence supporting this intervention, but meta-analysis has suggested this intervention may improve cognition and function in patients with schizophrenia.

CONCLUSION

The history of schizophrenia is rich and filled with mystery. Though current understanding of schizophrenia, including its etiology, pathogenesis, and treatment, has evolved considerably over the past 100 years, many puzzles remain. In sum, evidence points to schizophrenia as a complex, and likely heterogeneous, disease of the brain, resulting from a complex interaction of innate susceptibility and environmental factors, involving multiple neurotransmitter systems and virtually all brain structures. As research in neurobiology, genetics, and epidemiology continues to progress at an astonishing rate, application of such knowledge may usher in newer and better interventions, ultimately reducing global burden and improving outcomes of schizophrenia.

REFERENCES

American Psychiatric Association. (2013). *DSM-5. Diagnostic and statistical manual of mental disorders* (5th edition). Arlington, VA: American Psychiatric Publishing.

Andreasen, N. C. (1989). The American concept of schizophrenia. *Schizophrenia Bulletin, 15*(4), 519–531.

Angst, J. (2002). Historical aspects of the dichotomy between manic-depressive disorders and schizophrenia. *Schizophrenia Research, 57*(1), 5–13.

Caspi, A., Moffitt, T. E., Cannon, M., McClay, J., Murray, R., Harrington, H., . . . Craig, I. W. (2005). Moderation of the effect of adolescent-onset cannabis use on adult psychosis by a functional polymorphism in the catechol-O-methyltransferase gene: longitudinal evidence of a gene X environment interaction. *Biological Psychiatry, 57*(10), 1117–1127.

Chesney, E., Goodwin, G., & Fazel, S. (2014). Risks of all-cause and suicide mortality in mental disorders: a meta-review. *World Psychiatry, 13*, 153–160.

Green, M. (1996). What are the functional consequences of neurocognitive deficits in schizophrenia? *The American Journal of Psychiatry* (March), 321–330.

Hafner, H. & Heiden, W. (1997). Epidemiology of schizophrenia. *The Canadian Journal of Psychiatry, 42,* 139–151.

Heinrichs, R. W. (2003). Historical origins of schizophrenia: two early madmen and their illness. *Journal of the History of the Behavioral Sciences, 39*(4), 349–363.

Howard, R. (2001). Psychiatry in pictures. *The British Journal of Psychiatry, 179*(3), 0–1.

Jablensky, A. (1997). The 100-year epidemiology of schizophrenia. *Schizophrenia Research, 28*(2–3), 111–125.

Jablensky, A. (1999). The conflict of the nosologists: views on schizophrenia and manic-depressive illness in the early part of the 20th century. *Schizophrenia Research, 39*(2), 95–100.

Jablensky, A. (2010). The diagnostic concept of schizophrenia: its history, evolution, and future prospects. *Dialogues in Clinical Neuroscience,* 271–287.

Kendell, R. E., Cooper, J. E., Gourlay, A. J., Copeland, J. R., Sharpe, L., & Gurland, B. J. (1971). Diagnostic criteria of American and British psychiatrists. *Archives of General Psychiatry, 25*(2), 123–130.

Kety, S. S., Rosenthal, D., Wender, P. H., & Schulsinger, F. (1976). Studies based on a total sample of adopted individuals and their relatives: why they were necessary, what they demonstrated and failed to demonstrate. *Schizophrenia Bulletin, 2*(3), 413–428.

Kishimoto, T., Robenzadeh, A., Leucht, C., Leucht, S., Watanabe, K., Mimura, M., . . . Correll, C. U. (2014). Long-acting injectable vs oral antipsychotics for relapse prevention in schizophrenia: a meta-analysis of randomized trials. *Schizophrenia Bulletin, 40*(1), 192–213.

Knable, M. B., & Weinberger, D. R. (1995). Are mental diseases brain diseases? The contribution of neuropathology to understanding of schizophrenic psychoses. *European Archives of Psychiatry and Clinical Neuroscience, 245*(4–]5), 224–230.

Mayes, R., & Horwitz, A. V. (2005). *DSM-III* and the revolution in the classification of mental illness. *Journal of the History of the Behavioral Sciences, 41*(3), 249–267.

McGrath, J., Saha, S., Chant, D., & Welham, J. (2008). Schizophrenia: a concise overview of incidence, prevalence, and mortality. *Epidemiologic Reviews, 30,* 67–76.

Moskowitz, A., & Heim, G. (2011). Eugen Bleuler's Dementia praecox or the group of schizophrenias (1911): a centenary appreciation and reconsideration. *Schizophrenia Bulletin, 37*(3), 471–479.

Nordgaard, J., Arnfred, S. M., Handest, P., & Parnas, J. (2008). The diagnostic status of first-rank symptoms. *Schizophrenia Bulletin, 34*(1), 137–154.

Padma, T. (2014). Developing countries: The outcomes paradox. *Nature, 508*(7494).

Polari, A., Lavoie, S., Sarrasin, P., Pellanda, V., Cotton, S., & Conus, P. (2011). Duration of untreated psychosis: a proposition regarding treatment definition. *Early Intervention in Psychiatry, 5*(4), 301–308.

Saha, S., Chant, D., & McGrath, J. (2007). A systematic review of mortality in schizophrenia: is the differential mortality gap worsening over time? *Archives of General Psychiatry, 64*(10), 1123–1131.

Trimble, M. R. (1990). First-rank symptoms of Schneider. A new perspective? *The British Journal of Psychiatry, 156*(2), 195–200.

Van Os, J., & Kapur, S. (2009). Schizophrenia. *Lancet, 374*(9690), 635–645.

Weinberger, D. R., Wagner, R. L., & Wyatt, R. J. (1983). Neuropathological studies of schizophrenia: a selective review. *Schizophrenia Bulletin, 9*(2), 193–212.

Whiteford, H. a, Degenhardt, L., Rehm, J., Baxter, A. J., Ferrari, A. J., Erskine, H. E., . . . Vos, T. (2013). Global burden of disease attributable to mental and substance use disorders: findings from the Global Burden of Disease Study 2010. *Lancet, 382*(9904), 1575–1586.

Wykes, T., Steel, C., Everitt, B., & Tarrier, N. (2008). Cognitive behavior therapy for schizophrenia: effect sizes, clinical models, and methodological rigor. *Schizophrenia Bulletin, 34*(3), 523–537.

/// 2 /// CLINICAL DIAGNOSIS AND DIFFERENTIAL DIAGNOSIS OF SCHIZOPHRENIA

OLIVER FREUDENREICH

In this chapter, we will review the clinical approach to the diagnosis of schizophrenia or a related schizophrenia spectrum disorder. We will discuss the differential diagnosis of psychosis and the diagnostic assessments needed to distinguish between primary and secondary causes of psychosis. This chapter contains guidance about how to comprehensively evaluate patients beyond the bare bones of establishing that diagnostic criteria for schizophrenia have been met. Diagnostic criteria such as those of the American Psychiatric Association (i.e., *DSM-5;* 2013) or the World Health Organization (i.e., *ICD-10;* 1993) are important for physicians in order to speak a common language; they cannot capture the heterogeneity of schizophrenia as a syndrome, with regard to either psychiatric symptomatology and societal function or medical and psychiatric comorbidities.

CLINICAL APPROACH TO DIAGNOSIS

The basis for a diagnosis of schizophrenia is a comprehensive history, the physical examination, and ancillary laboratory studies. In addition to the cross-sectional patient interview and examination, collateral information from friends, family members, or other sources is needed to determine how symptoms evolved over time and to obtain a complete symptom inventory. The longitudinal history combined with cross-sectional data provides the clinical information needed for a differential diagnosis and a working diagnosis of schizophrenia. Although schizophrenia is often referred to as a diagnosis of exclusion (i.e., it is only diagnosed in the absence of medical diseases or substances that could account for the psychosis), it is still diagnosed based on the presence of characteristic psychiatric symptoms and illness course, just like any other medical-neurological disease. However, merely making a categorical diagnosis of schizophrenia without further delineating relevant symptom dimensions, functional abilities, and medical comorbidities is insufficient for treatment planning. The next sections of this chapter will provide details regarding the differential diagnosis of psychosis and the comprehensive assessment of schizophrenia.

DIFFERENTIAL DIAGNOSIS OF PSYCHOSIS

In constructing a differential diagnosis for psychosis clinicians can make a broad distinction between primary and secondary psychosis (see Figure 2.1). In secondary psychosis, the psychotic symptoms (i.e., psychosis and/or hallucinations) are viewed as being the direct result of medical–surgical illness or substances and drugs (i.e., "organic" to use an older term), and in primary psychosis, the psychosis is thought to be the result of a psychiatric illness. Unfortunately, the psychopathological picture on exam alone does not help distinguish between primary and secondary psychosis. One hundred years ago, the father of "organic psychiatry," Karl Bonhoeffer already recognized that there was no specific clinical picture or pathognomonic symptom that reliably pointed to a specific medical condition (Neumarker, 2001). Clinical presentations that are atypical for primary psychiatric illnesses

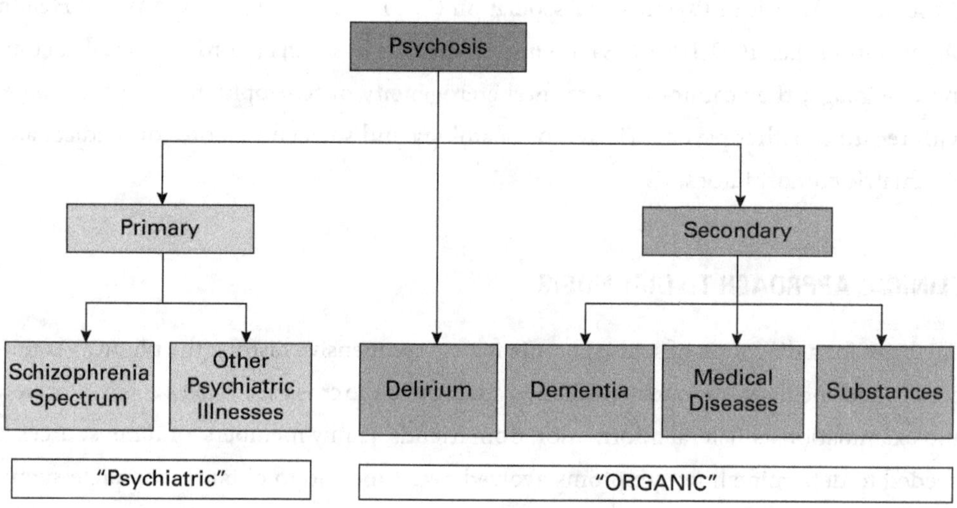

FIGURE 2.1 Differential diagnosis of psychosis

with regard to age of onset, illness course, symptom combinations, and treatment response should alert clinicians to the possibility of secondary psychosis. It is important to consider a secondary psychosis in patients with a known primary psychotic disorder (e.g., a patient with schizophrenia who develops a delirium from an infection). Also, the mere presence of a potential cause of secondary psychosis (e.g., a positive urine drug screen for cannabis or a diagnosis of hyperthyroidism) does not prove causation. A temporal relationship between the onset and severity of psychosis and the onset and severity of a medical illness or use of a substance is consistent with causation. Serial examinations and long-term follow-up can usually establish the correct diagnosis in cases that are confusing at initial presentation.

SECONDARY PSYCHOSIS

Secondary psychosis (i.e., delusions and hallucinations) can occur in any of those four categories: delirium, dementia, medical and neurological diseases, and substances (illicit drugs and alcohol, medication-induced toxidromes, and environmental toxins).

Delirium

A delirium is accompanied by psychosis in about 50 percent of cases (Meagher et al., 2007). However, prominent psychosis can overshadow the hallmark finding of delirium (i.e., inattention). Missing a delirium, which *always* has a medical cause and is frequently treatable, is a grave mistake. The clinical situation usually helps to identify patients who are at high risk for a delirium. For example, an older patient in a nursing home who develops psychosis should be considered to have developed a delirium until proven otherwise.

Dementia

For a comprehensive diagnostic review, it is helpful to consider dementia and other cognitive disorders in their own category. First, dementia is a risk factor for a delirium. Second, many dementias are accompanied by psychosis, including Alzheimer's disease and Lewy body dementia. A competent cognitive exam is thus needed in all patients presenting with psychosis to exclude a dementia.

Medical and Neurological Diseases

The potential medical causes for psychosis are legion. Box 2.1 provides a summary of medical causes that can be present with psychosis. In many cases, however, psychosis is

BOX 2.1

MEDICAL DIFFERENTIAL DIAGNOSIS OF PSYCHOSIS*

- Neurological: Strokes, seizures, demyelinating diseases, brain tumors, basal ganglia diseases (Huntington's disease, Wilson's disease, Parkinson's disease), dementias, head injury.
- Autoimmune diseases: Systemic lupus erythematosus (SLE), paraneoplastic syndromes, N-methyl-D-aspartate (NMDA) receptor encephalitis.
- Infections: Human immunodeficiency virus (HIV) infection, neurosyphilis, neuroborreliosis (Lyme disease), herpes simplex encephalitis, tuberculosis, toxoplasmosis, neurocysticercosis, cerebral malaria.
- Endocrine diseases: hypoglycemia, hyper/hypothyroidism, Addison's disease, Cushing's disease, hypo/hyperparathyroidism.
- Genetic diseases: velo-cardio-facial syndrome (VCFS).
- Vitamin deficiencies: B12/folate, pellagra.
- Other: narcolepsy, metabolic disorders (e.g., adrenoleukodystrophy).

**This list emphasizes medical diseases that may present with psychosis outside a delirium*

Adapted from (Freudenreich, 2008b)

an atypical feature of the clinical presentation. For example, although psychosis can occur in patients with hyperthyroidism, this would be very unusual.

Drugs of Abuse, Medications, and Toxins

Alcohol and sedative-hypnotics are important drug-induced causes of psychosis, both during intoxication but particularly during withdrawal states (including delirium tremens). Patients with chronic, heavy alcohol use can develop persistent alcoholic hallucinosis or pathological jealousy (the Othello syndrome). Illicit drugs that can cause psychosis are cannabis and stimulants (e.g., cocaine and methamphetamine) and particularly psychotomimetics where alterations in perception are expected (e.g., lysergic acid diethylamide [LSD], hallucinogenic mushrooms, phencyclidine [PCP]). Potent designer drugs purchased over the Internet have become a significant cause of psychosis. Many of those drugs are not detected by standard urine drug screens and can cause severe and prolonged psychosis lasting for more than a week. Considering the clinical and geographic context is critical to making a diagnosis of a drug-induced psychosis. Examples are college students using stimulants for "cramming" before an exam or using party drugs on the weekend after an exam.

Only a few medications are an important likely cause of psychosis. Examples include corticosteroids, stimulants, dopaminergic drugs like L-dopa, and interferon. Anticholinergics are also associated with psychosis but usually cause a delirium and not only psychosis. Many other medications have been associated with psychosis in rare cases (e.g., mefloquine for malaria prophylaxis).

Poisoning with environmental toxins requires a high-index of suspicion if psychosis is the presenting symptoms. Toxins to consider include carbon monoxide, organophosphates, and heavy metals (e.g., arsenic, manganese, mercury, and thallium).

Medical Work-up of Psychosis

The patient's history and the physical exam with emphasis on the neurological and cognitive parts is the cornerstone of making the correct diagnosis. There is no one agreed-upon laboratory work-up for psychosis. Laboratory tests need to be selected judiciously to avoid false-positive and false-negative results (Freudenreich, Schulz, & Goff, 2009). The selection of tests (see Box 2.2) should emphasize eliminating major organ failure and a delirium or other life-threatening causes of psychosis as well as treatable causes of psychosis (the prototypes for the latter would be hyperthyroidism, vitamin B12 deficiency, or neurosyphilis). The role of *routine* brain imaging without abnormal findings on a neurological exam is controversial because the yield in otherwise healthy young patients with psychosis is low (Khandanpour, Hoggard, & Connolly, 2013).

PRIMARY PSYCHOSIS

There are many psychiatric reasons for psychosis that psychiatrists will consider. Schizophrenia is the major psychiatric cause of psychosis but psychotic symptoms or psychosis-like experiences occur in many other psychiatric conditions (see Box 2.3). The main distinction to be made is between schizophrenia spectrum conditions and episodic mood disorders where psychosis occurs only at the height of mania or the depth of depression. Delusional beliefs can also occur in obsessive disorders (e.g., body dysmorphic disorder) or anxiety disorders (e.g., the olfactory reference syndrome).

One major, unresolved issue in our current psychiatric nosology is the relationship between schizophrenia and bipolar spectrum conditions. Ever since

BOX 2.2

MEDICAL WORK-UP FOR SECONDARY PSYCHOSIS

SCREEN BROADLY

- Complete blood count (CBC), glucose, full chemistry including calcium, liver function tests, erythrocyte sedimentation rate (ESR), antinuclear antibody (ANA).
- Urine analysis (UA) and urine drug screen (UDS).
- Consider brain imaging with CT or MRI.*

EXCLUDE SPECIFICALLY

- Thyroid stimulating hormone (TSH), vitamin B12 and folate, human immunodeficiency virus (HIV), fluorescent treponemal antibody absorption (FTA-Abs).

INVESTIGATE FURTHER AS CLINICALLY INDICATED**

- Electroencephalogram.
- Chest radiography, lumbar puncture, blood and urine cultures, arterial blood gases.
- Serum cortisol levels.
- NMDA receptor antibodies.
- Serum cortisol levels.
- Drug levels.
- Genetic testing.

**Low yield in first-episode patients with no indication of a neurological or medical problem based on history and exam.*

***A broader search is indicated if delirium is suspected. Epidemiological considerations, the clinical picture, and the immune status guide the extent of the work-up.*

Kraepelin proposed to broadly divide the major psychiatric disorders into schizophrenia and manic-depressive illness (bipolar disorder in today's terminology), his dichotomy has influenced clinical care, education, and research (Craddock & Owen, 2010). Arguments for and against Kraepelin's classification can be made. For clinicians, the Kraepelinian dichotomy holds up for many patients who appear typical for either category and guides treatment (e.g., lithium works well for the prevention of mood episodes but is ineffective for acute psychosis of schizophrenia). However, a significant minority of patients seem to straddle the two categories, with symptoms from both schizophrenia and bipolar disorder, leading to the unreliable and yet clinically needed diagnosis of schizoaffective disorder. More problematic is the overlap between schizophrenia and bipolar disorder at the biological level where they share risk factors, genetic risk loci (Smoller

BOX 2.3

DIFFERENTIAL DIAGNOSIS OF PSYCHIATRIC DISORDERS WITH PSYCHOSIS

MAJOR CAUSES

Schizophrenia spectrum disorders

- Schizophrenia.
- Schizoaffective disorder.
- Schizotypal (personality) disorder.
- Delusional disorder.*

Psychotic mood disorders

- Bipolar disorder with psychotic mood episodes.
- Recurrent psychotic depression.

Third group of psychosis

- Brief psychotic disorder.
- Schizophreniform disorder.
- Acute and transient psychotic disorders (ATPD).

MINOR CAUSES

Psychosis-like experiences or subclinical psychosis

- Borderline personality disorder.
- Post-traumatic symptom disorder.
- Autism spectrum disorder.
- Attenuated psychosis syndrome (including prodrome of schizophrenia).

Obsessive compulsive disorder
Body dysmorphic disorder
Paranoid personality disorder

**Not always included in schizophrenia spectrum disorders*

et al., 2013), and abnormalities in neural circuitry (Baker et al., 2014), throwing into doubt the validity of current diagnostic categories based on Kraepelin's disease entities.

Schizophrenia

As the prototypical psychotic disorder, schizophrenia is defined by two clinical features: psychotic symptoms (i.e., delusions and hallucination, disorganized thinking (formal thought disorder), and grossly disorganized or catatonic behavior) during the acute phases of the illness and a chronic disease course. For most patients, the course, although chronic, follows a relapsing-remitting pattern with accrued disability over time. When not acutely psychotic, patients struggle with negative symptoms and cognitive symptoms, which together account for the disability that is typical for most patients. A criteria-based diagnosis of schizophrenia requires the presence of characteristic symptoms; impairment in functioning; and the exclusion of secondary causes of psychosis. There are no symptoms that are pathognomonic for schizophrenia.

Comprehensive Assessment of Schizophrenia

A purely criteria-based diagnosis of schizophrenia does not provide the rich understanding of the clinical syndrome needed to guide treatment decisions. Using eight symptom dimensions to characterize patients can add valuable information to the assessment: five dimensions to better describe the characteristic symptoms of schizophrenia (i.e., motor symptoms [abnormal motor phenomena including catatonia], positive symptoms broken up into delusions, hallucinations, and formal thought disorder, and negative symptoms [restricted emotional expressivity and avolition-apathy]); one dimension to describe cognition; and two dimensions to describe mania and depression (Barch et al., 2013). Clinicians can rate each of the eight symptom dimensions on a five-point Likert scale, ranging from not present to present and severe. A dimensional approach highlights the importance of considering cognitive problems, which are not a diagnostic criterion. Eighty-five percent of patients with schizophrenia have significant cognitive impairment associated with schizophrenia (CIAS), particularly in the realms of working memory, verbal memory, and executive function (Heinrichs & Zakzanis, 1998). The relationship between cognitive difficulties and poor function is well established. Viewing schizophrenia as a neurocognitive disorder reminds clinician to keep their cognitive abilities in mind when treating schizophrenia patients (Kahn & Keefe, 2013). Verbal and complex instructions, for example, are not a good way to communicate treatment plans to patients with a significant degree of CIAS. This cognitive impairment persists and does not respond to treatment with antipsychotics (Keefe et al., 2007). Similarly, lack of insight into the nature of illness is common and probably at least in part due to higher-order cognitive problems (Nair, Palmer, Aleman, & David, 2014).

In addition to these eight symptom dimensions, functional abilities and limitations need to be better delineated, and a risk assessment needs to be conducted. Additional assessments are summarized in Box 2.4. Clinicians need to appreciate a patient's quality

BOX 2.4

COMPREHENSIVE ASSESSMENT OF SCHIZOPHRENIA

Diagnostic psychiatric assessment

- Presence of psychosis (positive symptoms).
- Nonpsychotic symptom clusters (negative symptoms, affective symptoms).
- Neurocognitive examination (executive function, working memory, verbal memory, abstraction).
- Insight into illness, including capacity to accept or reject treatment.
- Psychiatric comorbidities including substance use.

Assessment of functional capacities (strengths and weaknesses)

- Treatment motivation.
- Functional ability to participate in treatment and rehabilitation.

Assessment of psychosocial adjustment

History of psychosocial adversity (homelessness; trauma; poverty)

- Work history and potential.
- Relationships with family members and friends.
- Estimate of financial security.
- Meaningful community activities.

Assessment of quality of life

- Physical pain; medical illness burden; depression, and demoralization.
- Side-effect burden from psychotropics.

Assessment of adherence

- Attitude toward treatment; barriers; actual adherence behavior.

Risk assessment: violence and suicide

- History of suicide attempts; chronic suicidality; depression and demoralization.
- History of violence and legal problems; impulsivity; anger.

Adapted from (Freudenreich, Viron, & Shtasel, 2015)

of life, particularly with regard to the side effects from psychotropics (e.g., sedation) but also their lack of efficacy for some domains (e.g., cognitive impairment leading to difficulties completing college after an episode of psychosis). The patient's view of his quality of life combined with lack of insight influences adherence to treatment. Adherence needs to be understood both as an attitude and as an actual behavior (Freudenreich & Tranulis, 2009): if there are barriers, even motivated patients will not be able to be adherent. For example, some patients who are not opposed to taking medications might not be able to pay for the medicine.

Schizoaffective Disorder

The core features of schizoaffective disorder are those of schizophrenia. Its characteristic symptoms must be present for some time without significant mood symptoms. However, in addition to the symptoms of schizophrenia, patients with schizoaffective disorder experience a substantial burden of mood symptoms (in the form of full manic or depressive episodes) over the course of their illness (Malaspina et al., 2013). The diagnosis can be difficult to make with certainty unless clinicians have longitudinal information. In clinical practice, schizoaffective disorder is often used for patients in whom psychosis and serious mood symptoms are present to an extent no longer well explained by bipolar disorder or a psychotic mood disorder. In terms of function, patients with schizoaffective disorder fall between patients with schizophrenia and patients with bipolar disorder. However, schizoaffective disorder resembles schizophrenia more than bipolar disorder (Pagel, Baldessarini, Franklin, & Baethge, 2013) and is, therefore, considered part of the schizophrenia spectrum. It should be emphasized that many patients with schizophrenia experience subclinical depressive symptoms and demoralization. Those mood symptoms are entirely consistent with schizophrenia and do not require a diagnosis of schizoaffective disorder.

Schizotypal Personality Disorder

Patients with schizotypal personality disorder resemble patients with schizophrenia in that they have odd ideas or describe unusual perceptual experiences (e.g., believing in extrasensory perception) (Rosell, Futterman, McMaster, & Siever, 2014). In contrast to schizophrenia, however, they are not psychotic at the syndromal level. They are usually described as "eccentric" by others and live isolated lives on the fringes of society where they struggle to connect with other people, similar to patients with schizophrenia. These difficulties emerge during adolescence and persist throughout life without much change, which is typical for personality disorders. However, muted features resembling schizophrenia (i.e., schizotypal traits) can also be viewed dimensionally as they exist in the general population (Esterberg & Compton, 2009). If schizotypal traits are severe enough, such patients can be said to have schizotypal disorder (the term used in ICD-10 instead of schizotypal personality disorder). Schizotypal disorder from a dimensional perspective represents a mild form of schizophrenia.

BOX 2.5

CLASSICAL EPONYMOUS DELUSIONAL DISORDERS*

- de Clérambault syndrome (erotomania)—delusion of being loved by somebody famous.
- Othello syndrome (morbid jealousy)—delusion of infidelity.
- Ekbom syndrome (delusional parasitosis)—somatic delusion of infestation.

**Delusions can occur in other psychiatric disorders or secondary psychosis*

Delusional Disorder

The core feature of delusional disorder is the presence of a delusional belief in the absence of other symptoms characteristic of schizophrenia. In delusional disorder, hallucinations are absent except if they are thematically related to the delusions. Smelling gas for example in somebody worried about getting poisoned would still be consistent with delusional disorder. Patients with delusional disorder are not thought disordered, they are interpersonally well related, and although they might be distressed about their situation, the delusion is not thought to be secondary to a mood disorder. Traditionally, delusional disorders were labeled by the theme of the delusions (e.g., grandiose or persecutory) or carried eponyms (see Box 2.5). Delusional disorder can be very difficult to diagnose if the delusional belief is plausible and not patently absurd or bizarre. Somatic delusions, infidelity, or persecutory delusions in a previous gang member are examples. A critical and not always easy distinction needs to be made between delusions and overvalued ideas, with only the former being evidence of psychosis. The circumscribed nature of the delusion can make it difficult to appreciate unless one stumbles on it during the interview. The delusions in delusional disorder can be rather fixed and impairing even if circumscribed in nature.

Brief Psychotic Disorders and Schizophreniform Disorders

Not all psychiatric patients with prominent psychotic symptoms have schizophrenia or a mood disorder. There appears to exist a third group of psychoses, composed of patients who experience episodes of recurrent psychosis (but not clearly bipolar disorder) and whose illness follows a favorable course. In the World Health Organization's International Classification of Diseases system, such good-prognosis patients are classified as having acute and transient psychotic disorders (ATPD) (Gaebel, 2012). As the name implies,

BOX 2.6
CATATONIC SYMPTOMS

- Hypokinetic symptoms: catalepsy/posturing, stupor, mutism.
- Hyperkinetic symptoms: agitation, mannerism, stereotypes.
- Signs on exam: waxy flexibility, negativism, echophenomena (echolalia and echopraxia).

Based on (Freudenreich, 2008a)

such patients have an acute onset of psychosis over one or two weeks that, after a brief duration, fully remits. During the episode of psychosis, patients are often described as "perplexed," which can raise clinical concerns for confusional states (Legesse, Freudenreich, Murray, & Price, 2011). The psychopathology is unstable, diverse, and fluctuates, hence the term *polymorphous psychopathology* to describe a patient during an episode. In some cases a stressor plausibly contributed to the psychotic episode. In the *DSM* system, such patients will get classified as either having a brief psychotic disorder (if symptoms are less than four weeks) or a schizophreniform disorder (if symptoms last longer than four weeks but resolve in less than six months). Some patients with schizophreniform disorder are in the early course of schizophrenia in which the duration criterion of six months for schizophrenia (according to *DSM*) has not yet been met.

Catatonia

Catatonic symptoms (see Box 2.6) can occur during the course of schizophrenia or its related disorders. In fact, the catatonic subtype of schizophrenia was one of the original forms of schizophrenia described by Kraepelin (Heckers, Tandon, & Bustillo, 2010). However, catatonic symptoms are not specific for schizophrenia but occur in other psychiatric disorders (notably mood disorders) and toxic-medical conditions (Tandon et al., 2013). The majority of patients presenting with catatonic symptoms will not have schizophrenia. Still, up to one-third of patients will and it is. Therefore, important to look for catatonic symptoms in a patient experiencing a psychotic episode because catatonic symptoms can easily be missed and go untreated (Fink & Taylor, 2006).

MEDICAL COMORBIDITY

Schizophrenia is a psychiatric illness with reduced life expectancy. Compared to their peers who do not have schizophrenia, patients with schizophrenia die a decade or more earlier (Colton & Manderscheid, 2006). Although some of the excess mortality can be attributed to psychiatric causes (i.e., suicide) the main medical causes of premature death is cardiovascular disease (Auquier, Lancon, Rouillon, & Lader, 2007; Ifteni, Correll, Burtea, Kane, & Manu, 2014). A major contributor to cardiovascular mortality in schizophrenia patients is a modifiable risk factor, namely smoking (Brown, Inskip, & Barraclough, 2000). Although the prevalence of smoking among people with psychiatric illness is twice as high as for people without mental illness (Lasser et al., 2000), the prevalence among patients with schizophrenia has been estimated to approach 80 percent in some surveys (Prochaska, Hall, & Bero, 2008). Smoking is a major contributor to death for patients with schizophrenia, accounting for over 50 percent of total mortality in one large cohort study (Callaghan et al., 2014). In addition to smoking, however, weight gain and the associated metabolic syndrome is a second major preventable cause of cardiovascular disease. Like smoking, obesity rates are high in patients with schizophrenia (Correll et al., 2010). Patients contribute to obesity via a sedentary life-style and poor eating habits but there is also an iatrogenic contribution: it has long been known that antipsychotics are associated with weight gain (Allison et al., 1999). Other weight-related problems include obstructive sleep apnea, which is often not recognized (Kalucy, Grunstein, Lambert, & Glozier, 2013). Blood-borne infections like hepatitis C and human immunodeficiency virus (HIV) occur at elevated rates compared to the general population (Blank et al., 2014) and screening for both should be considered. More recently, cancer as a cause of death for patients with schizophrenia has become a focus of attention (Crump, Winkleby, Sundquist, & Sundquist, 2013; Irwin, Henderson, Knight, & Pirl, 2014).

Assessment

The medical assessment should emphasize those conditions that contribute to morbidity and mortality in patients with schizophrenia. Priority should be given to identify modifiable cardiovascular risk factors with emphasis on smoking and obesity; conditions that have a negative impact on cognition; and iatrogenic problems related to the use of antipsychotics (see Box 2.7). Psychiatrists can play an active role in guideline-concordant

BOX 2.7
FOCUSED MEDICAL ASSESSMENT FOR A PATIENT WITH SCHIZOPHRENIA

History of head injuries

Iatrogenic problems from antipsychotics

- Neurological symptoms: extrapyramidal symptoms, tardive dyskinesia.
- Antipsychotic-associated weight gain.

Infectious diseases

- Human immunodeficiency virus, hepatitis, tuberculosis.

Risk factors for cardiovascular disease

- Hypertension, diabetes, dyslipidemia.
- Smoking history.
- Wellness assessment: physical activity, diet.

Adapted from (Freudenreich, O., Viron, M., & Shtasel, D. (2015)).

BOX 2.8
ANTIPSYCHOTIC SAFETY MONITORING (FOR ADULTS)

EVERY VISIT

- Weight/BMI/waist circumference.
- Blood pressure.
- Screening for tardive dyskinesia (e.g., AIMS).

PRE-TREATMENT, AFTER 3 MONTHS, AND THEN ANNUALLY*

- Fasting plasma glucose (or HbA1c).
- Fasting lipid profile.
- Prolactin level.**

BMI = Body Mass Index

AIMS = Abnormal Involuntary Movement Scale

**More frequent laboratory monitoring can be indicated*

***Not needed for prolactin-sparing antipsychotics*

HbA1c = Hemoglobin A1c

Based on (American Diabetes Association, 2004; Goff et al., 2005; Pringsheim, Panagiotopoulos, Davidson, & Ho, 2011).

screening for the metabolic syndrome and the early recognition of tardive dyskinesia (see Box 2.8).

CASE STUDY

Mr. B is a previously healthy 21-year-old college student who had been admitted to a psychiatric inpatient unit following an acute episode of psychosis. He was discharged five days ago from the inpatient unit after a 10-day stay during which he was started on risperidone 1 mg at night. He comes to your clinic to establish outpatient care.

What Assessments Are You Considering in Addition to the Standard Initial Interview?

- Dimensional assessment of psychopathology: this will help track treatment efficacy. At some point, more detailed neurocognitive testing should be considered.
- Risk assessment: is outpatient treatment appropriate?
- Assessment of function, quality of life and adherence: important because this patient is at high risk of discontinuing his medications.
- Weight/BMI/waist circumference, blood pressure, and AIMS to begin antipsychotic safety monitoring.

What Blood Work if Any Do You Order?

- Review the adequacy of the work-up for secondary psychosis.
- The patient needs antipsychotic safety monitoring. If not done in the hospital, a baseline assessment should be done which will need to be repeated in three months. The most basic panel includes a fasting blood sugar (or alternatively HbA1c) and a fasting blood sugar. Prolactin should be considered as the patient is on risperidone, which reliably increases prolactin levels.

REFERENCES

Allison, D. B., Mentore, J. L., Heo, M., Chandler, L. P., Cappelleri, J. C., Infante, M. C., . . . Weiden, P. J. . (1999). Antipsychotic-induced weight gain: a comprehensive research synthesis. *The American Journal ofPpsychiatry, 156*(11), 1686–1696.

American Diabetes Association. (2004). Consensus development conference on antipsychotic drugs and obesity and diabetes. *Diabetes Care, 27*(2), 596–601.

American Psychiatric Association. (2013). *DSM-5. Diagnostic and statistical manual of mental disorders* (5th ed.). Arlington, VA: American Psychiatric Publishing.

Auquier, P., Lancon, C., Rouillon, F., & Lader, M. (2007). Mortality in schizophrenia. *Pharmacoepidemiology and Drug Safety, 16*(12), 1308–1312.

Baker, J. T., Holmes, A. J., Masters, G. A., Yeo, B. T., Krienen, F., Buckner, R. L., . . . Ongur, D. (2014). Disruption of cortical association networks in schizophrenia and psychotic bipolar disorder. *JAMA Psychiatry, 71*(2), 109–118.

Barch, D. M., Bustillo, J., Gaebel, W., Gur, R., Heckers, S., Malaspina, D., . . . Carpenter, W. (2013). Logic and justification for dimensional assessment of symptoms and related clinical phenomena in psychosis: relevance to DSM-5. *Schizophrenia Research, 150*(1), 15–20.

Blank, M. B., Himelhoch, S. S., Balaji, A. B., Metzger, D. S., Dixon, L. B., Rose, C. E., . . . Heffelfinger, J. D. (2014). A multisite study of the prevalence of HIV with rapid testing in mental health settings. *American Journal of Public Health. 150*(12), 2377–2384.

Brown, S., Inskip, H., & Barraclough, B. (2000). Causes of the excess mortality of schizophrenia. *The British Journal of Psychiatry: the Journal of Mental Science, 177*, 212–217.

Callaghan, R. C., Veldhuizen, S., Jeysingh, T., Orlan, C., Graham, C., Kakouris, G., . . . Gatley, J. (2014). Patterns of tobacco-related mortality among individuals diagnosed with schizophrenia, bipolar disorder, or depression. *Journal of psychiatric research, 48*(1), 102–110.

Colton, C. W., & Manderscheid, R. W. (2006). Congruencies in increased mortality rates, years of potential life lost, and causes of death among public mental health clients in eight states. *Preventing Chronic Disease, 3*(2), A42.

Correll, C. U., Druss, B. G., Lombardo, I., O'Gorman, C., Harnett, J. P., Sanders, K. N., . . . Cuffel, B. J. (2010). Findings of a U.S. national cardiometabolic screening program among 10,084 psychiatric outpatients. *Psychiatric Services, 61*(9), 892–898.

Craddock, N., & Owen, M. J. (2010). The Kraepelinian dichotomy—going, going . . . but still not gone. *The British Journal of Psychiatry: the Journal of Mental Science, 196*(2), 92–95.

Crump, C., Winkleby, M. A., Sundquist, K., & Sundquist, J. (2013). Comorbidities and mortality in persons with schizophrenia: a Swedish national cohort study. *The American Journal of Psychiatry, 170*(3), 324–333.

Esterberg, M. L., & Compton, M. T. (2009). The psychosis continuum and categorical versus dimensional diagnostic approaches. *Current Psychiatry Reports, 11*(3), 179–184.

Fink, M., & Taylor, M. A. (2006). Catatonia: subtype or syndrome in DSM? *The American Journal of Psychiatry, 163*(11), 1875–1876.

Freudenreich, O. (2008a). Psychotic signs and symptoms. In O. Freudenreich (Ed.) *Psychotic disorders. Practical Guides in Psychiatry* (pp. 2–13). Philadelphia: Lippincott Williams & Wilkins.

Freudenreich, O. (2008b). Secondary schizophrenia. In O. Freudenreich (Ed.) *Psychotic disorders. Practical guides in psychiatry* (pp. 36–44). Philadelphia, PA: Lippincott Williams & Wilkins.

Freudenreich, O., Schulz, S. C., & Goff, D. C. (2009). Initial medical work-up of first-episode psychosis: a conceptual review. *Early Interventional Psychiatry, 3*(1), 10–18.

Freudenreich, O., & Tranulis, C. (2009). A prototype approach toward antipsychotic medication adherence in schizophrenia. *Harvard Review of Psychiatry, 17*(1), 35–40.

Freudenreich, O., Viron, M., & Shtasel, D. (2015). Serious mental illness. In T. A. Stern, M. Fava, T. E. Wilens & J. F. Rosenbaum (Eds.), *Massachusetts General Hospital comprehensive clinical psychiatry* (2nd ed.). Philadelphia, PA: Mosby/Elsevier.

Gaebel, W. (2012). Status of psychotic disorders in ICD-11. *Schizophrenia Bulletin, 38*(5), 895–898.

Goff, D. C., Cather, C., Evins, A. E., Henderson, D. C., Freudenreich, O., Copeland, P. M., . . . Sacks, F. M.(2005). Medical morbidity and mortality in schizophrenia: guidelines for psychiatrists. *Journal of Clinical Psychiatry, 66*(2), 183–194; quiz 147, 273–184.

Heckers, S., Tandon, R., & Bustillo, J. (2010). Catatonia in the DSM—shall we move or not? *Schizophrenia Bulletin, 36*(2), 205–207.

Heinrichs, R. W., & Zakzanis, K. K. (1998). Neurocognitive deficit in schizophrenia: a quantitative review of the evidence. *Neuropsychology, 12*(3), 426–445.

Ifteni, P., Correll, C. U., Burtea, V., Kane, J. M., & Manu, P. (2014). Sudden unexpected death in schizophrenia: autopsy findings in psychiatric inpatients. *Schizophrenia Research, 155*(1–3), 72–76.

Irwin, K. E., Henderson, D. C., Knight, H. P., & Pirl, W. F. (2014). Cancer care for individuals with schizophrenia. *Cancer, 120*(3), 323–334.

Kahn, R. S., & Keefe, R. S. (2013). Schizophrenia is a cognitive illness: time for a change in focus. *JAMA Psychiatry, 70*(10), 1107–1112.

Kalucy, M. J., Grunstein, R., Lambert, T., & Glozier, N. (2013). Obstructive sleep apnoea and schizophrenia—a research agenda. *Sleep Medicine Reviews, 17*(5), 357–365.

Keefe, R. S., Bilder, R. M., Davis, S. M., Harvey, P. D., Palmer, B. W., Gold, J. M., . . . Lieberman, J. A. Catie Investigators Neurocognitive Working, Group . (2007). Neurocognitive effects of antipsychotic medications in patients with chronic schizophrenia in the CATIE Trial. *Archives of General Psychiatry, 64*(6), 633–647.

Khandanpour, N., Hoggard, N., & Connolly, D. J. (2013). The role of MRI and CT of the brain in first episodes of psychosis. *Clinical Radiology, 68*(3), 245–250.

Lasser, K., Boyd, J. W., Woolhandler, S., Himmelstein, D. U., McCormick, D., & Bor, D. H. (2000). Smoking and mental illness: A population-based prevalence study. *JAMA: the Journal of the American Medical Association, 284*(20), 2606–2610.

Legesse, B., Freudenreich, O., Murray, E., & Price, B. (2011). A case report of confusional psychosis with abrupt onset and rapid resolution of symptoms. *Psychosomatics, 52*(5), 468–471.

Malaspina, D., Owen, M. J., Heckers, S., Tandon, R., Bustillo, J., Schultz, S., et al. (2013). Schizoaffective Disorder in the *DSM-5*. *Schizophrenia Research, 150*(1), 21–25.

Meagher, D. J., Moran, M., Raju, B., Gibbons, D., Donnelly, S., Saunders, J., . . . Trzepacz, P. T. (2007). Phenomenology of delirium. Assessment of 100 adult cases using standardised measures. *The British Journal of Psychiatry: the Journal of Mental Science, 190*, 135–141.

Nair, A., Palmer, E. C., Aleman, A., & David, A. S. (2014). Relationship between cognition, clinical and cognitive insight in psychotic disorders: a review and meta-analysis. *Schizophrenia Research, 152*(1), 191–200.

Neumarker, K. J. (2001). Karl Bonhoeffer and the concept of symptomatic psychoses. *History of Psychiatry, 12*(46 Pt 2), 213–226.

Pagel, T., Baldessarini, R. J., Franklin, J., & Baethge, C. (2013). Characteristics of patients diagnosed with schizoaffective disorder compared with schizophrenia and bipolar disorder. *Bipolar Disorders, 15*(3), 229–239.

Pringsheim, T., Panagiotopoulos, C., Davidson, J., & Ho, J. (2011). Evidence-based recommendations for monitoring safety of second generation antipsychotics in children and youth. *Journal of the Canadian Academy of Child and Adolescent Psychiatry = Journal de l'Academie canadienne de psychiatrie de l'enfant et de l'adolescent, 20*(3), 218–233.

Prochaska, J. J., Hall, S. M., & Bero, L. A. (2008). Tobacco use among individuals with schizophrenia: what role has the tobacco industry played? *Schizophrenia Bulletin, 34*(3), 555–567.

Rosell, D. R., Futterman, S. E., McMaster, A., & Siever, L. J. (2014). Schizotypal personality disorder: a current review. *Current Psychiatry Reports, 16*(7), 452.

Smoller, J. W., Craddock, N., Kendler, K., Lee, P. H., Neale, B. M., Nurnberger, J. I., . . . Sullivan, P. F. (2013). Identification of risk loci with shared effects on five major psychiatric disorders: a genome-wide analysis. *Lancet, 381*(9875), 1371–1379.

Tandon, R., Heckers, S., Bustillo, J., Barch, D. M., Gaebel, W., Gur, R. E., . . . Carpenter, W. (2013). Catatonia in DSM-5. *Schizophrenia research, 150*(1), 26–30.

World Health Organization. (1993). *The ICD-10 classification of mental and behavioural disorders: diagnostic criteria for research*. Geneva: World Health Organization.

/// 3 /// EPIDEMIOLOGY AND RISK FACTORS INFLUENCING SCHIZOPHRENIA

ERIC A. EPPING and DONALD W. BLACK

INTRODUCTION

Schizophrenia affects millions worldwide. The most commonly reported rate of individuals diagnosed with the disorder is 0.5–1 percent of the adult population. There has been a significant amount of research that indicates differences in the prevalence of schizophrenia depending on several variables including location, age, and gender. The heterogeneity of symptoms and changing diagnostic criteria over time for schizophrenia adds additional challenges in diagnosis and evaluation of its epidemiology. The reliability of diagnosing mental disorders including schizophrenia has improved with the development of structured diagnostic assessments, including the Present State Examination Schedules for Clinical Assessment in Neuropsychiatry (SCAN), the Composite International Diagnostic Interview, and the Diagnostic Interview Schedule, (DIS), as well as the more formal criteria starting with *DSM-III* (Eaton & Chen, 2007).

INCIDENCE AND PREVALENCE OF SCHIZOPHRENIA WORLDWIDE

Incidence is defined as the number of new cases identified over a specific time period in a unit of the population. The incidence rate of schizophrenia estimated from several studies around the world in the 1960s and 1970s was 0.20 per 1000 per year with a range between 0.11 and 0.70 per 1000 (Messias, Chen, & Eaton, 2007). A study from the World Health Organization conducted in the 1980s at 10 different sites reported similar incidence rates around the world (Jablensky et al., 1992). However, the preponderance of studies shows variation of incidence rates depending on location. A systematic review of 55 studies with 170 different incidence rates estimated median incidence to be 15.2 per 100,000, with a 10-90 percent range of 7.7-43.0 (McGrath, Saha, Chant, & Welham, 2008). These authors concluded that incidence rates are variable around the world. One consistent finding from this review was that incidence rates were higher in older studies. Although some have argued that this may suggest a decline in the number of new cases over time, this change of incidence rates also coincides with the transition to stricter diagnostic criteria. Even in studies done with the most up-to-date methods, differences in methodologies still contribute to at least some of the variation in reported rates, whether incidence or prevalence.

Prevalence measures the total number of cases in a population over a defined time, represented as the number per unit of population. The most comprehensive review of schizophrenia prevalence included data from 188 studies from 46 countries around the world. The overall point prevalence (measured over one month or less) of schizophrenia was estimated to be 4.6 per 1000, with a 10–90 percent range from 1.9 to 10.0 per 1000. Period prevalence (measured between 1 and 12 months) was 3.3 per 1000 (10–90 percent range from 1.3–8.2) and lifetime prevalence was also reported to be similar to point prevalence at 4.0 per 1000 (10–90 percent range from 1.6–12.1), consistent with the chronic nature of the illness (Saha, Chant, Welham, & McGrath, 2005).

AGE OF ONSET AND GENDER DIFFERENCES

The peak incidence of schizophrenia is in late adolescence/early adulthood, although the illness can develop at any age, including childhood or during senescence (Abidi, 2013; Eaton & Chen, 2007). The peak age of onset has been reported to be highest between the ages of 15–24 years. A second, though much smaller peak of onset has been identified in women age 55 to 64 years, but not for older men (Eaton & Chen, 2007). Many studies have found an earlier age of onset for men than women, but more recent findings have challenged this view. A meta-analysis of 46 studies that included over 29,000 men and over 19,000 women found male onset overall was only one year earlier than for females using the definition of onset as first hospital admission; this was only observed among studies that used *DSM III, III-R,* or *IV*. Results from studies that used the *International Classification of Disease (ICD)* found no differences in age of onset between men and women (Eranti, MacCabe, Bundy, & Murray, 2013). These results illustrate the methodological challenges in conducting epidemiology studies in schizophrenia.

Older studies initially reported an equal distribution in the rate of schizophrenia between men and women, but more recent studies using modern diagnostic criteria report a higher ratio for men versus women (men: women ratio of 1.4) (McGrath et al., 2008). Older studies may have included women who would now be diagnosed with a mood rather

BOX 3.1

OVERVIEW OF EPIDEMIOLOGY AND DEMOGRAPHICS OF SCHIZOPHRENIA

Median worldwide incidence estimated at 15.2 per 100,000 (10–90 percent interval of 7.7–43.0)

Point prevalence worldwide estimated at 4.6 per 1000 (10–90 percent interval of 1.9–10.0)

Lifetime prevalence worldwide estimated at 4.0 per 1000 (10–90 percent interval of 1.6–12.1)

Peak age of onset between ages 15–24

Males may have a slightly earlier age of onset (1 year or less)

Men to women ratio estimated to be 1.4: 1.0

than a psychotic disorder. One systematic review of prevalence rates found no difference in rates between genders (Saha et al., 2005). Additional work is needed to understand the differences in the results of these studies comparing incidence versus prevalence. There may be gender-specific biological factors interacting with environmental exposures that contribute to differences in incidence and age of onset between males and females. See Box 3.1 for a summary of incidence, prevalence and demographics of schizophrenia.

FACTORS THAT CONTRIBUTE TO THE RISK OF DEVELOPING SCHIZOPHRENIA

The pathophysiology of schizophrenia, including its genetics, will be discussed elsewhere in this book. This section will focus on environmental factors that have evidence for association with schizophrenia and may contribute to illness risk. These factors are summarized in Box 3.2. An important aspect of all these factors is that, although the exposure may significantly increase the risk of schizophrenia, the increase remains small relative to the total population at risk. Most individuals with these exposures do not develop the disorder, which suggests that underlying genetic risk factors interacting with environmental exposures are critical to its development.

Socioeconomic Status

There is a significant association between socioeconomic status and schizophrenia, prevalence, with less developed countries having higher rates than more developed countries (Saha et al., 2005). Within more developed countries, there is no consistent evidence that socioeconomic status at birth is associated with differences in the risk of developing the

BOX 3.2

FACTORS CONTRIBUTING TO SCHIZOPHRENIA RISK

Socioeconomic Status:
Status at birth not consistently associated with illness.
Patients more likely to fall into lower status due to illness.
Ethnicity:
Isolated populations with increased rates (Sweden, Finland, Palau Islands, Dagestan) and decreased rates (Hutterites in United States).
Increase in rates for ethnic minorities in United States and England.
Immigrants:
Migrants from one part of the world to another have higher rates than in the country of origin and destination.
Population Density:
More densely populated regions have increased risk.
Infections:
Increased risk from *in utero* infections (influenza in second trimester, rubella, measles, varicella-zoster, polio, and herpes).
Increased risk from postnatal infections (*Toxoplasma gondii,* meningitis).
Birth Season:
Birth during winter months increases risk.
Pregnancy/Delivery:
Increased risk with pregnancy complications.
Increased risk due to abnormal fetal development.
Delivery complications including asphyxia, emergency Caesarian section.
Parental age:
Older paternal or maternal age may increase risk in offspring.
Drug use:
Some evidence for marijuana, cocaine and stimulant use increasing risk, but may depend on susceptibility, age of use, and other factors.

illness (Kwok, 2014). Patients diagnosed and treated for schizophrenia are more likely to come from the lowest socioeconomic class, although there is some evidence that the parents of offspring who develop schizophrenia are more likely to be from a higher socioeconomic class. The most likely explanation for this finding is that patients with schizophrenia decline in social status because of the effects of the symptoms of the illness on their social and occupational functioning (Messias et al., 2007).

Ethnicity and Immigration

Significant differences in prevalence have been reported in isolated regions, with lower prevalence reported among the Hutterites in the United States, and higher rates in north

Sweden, parts of Finland, the Palau Islands in the Pacific, and Dagestan in the North Caucasus Mountains (Jablensky, Kirkbride, & Jones, 2011). The heterogeneity of the illness is also complicated by cultural differences in symptom presentation, and variations in assessment across studies all confound obtaining clearly apparent differences in ethnicity (Kalra, Bhugra, & Shah, 2012).

Several studies have consistently reported higher prevalence of schizophrenia in African Americans (Kalra et al., 2012), even after controlling for socioeconomic status. Increased incidence in African and ethnic minorities was also found in a study from England (Kirkbride et al., 2006). Some argue that the difference is due to health disparities in minorities, which increase risk of developing schizophrenia (Kalra et al., 2012). Others have found that there may be a bias in overdiagnosis of schizophrenia, at least in African American populations (Gara et al., 2012).

One consistent finding related to ethnicity is evidence for higher rates of schizophrenia in people who migrate from part of the world to another. The relationship of schizophrenia to immigration has been reported as far back as the first half of the twentieth century in the United States (Kalra et al., 2012). First- and second-generation immigrants from Africa or the Caribbean to the United Kingdom have been found to have rates of schizophrenia several times higher than the general population. This phenomenon has also been observed in Surinam immigrants to the Netherlands. These rates are much higher than their country of origin, indicating that factors related to immigration but also other factors that persist into the second generation may contribute to increased risk.

Urban/Rural Differences

Research has shown a higher risk of schizophrenia for those born in more densely populated regions (Kirkbride et al., 2006). The increase in relative risk from this variable has been estimated to be between 2 and 4 times higher than in nonurban areas. Several factors related to urban living may contribute to this increase in risk, such as environmental exposures to toxins or infectious agents or stressful life experiences specific to city life (Messias et al., 2007). However, there is no clear understanding of the extent to which these factors contribute to etiology. Some of these are discussed in more detail next.

Infections

Exposure to infectious agents, either in utero or early life has been implicated in increasing the risk of schizophrenia. These exposures are thought to affect normal neurodevelopmental pathways, and they must occur during specific windows of development.

Offspring of mothers exposed to influenza during the second trimester of pregnancy have increased risk of schizophrenia. Evidence of *in utero* infections from rubella, measles, varicella-zoster, polio, and herpes has also been reported as increasing risk (Hagberg, Gressens, & Mallard, 2012). Postnatal infections may also be risk factors. Several studies have shown that individuals exposed to *Toxoplasma gondii,* a parasite that infects cats have increased prevalence of the illness. Acute infection with the organism can also cause psychotic symptoms, supporting a possible link to schizophrenia (Severance, Yolken, & Eaton, 2014). Based on data from a meningitis outbreak in Brazil in the early 1970s, children who contracted meningitis had five times the prevalence of psychotic illness than uninfected siblings when assessed as adults (Gattaz, Abrahão, & Foccacia, 2004).

Birth Seasonality and Complications During Pregnancy/Delivery

Individuals born in the winter are at increased risk for schizophrenia, and this observation has been replicated over the years (Messias et al., 2007). The increase in risk is only estimated to be 10 percent, but it is consistent in the Northern and Southern Hemispheres. The seasonal effect may be related to increased maternal infections from agents such as influenza during the winter.

Complications during pregnancy and at the time of birth have been shown to increase schizophrenia risk by about twofold (Schmitt, Malchow, Hasan, & Falkai, 2014). A comprehensive meta-analysis of studies in this area identified three types of complications associated with schizophrenia: (1) complications during pregnancy such as diabetes, bleeding, pre-eclampsia and Rh incompatibility; (2) abnormalities in fetal growth or development, including congenital malformations, low birth weight, and smaller head circumference; and (3) delivery complications such as uterine atony, emergency Caesarian section, and asphyxia (Cannon, Jones, & Murray, 2002). In a sample of individuals initially identified at increased risk of schizophrenia, then followed over time prospectively, those who eventually developed schizophrenia were found to have significantly higher rates of obstetric complications (Mittal et al., 2009).

Parental Age

Older parental age has been linked to schizophrenia. Starting from age 25 years and stratifying into 5-year periods increasing until age 50 years, schizophrenia risk increases in each older age group of fathers, with the highest in the 50 years and older group (Malaspina et al., 2001). One study reported increased risk from the age of the father only after age 50 years when controlling for socioeconomic factors and family history.

They also identified paternal age differences depending on gender of the offspring, with the increased risk in females from paternal age of 50 years or greater, but only from paternal age of 55 years and older when the offspring was male (Byrne, Agerbo, Ewald, Eaton, & Mortensen, 2003). This finding was in a cohort from Denmark, but it was not observed in a more recent meta-analysis that did support the association between increased paternal age with increased risk (Miller et al., 2011).

These observations are biologically plausible as advanced male age is known to increase the number of new mutations in germline cells as errors in DNA replication accumulate as the cells divide, however, findings to date do not consistently support the idea that increased paternal de novo germline mutations alone increase the risk of schizophrenia. A study of over two million individuals in Denmark born between 1955 and 1992 found that older paternal age only increased schizophrenia risk with the firstborn child (Petersen, Mortensen, & Pedersen, 2011). This implies that other factors are contributing to risk rather than de novo mutations, because the risk of schizophrenia should increase with each subsequent child born. The National Institute of Health Schizophrenia Sibling Study found that older age of the mother (versus older age in the father) was more highly correlated with an offspring affected by schizophrenia being later in the birth order compared to other siblings in the family. This also argues against de novo mutations from the father as a significant causal factor because mothers do not have increased de novo mutations with older age. In contrast, another study with 90 percent of the population of Sweden born between 1973 and 2001 found advanced paternal age was associated with increased risk of schizophrenia and other psychiatric disorders. This latter study used a broader diagnostic criteria for schizophrenia (D'Onofrio et al., 2014).

Cannabis and Other Drug Use

Multiple studies have examined the relationship between cannabis use and psychosis (D'Souza, 2007). A recent meta-analysis of 83 studies concluded that the age of schizophrenia onset for cannabis users was 2.7 years earlier compared with those who did not use cannabis. Substance users in general (which included cannabis use) were found to have onset 2.0 years earlier, but alcohol use did not show any effect on age of onset (Large, Sharma, Compton, Slade, & Nielssen, 2011). As summarized by Giordano and colleagues (Giordano, Ohlsson, Sundquist, Sundquist, & Kendler, 2014), cannabis use can cause acute and temporary symptoms of psychosis, individuals who are either susceptible to or have already manifest psychotic disorders are more likely to smoke cannabis, and cannabis is postulated to be a causal factor for psychotic disorders. This recent paper from a Swedish sample concluded that there is a modest association between cannabis abuse and later diagnosis of schizophrenia, but a large portion of the association is confounded by other shared factors within families, such as common genetics and environment. They conclude that uncorrected measures of association that are reported in most studies overestimate the link between cannabis use and subsequent manifestation of schizophrenia. The authors also examined the relationship between other drug use and schizophrenia and found cocaine and stimulant use was associated with increased risk of schizophrenia. There was also no causal relationship between cannabis use and affective disorders. More information on the consequences of substance abuse in schizophrenia patients is provided below.

CONSEQUENCES AND OUTCOMES OF SCHIZOPHRENIA

Just as the signs and symptoms of schizophrenia are heterogeneous, the development, course, and outcome of illness are highly variable. Overall, the chronic nature often leads to significant morbidity and early mortality, although some patients diagnosed with schizophrenia are considered to have recovered from the illness. These outcomes are summarized in Box 3.3.

Onset and Course of Illness

Many patients with schizophrenia have subtle signs and symptoms present from childhood for years before diagnosis. These can include mild cognitive deficits, delays in developmental milestones, social difficulties, minor physical anomalies of the face, head, or extremities, and soft neurological signs. These findings also support the idea that schizophrenia is a neurodevelopmental disorder. Negative symptoms are more likely to occur

BOX 3.3
SCHIZOPHRENIA OUTCOMES

One-third have milder symptoms and a better outcome, 1 of 7 may show full recovery.
Poor outcome associated with more negative symptoms, low IQ, younger age of onset.
Some evidence supports better outcomes in developing countries.
Less likely to be married.
Lower rates of fertility/reproduction.
Greatest individual disability of all diseases/disorders.
Increased mortality rates nearly three times the general population.

first, and they occur on average five years before the first psychotic episode (Messias et al., 2007). Evaluation of signs and symptoms in the prodrome of schizophrenia has been of intense interest due to the potential benefit of identifying and treating individuals prior to full development of the illness as a preventive measure. The prodrome is discussed in a separate chapter in this textbook.

The long-term course and outcome of schizophrenia are also variable. Longitudinal data show that one-third of patients have a better outcome with milder symptoms, and the remaining two-thirds have more severe symptoms with poor functioning (Perkins, Miller-Andersen, & Lieberman, 2007). Antipsychotic treatment has had the greatest benefit in reducing positive symptoms in the active phase, but negative symptoms often persist, resulting in a residual phase that persists with periods of acute exacerbations (Black & Andreasen, 2014). Cognitive impairment, which develops during the prodrome, tends to persist over time, and does not respond to treatments (Keefe, 2014). Some features of the disorder are associated with either a good or poor outcome. Gradual onset, prominent negative symptoms, low IQ, and younger age of onset are some of the variables that predict poor outcome (Black & Andreasen, 2014).

Approximately 1 out of 7 patients appear to recover from schizophrenia, defined as at least two years of mild to no symptoms and normal psychosocial functioning (Jaaskelainen et al., 2013). Zipursky recently discussed the disconnect between potential and actual outcomes in schizophrenia patients, arguing that because schizophrenia is not considered a progressive brain disease, outcomes should be better (Zipursky, 2014). Factors such as poor adherence and response to treatment, cognitive deficits, substance use, and other comorbid mental disorders, and limits in access to treatment all contribute to overall poor outcomes. Research suggests that patients in developing countries have better outcomes (Messias et al., 2007), but not all researchers agree (Rangaswamy & Greeshma, 2012). Several theories have been proposed to explain this possible difference, such as less severity of psychosis and fewer residual symptoms (possibly due to a selection bias of those with in utero or birth complications less likely to survive gestation or delivery) or a better environment that supports recovery with more family support and less economic competition or stigma.

Marriage/Reproduction

Patients diagnosed with schizophrenia are less likely to be married before, at the time of diagnosis, and afterward (Agerbo, Byrne, Eaton, & Mortensen, 2004). They are also more likely to be single as early as 20 years before diagnosis, with the likelihood of being single highest at the time of first hospitalization. Men with schizophrenia are also more likely to be single than women, which may be due to differences in age of onset. Women, who develop the illness later than men, may be more likely to already be married prior to development of prominent symptoms compared to men. These findings may indicate that individuals who develop schizophrenia face more difficulties developing relationships and achieving intimacy.

Low rates of fertility and reproduction have long been observed in schizophrenia patients. Factors related to the illness, such as apathy, decreased interest in socialization, low sex drive, and chronic hospitalization or institutionalization may all contribute to schizophrenia patients having fewer children. Lower fertility in men has also been reported (Nimgaonkar, 1998), again possibly with younger age of onset in men contributing. Despite this, rates of the disorder have persisted over time, indicating that other environmental and genetic factors (such as de novo mutations) may contribute to persistence of the illness.

Morbidity/Mortality

Schizophrenia causes significant morbidity and early mortality. The 2010 Global Burden of Disease Study reported that schizophrenia accounted for between 5.0 and 9.8 million disability adjusted life years lost to mortality or morbidity worldwide (Whiteford et al., 2013). Although this is proportionally small due to the lower prevalence of the illness, acute schizophrenia had the largest disability weight in the GBD survey, indicating that the illness has the largest individual disability of *all* diseases and disorders.

Increased mortality has long been observed (Black & Fisher, 1992). A systematic review of 37 studies from 25 countries estimated increased all-cause mortality in patients with schizophrenia by estimating a median standardized mortality ratio (SMR) of 2.58 (Saha, Chant, & McGrath, 2007). In a study from Denmark, about one-fourth of deaths in patients with psychotic disorders over 20 years were due to non-natural causes, such as suicide, homicide, and accidents (Hiroeh, Appleby, Mortensen, & Dunn, 2001). Suicide, suicide attempts, and self-harm behaviors are all increased in schizophrenia patients, and these are discussed in more detail in a separate chapter.

The overall causes of death in schizophrenia patients appear to have changed over the decades (Bushe, Taylor, & Haukka, 2010). In 1980, leading causes of mortality were suicide, accidents, and infectious disease. The overall mortality appears to have reached its peak in 1995 and slightly declined since then. Today the more common causes of mortality remain suicide and accidents in younger patients, but also natural causes, mainly from cardiovascular disease and cancer that occur at younger ages than the general population. Schizophrenia patients have a higher rate of smoking, engage in other unhealthy lifestyle

BOX 3.4

CHRONIC ILLNESSES WITH SIGNIFICANTLY HIGHER INCIDENCE IN SCHIZOPHRENIA PATIENTS

AIDS
Liver disease.
Any tumor.
Diabetes.
Moderate to severe renal disease.
Hemiplegia.
Ulcer disease.
Chronic pulmonary disease.
Dementia.
Cerebrovascular disease.
Peripheral vascular disease.
Congestive heart failure.
Myocardial infarction.

Source: Laursen, T. M., Munk-Olsen, T., & Gasse, C. (2011). Chronic somatic comorbidity and excess mortality due to natural causes in persons with schizophrenia or bipolar affective disorder. PLoS ONE, 6(9), e24597.

behaviors, and have inconsistent medical care, which increase risk of morbidity and mortality from illnesses such as heart disease and cancer (von Hausswolff-Juhlin, Bjartveit, Lindström, & Jones, 2009). Schizophrenia patients also have a higher incidence rate of several chronic medical conditions compared to the general population, and these are listed in Box 3.4. It is estimated that these comorbid conditions account for half of the excess mortality in schizophrenia patients (Laursen, Munk-Olsen, & Gasse, 2011). There is also concern that side effects of newer antipsychotics, such as weight gain, diabetes, and hypertension, may also contribute to increased morbidity and mortality now and in the future. Recent health care reform with requirements for integrated care in the United States may improve these health outcomes.

Violence and Criminal Behavior

Most patients with schizophrenia do not commit violent acts, but they are more likely to commit acts of violence than people in the general population (Fazel, Gulati, Linsell, Geddes, & Grann, 2009). Men with schizophrenia are four to five times more likely to commit a violent act, whereas women have an eightfold risk. Fazel et al. found that most of the increased risk was due to comorbid substance abuse, and the risk for individuals with psychosis was similar to individuals who have substance abuse without psychosis. Comorbid substance use and antisocial personality disorder were also major factors responsible for increased criminal behavior in persons with schizophrenia, and a significant portion of the incarcerated population in the United States has severe mental illness, with estimates ranging from 10 percent-18 percent (McCabe, Christopher, Druhn, Roy-Bujnowski, Grudzinskas, & Fisher, 2012). Other risk factors associated with violence in individuals with schizophrenia include hostile behavior, non-adherence to treatments, poor impulse control, and criminal history (Witt, van Dorn, & Fazel, 2013). Individuals with schizophrenia also have increased risk of being victims of violence, and that risk is higher than the risk of committing violence (Choe, Teplin, & Abram, 2008).

REFERENCES

Abidi, S. (2013). Psychosis in children and youth: Focus on early-onset schizophrenia. [Review]. *Pediatrics in Review / American Academy of Pediatrics, 34*(7), 296–305.

Agerbo, E., Byrne, M., Eaton, W. W., & Mortensen, P. B. (2004). Marital and labor market status in the long run in schizophrenia. *Archives of General Psychiatry, 61*(1), 28–33.

Black, D. W., & Andreasen, N. C. (2014). Schizophrenia spectrum and other psychotic disorders In D. W. Black & N. C. Andreasen (Eds.) *Introductory textbook of psychiatry* (6th ed.) pp. 125–154). Arlington, VA: American Psychiatric Publishing.

Black, D. W., & Fisher, R. (1992). Mortality in *DSM-IIIR* schizophrenia. *Schizophrenia Research, 7*(2), 109–116.

Bushe, C. J., Taylor, M., & Haukka, J. (2010). Review: Mortality in schizophrenia: a measurable clinical endpoint. *Journal of Psychopharmacology (Oxford, England), 24* (Suppl 4), 17–25.

Byrne, M., Agerbo, E., Ewald, H., Eaton, W. W., & Mortensen, P. B. (2003). Parental age and risk of schizophrenia: A case-control study. *Archives of General Psychiatry, 60*(7), 673–678.

Cannon, M., Jones, P. B., & Murray, R. M. (2002). Obstetric complications and schizophrenia: historical and meta-analytic review. [Historical Article]. *The American Journal of Psychiatry, 159*(7), 1080–1092.

Choe, J., Teplin, L., & Abram, K. (2008). Perpetration of violence, violent victimization, and severe mental illness: Balancing public health concerns. *Psychiatric Services, 59*(2), 153–164.

D'Onofrio, B. M., Rickert, M. E., Frans, E., Kuja-Halkola, R., Almqvist, C., Sjölander, A.,. . .Lichtenstein, P. (2014). Paternal age at childbearing and offspring psychiatric and academic morbidity. *JAMA Psychiatry, 71*(4), 432–438.

D'Souza, D. C. (2007). Cannabinoids and Psychosis. *International Review of Neurobiology, 78*, 289–326.

Eaton, W. W., & Chen, C.-Y. (2007). Epidemiology. In J. A. Lieberman, T. S. Stroup & D. O. Perkins (Eds.), *The American psychiatric publishing textbook of schizophrenia* (pp. 17–38). Arlington, VA: American Psychiatric Publishing.

Eranti, S. V., MacCabe, J. H., Bundy, H., & Murray, R. M. (2013). Gender difference in age at onset of schizophrenia: A meta-analysis. *Psychological Medicine, 43*(1), 155–167.

Fazel, S., Gulati, G., Linsell, L., Geddes, J. R., & Grann, M. (2009). Schizophrenia and violence: Systematic review and meta-analysis. *PLoS Medicine, 6*(8), e1000120.

Gara, M. A., Vega, W. A., Arndt, S., Escamilla, M., Fleck, D. E., Lawson, W. B.,. . .Strakowski, S.M. (2012). Influence of patient race and ethnicity on clinical assessment in patients with affective disorders. [Comparative Study]. *Archives of General Psychiatry, 69*(6), 593–600.

Gattaz, W. F., Abrahão, A. L., & Foccacia, R. (2004). Childhood meningitis, brain maturation and the risk of psychosis. *European Archives of Psychiatry and Clinical Neuroscience, 254*(1), 23–26.

Giordano, G. N., Ohlsson, H., Sundquist, K., Sundquist, J., & Kendler, K. S. (2014). The association between cannabis abuse and subsequent schizophrenia: a Swedish national co-relative control study. *Psychological Medicine.*

Hagberg, H., Gressens, P., & Mallard, C. (2012). Inflammation during fetal and neonatal life: implications for neurologic and neuropsychiatric disease in children and adults. *Annals of Neurology, 71*(4), 444–457.

Hiroeh, U., Appleby, L., Mortensen, P. B., & Dunn, G. (2001). Death by homicide, suicide, and other unnatural causes in people with mental illness: a population-based study. *The Lancet, 358*(9299), 2110–2112.

Jaaskelainen, E., Juola, P., Hirvonen, N., McGrath, J. J., Saha, S., Isohanni, M., . . .Miettunen, J.. .. (2013). A Systematic Review and Meta-Analysis of Recovery in Schizophrenia. *Schizophrenia Bulletin, 39*(6), 1296–1306.

Jablensky, A., Kirkbride, J. B., & Jones, P. (2011). Schizophrenia: The epidemiological horizon. In D. R. Weinberger & P. J. Harrison (Eds.), *Schizophrenia* (3rd ed., pp. 185–225). Chichester, West Sussex, UK; Hoboken, NJ: Wiley-Blackwell.

Jablensky, A., Sartorius, N., Ernberg, G., Anker, M., Korten, A., Cooper, J. E.,. . . Bertelsen, A. (1992). Schizophrenia: manifestations, incidence and course in different cultures. A World Health Organization ten-country study. *Psychological Medicine. Monograph supplement, 20*, 1–97.

Kalra, G., Bhugra, D., & Shah, N. (2012). Cultural aspects of schizophrenia. *International Review of Psychiatry (Abingdon, England), 24*(5), 441–449.

Keefe, R. S. E. (2014). The longitudinal course of cognitive impairment in schizophrenia: an examination of data from premorbid through posttreatment phases of illness. *The Journal of Clinical Psychiatry, 75*(Suppl 2), 8–13.

Kirkbride, J. B., Fearon, P., Morgan, C., Dazzan, P., Morgan, K., Tarrant, J.,. . .Jones, P.B. (2006). Heterogeneity in Incidence Rates of Schizophrenia and Other Psychotic Syndromes: Findings From the 3-Center ÆSOP Study. *Archives of General Psychiatry, 63*(3), 250–258.

Kwok, W. (2014). Is there evidence that social class at birth increases risk of psychosis? A systematic review. *The International Journal of Social Psychiatry., 60*(8), 801–808.

Large, M., Sharma, S., Compton, M. T., Slade, T., & Nielssen, O. (2011). Cannabis use and earlier onset of psychosis: A systematic meta-analysis. *Archives of General Psychiatry, 68*(6), 555–561.

Laursen, T. M., Munk-Olsen, T., & Gasse, C. (2011). Chronic somatic comorbidity and excess mortality due to natural causes in persons with schizophrenia or bipolar affective disorder. *PLoS ONE, 6*(9), e24597.

Malaspina, D., Harlap, S., Fennig, S., Heiman, D., Nahon, D., Feldman, D., & Susser, E.S.(2001). Advancing paternal age and the risk of schizophrenia. *Archives of General Psychiatry, 58*(4), 361–367.

McCabe, P. J., Christopher, P. P., Druhn, N., Roy-Bujnowski, K. M., Grudzinskas, A. J., & Fisher, W. H. (2012). Arrest types and co-occurring disorders in persons with schizophrenia or related psychoses. *The Journal of Behavioral Health Services & Research, 39*(3), 271–284.

McGrath, J., Saha, S., Chant, D., & Welham, J. (2008). Schizophrenia: A concise overview of incidence, prevalence, and mortality. *Epidemiologic Reviews, 30*(1), 67–76.

Messias, E. L., Chen, C.-Y., & Eaton, W. W. (2007). Epidemiology of schizophrenia: Review of findings and myths. *Psychiatric Clinics of North America, 30*(3), 323–338.

Miller, B., Messias, E., Miettunen, J., Alaräisänen, A., Järvelin, M.-R., Koponen, H., .. . Kirkpatrick, B. (2011). Meta-analysis of paternal age and schizophrenia risk in male versus female offspring. [Comparative Study]. *Schizophrenia Bulletin, 37*(5), 1039–1047.

Mittal, V. A., Willhite, R., Daley, M., Bearden, C. E., Niendam, T., Ellman, L. M., & Cannon, T. D. (2009). Obstetric complications and risk for conversion to psychosis among individuals at high clinical risk. *Early Intervention in Psychiatry, 3*(3), 226–230.

Nimgaonkar, V. L. (1998). Reduced fertility in schizophrenia: here to stay? *Acta Psychiatrica Scandinavica, 98*(5), 348–353.

Perkins, D. O., Miller-Andersen, L., & Lieberman, J. A. (2007). Natural History and Predictors of Clinical Course. In J. A. Lieberman, T. S. Stroup & D. O. Perkins (Eds.), *The American psychiatric publishing textbook of schizophrenia* (pp. 289–301). Arlington, VA: American Psychiatric Publishing.

Petersen, L., Mortensen, P. B., & Pedersen, C. B. (2011). Paternal age at birth of first child and risk of schizophrenia. *The American Journal of Psychiatry, 168*(1), 82–88.

Rangaswamy, T., & Greeshma, M. (2012). Course and outcome of schizophrenia. *International Review of Psychiatry (Abingdon, England), 24*(5), 417–422.

Saha, S., Chant, D., & McGrath, J. (2007). A Systematic review of mortality in schizophrenia: Is the differential mortality gap worsening over time? *Archives of General Psychiatry, 64*(10), 1123–1131.

Saha, S., Chant, D., Welham, J., & McGrath, J. (2005). A systematic review of the prevalence of schizophrenia. *PLoS Medicine, 2*(5), e141.

Schmitt, A., Malchow, B., Hasan, A., & Falkai, P. (2014). The impact of environmental factors in severe psychiatric disorders. *Frontiers in Neuroscience, 8*, 19.

Severance, E. G., Yolken, R. H., & Eaton, W. W. (2014). Autoimmune diseases, gastrointestinal disorders and the microbiome in schizophrenia: More than a gut feeling. *Schizophrenia Research*, epub ahead of print. Retrieved from http://www.sciencedirect.com/science/article/pii/S0920996414003193.

von Hausswolff-Juhlin, Y., Bjartveit, M., Lindström, E., & Jones, P. (2009). Schizophrenia and physical health problems. *Acta Psychiatrica Scandinavica, 119*, 15–21.

Whiteford, H. A., Degenhardt, L., Rehm, J., Baxter, A. J., Ferrari, A. J., Erskine, H. E., . . .Vos, T. (2013). Global burden of disease attributable to mental and substance use disorders: findings from the Global Burden of Disease Study 2010. *The Lancet, 382*(9904), 1575–1586.

Witt, K., van Dorn, R., & Fazel, S. (2013). Risk factors for violence in psychosis: Systematic review and meta-regression analysis of 110 studies. *PLoS ONE, 8*(2), e55942.

Zipursky, R. B. (2014). Why are the outcomes in patients with schizophrenia so poor? *The Journal of Clinical Psychiatry, 75*(Suppl 2), 20–24.

/// 4 /// THE PSYCHOSIS PRODROME AND ITS IMPLICATIONS

PATRICK D. MCGORRY
and SHERILYN GOLDSTONE

INTRODUCTION

The outlook for a young person experiencing the early stages of a psychotic illness today can—and should—be very different from that of just two decades ago. Over this time, basic research into the epidemiology and neurobiology of the psychotic illnesses has allowed the development of improved medical treatments, and innovative clinical research has led to the development of better services that are specifically designed around the unique needs of this particularly vulnerable group. This has led to a shift in focus from the historical, and largely palliative, approach to the care of those living with psychosis, to an emphasis on early intervention with evidence-based care delivered within an optimistic, recovery-oriented framework.

We now know that the course of the psychotic disorders is not fixed, with deterioration in social and occupational functioning and a poor prognosis inevitable, but, rather, it is fluid and can potentially be altered by appropriate interventions that target specific risk factors known to influence outcome (Alvarez-Jimenez et al., 2012; Bertelsen et al., 2008; Crumlish et al., 2009; Hegelstad et al., 2012; Henry et al., 2010; Larsen et al., 2011; Menezes et al., 2009; Morgan et al., 2014; Norman et al., 2011). This has created an explosion of interest in early intervention and phase-specific, recovery-focused treatment for early psychosis, in a paradigm shift towards a more preemptive, personalized approach to psychiatry (Insel, 2007). Here, we will give an overview of the importance of the concept of the prodrome, as established by the early psychosis paradigm, and its broader implications for our understanding of the evolution of serious mental illness more generally.

The Prodrome: An Opportunity for Preemptive Intervention

In medicine, a "prodrome" is defined as an early symptom or set of symptoms that indicate the onset of an illness, prior to its full development. Although it has long been recognized that the major mental disorders develop from a pre-onset period marked by increasing levels of relatively nonspecific symptomatology and distress, associated with a corresponding decline in functioning (Fava & Tossani, 2007; Hafner et al., 2003; Hafner, Maurer, Trendler, an der Heiden, & Schmidt, 2005; Hetrick, Parker, Hickie, Purcell, Yung, & McGorry, 2008; Yung, et al., 1998), the idea of intervening during this prodromal period with the aim of preventing the onset of full-threshold illness was first proposed just over two decades ago (Eaton, Badawi, & Melton, 1995; Mrazek & Haggerty, 1994; American Psychiatric Association, 1997). This represented a dramatic shift in thinking in psychiatry, which had been slow to adopt the preventive framework that had been accepted decades earlier in physical medicine, largely due to the widespread pessimism associated with the diagnosis of schizophrenia, as well as a lack of predictive markers able to identify those at risk of developing a psychotic disorder. Over the last several decades, this has slowly been changing, primarily as a result of careful research that has identified clinical criteria that indicate an ultrahigh risk of transition to psychosis, and the demonstration that early intervention prior to the onset of illness has the potential to prevent the development of full-threshold psychosis, or at the very least, to modify the course of illness by minimizing the accumulation of secondary disability.

DEFINING THE PSYCHOSIS PRODROME

Defining the clinical features of the prodromal period was a key advance in our understanding and treatment of the psychotic illnesses, because this has opened the way for the development of potentially preemptive interventions. Careful retrospective studies of first-episode psychosis patients have shown that, in general, negative symptoms such as decreased concentration, reduced drive, lack of energy, and social withdrawal predominate early in this phase, accompanied by general symptoms such as sleep disturbance, anxiety, and irritability. Affective symptoms, particularly anxiety and depression, and relationship difficulties are also common. These symptoms tend to accumulate and increase in severity until relatively late in the prodrome, when subthreshold psychotic symptoms emerge (Hafner et al., 2003; Yung & McGorry, 1996a, 1996b). Ultimately, these positive symptoms intensify and may culminate in a transition to frank psychosis. Typically, increasing levels of social and vocational disability accompany the increase in symptomatology, and this phase is also characterized by high levels of self-harm and suicidal behavior (Phillips et al., 2009). Early intervention is paramount, first because much of the disability associated with the psychotic disorders develops well before the onset of frank psychosis and is difficult to reverse, even if the first psychotic episode is successfully treated (Hafner et al., 2003). Furthermore, the most important risk factor for poor outcome is a long duration of untreated illness (Marshall et al., 2005; Perkins, Gu, Boteva, & Lieberman, 2005).

However, because these symptoms, including subthreshold psychotic-like experiences, are common in the general population, particularly in adolescents and young adults (Wigman et al., 2012), they cannot be considered as diagnostic of a prepsychotic state in their own right (van Os, Hanssen, Bijl, & Vollebergh, 2001; Yung et al., 2006). Additional risk factors and specific criteria are necessary to exclude false positive cases to avoid unnecessary treatment and the stigma associated with the diagnosis of a mental illness. In the mid-1990s, our research group operationalized criteria for the prospective identification of individuals at increased risk of progressing to a first episode of psychosis—that is, as being in the prodromal phase of illness. These "ultrahigh risk" or "clinical high risk" criteria are based on a combination of epidemiological evidence and known trait and state risk factors for psychosis (Yung & McGorry, 1996a; Yung et al., 2003). They can be divided into three groups on the basis of the young person's presenting symptoms: attenuated psychotic symptoms; brief, self-limiting intermittent psychotic symptoms; and genetic risk of schizophrenia (a first-degree relative with schizophrenia/schizoaffective disorder) with a recent significant decrease in functioning.

Although early studies showed that up to 40 percent of the young people who met these criteria made a transition to psychosis within the following year (Yung & McGorry, 1996a), more recent data has revealed that the 12-month transition rate has fallen to around 22 percent in recent cohorts, yet over a three-year period it remains at around 36 percent (Fusar-Poli, Bonoldi, Yung, & van Os, 2012; Nelson et al., 2013). By comparison, in a meta-analysis of six prospective studies of the non-help-seeking general population, Kaymaz and colleagues (Kaymaz et al., 2012) have calculated the 12-month rate of transition to psychotic illness in those reporting psychotic-like experiences as 0.56 percent, compared to 0.16 percent in those who did not report such symptoms. This provides a useful baseline against which to compare the rate of transition in those considered to be at ultrahigh risk of psychosis.

Although the ultrahigh-risk criteria show good relative specificity for transition to psychosis, the majority of young people who fulfil these criteria do not develop a full-threshold psychotic disorder, and a significant proportion (up to approximately 50 percent) experience remission of their psychotic symptoms within a year of seeking help (Addington et al., 2011; Simon et al., 2013). However, most of these young people continue to report clinically relevant symptoms, primarily a blend of anxiety and depression, as well as difficulties in social and occupational functioning, highlighting their need for ongoing care (Nelson et al., 2013). Moreover, long-term follow-up has shown that transition to psychosis can occur up to 10 years following initial diagnosis, clearly indicating that these young people may remain vulnerable for long periods of time (Nelson et al., 2013), and again emphasizing the need for careful monitoring and clinical care.

INTERVENTIONS IN THE PRODROMAL PHASE

The aim of treatment in the prodromal phase is to provide comprehensive clinical care designed to reduce distressing symptoms and improve functioning, and, if possible, to prevent these symptoms from worsening and developing into full-threshold sustained psychosis. If psychosis does occur, the aim of treatment becomes to minimize the duration of untreated psychosis, attain and maintain remission of symptoms, and promote the best possible functional recovery (McGorry, Nelson, & Goldstone, 2012). The prodromal interventions that have been trialed to date include psychologically based strategies, such as psychoeducation, supportive psychotherapy, cognitive behavioral therapy (CBT) and family work; biologically based strategies, including symptomatic treatment for depression, anxiety, and subthreshold psychotic symptoms, through to experimental neuroprotective approaches.

Ten intervention studies have now been conducted in these young people, investigating the use of medications (low-dose antipsychotics and/or antidepressants), psychosocial treatments, or both, to prevent the onset of psychosis. A recent meta-analysis of these trials has shown that each of these treatments are effective, with an overall number needed to treat of 9 (95 percent, confidence interval 6–15) and an overall risk reduction at 12 months of 54 percent (Van Der Gaag et al., 2013). However, risk–benefit concerns related to the use of antipsychotic medication, even at low doses, means that psychosocial interventions, including supportive therapy and CBT, and other benign interventions, such as treatment with omega-3 fatty acids (Amminger et al., 2010), or glycine, which has shown some promise in a recent pilot study (Woods, Walsh, Pearlson, & McGlashan, 2006), are currently recommended as first-line therapies in this patient group (McGorry et al., 2012). Drug therapies should only be considered if distressing symptoms *and* impairment persist or worsen. Antipsychotic medication may have a place in the treatment of those who fail to respond to initial intervention with psychosocial therapies;

symptom severity alone may not be a perfect guide for the need for antipsychotic medication, because the definition of "full-threshold psychosis" may vary. Other factors, such as symptom type and pattern, and other clinical phenomena, including patient choice, comorbid substance use, triggers and stressors, genetic and other biomarkers, and so forth will also determine the optimal treatment for a given patient. When antipsychotics are prescribed, the best candidates are those with a more favorable metabolic and neurological safety profile, such as aripiprazole (Kahn et al., 2008).

The results of the intervention trials to date are promising, but there is a need to carefully study other strategies such as cognitive remediation and benign biotherapies targeting candidate neurobiological mechanisms such as inflammation and oxidative stress. Determination of the optimal sequence of interventions and definition of therapeutically relevant subgroups via sophisticated clinical trial designs is necessary to build a solid evidence base to inform future therapeutic strategies for this particularly vulnerable patient group.

THE PSYCHOSIS PRODROME OR A PLURIPOTENTIAL RISK SYNDROME?

Although subthreshold psychotic phenomena are universally present prior to the onset of schizophrenia, transient subthreshold psychotic experiences are common in healthy young people from the general population (van Os & Linscott, 2012; van Rossum, Dominguez, Lieb, Wittchen, & van Os, 2011; Varghese et al., 2011), although only a minority of these cases evolve into a diagnosable mental illness each year. A significant proportion (approximately 27 percent) of young people with depressive or anxiety disorders also report psychotic-like experiences (van Rossum et al., 2011; Wigman et al., 2011), with the presence of psychotic symptoms being associated with a poorer course of illness (van Rossum et al., 2011; Wigman et al., 2011). Furthermore, the vast majority of young people who fulfil the ultrahigh-risk criteria also have at least one diagnosable Axis 1 disorder (Fusar-Poli, Yung, McGorry, & van Os, 2014). There may also be other pathways to psychosis onset, with this occurring not only via the ultrahigh-risk route (Schultze-Lutter, 2009; Schultze-Lutter, Ruhrmann, Berning, Maier, & Klosterkotter, 2010).

Thus, there is considerable overlap between the psychopathological dimensions represented in the at-risk state, and it is increasingly evident that the concept of "ultrahigh risk" might usefully be broadened to one of a "pluripotential risk state," rather than being considered specific to psychosis alone (McGorry, 2010). Psychotic phenomena may be considered an indication of severity of illness, rather than a specific indicator of imminent risk of a full-threshold psychotic illness (Foulds & Bedford, 1975; Kelleher et al., 2012; Stochl et al., 2014). This has obvious implications for the treatment approach for these young people, as well as for our understanding of the evolution of the early stages of mental illness. In terms of therapeutic intervention, the presence of psychotic phenomena per se should not be the primary determinant of treatment selection (i.e., prescription of antipsychotic medication); instead, first-line treatment should favor supportive psychosocial interventions, in line with the clinical staging model (McGorry et al., 2012), with careful ongoing monitoring of the young person's mental state.

RISK SYNDROMES IN PSYCHIATRY

The idea of a pluripotential risk syndrome has much to offer in psychiatry, in that it opens real possibilities for preventive, or at least pre-emptive intervention (McGorry, 2010). Preventive medicine relies on the idea of risk and benefit, where the risk and costs associated with the intervention are considered in the light of the potential benefits to the target population and the costs associated with managing the illness or health condition in that population. Universal prevention offers interventions (such as vaccination) to the entire population, with the aim of benefiting all and minimizing the impact and costs associated with the illness in the whole population. Selective prevention involves interventions being offered to a subgroup of people considered to be at particular risk of illness or to maintain optimum health in that population (for example, smoking cessation programs for smokers; antenatal screening of pregnant women), whereas indicated prevention targets individuals identified as being at high risk (for example, statin therapy for those with high cholesterol to prevent heart attacks or stroke).

As is the case for physical illness, many of the risk factors for poor mental health are universal, and largely environmental or social in nature. These include poverty, deprivation, social isolation, conflict, and powerlessness, among many others, and require a broad societal approach with a human rights agenda to tackle them. Higher-level prevention is more complex, in that it requires the identification of subpopulations and individuals who are at risk of developing a mental illness. Predicting any individual's risk of the onset of a mental illness, its likely course, or their response to a particular therapy, requires a detailed knowledge of the environmental, social and neurobiological risk factors that influence these aspects, as well as the availability of suitable markers that can be tested to determine their specific risk profile (McGorry, 2013b). Although this predictive, personalized approach to diagnosis and treatment is now routine in many areas of physical medicine, it remains largely aspirational in psychiatry today. This is because as yet we have a relatively poor knowledge of the causal and/or malleable risk factors for the onset of mental illness, though advances in our understanding of neurobiology, genetics, and computational biology, as well as the complexity of the interactions between the biological, psychological, and social factors that contribute to the development of mental illness, are making rapid headway in this area (McGorry, Keshavan, et al., 2014). In the last few years we have begun moving closer to a more personalized approach to detection and treatment on the basis of sophisticated analyses of combinations of immune/inflammatory markers (Perkins et al., 2015) and neurobiological markers (McGorry, Keshavan, et al., 2014; Perkins et al., 2015; Pettersson-Yeo et al., 2013) associated with risk of transition to psychosis.

However, given the lack of definitive biomarkers for individual risk, and the evidence suggesting that subthreshold symptoms strongly predict future disorder (Eaton et al., 1995; Harrington & Clark, 1998; Hetrick et al., 2008; Seeley, Stice, & Rohde, 2009; Yung, Phillips, Yuen, & McGorry, 2004), it has been suggested that these subthreshold syndromes can be considered as risk factors, and that these can be targeted by specific interventions to reduce the risk of fully-fledged illness (Bell, 1992; Eaton et al., 1995; Mrazek & Haggerty, 1994). Here, a focus on the very early stages of illness, or prodromal period, has great potential (van Os, 2013) in terms of possibilities for preventive or preemptive intervention, and is central to the clinical staging model (McGorry, 2013a; McGorry, 2007a; McGorry, Nelson, Goldstone, & Yung, 2010).

PARADIGM SHIFT: FROM PALLIATIVE TO PREVENTIVE PSYCHIATRY

The evolution of the mental disorders is perhaps more usefully described within the context of a clinical staging model (McGorry, 2007a; McGorry et al., 2010). Clinical staging differs from conventional diagnostic practice in that it defines the extent of progression of a disorder at a particular point in time and where a person lies along the course of their illness. The differentiation of early, milder clinical phenomena from those that accompany illness extension, progression, and chronicity lies at the heart of the concept. Staging frameworks are central to preemptive medicine, since they enable clinicians to select treatments relevant to the earlier stages of an illness, and generally assume that such interventions will be both more effective and less harmful than treatments delivered at later stages. They also offer the possibility that early, successful intervention may change the expected course of a disorder by preventing progression to subsequent stages, and such early intervention may result in remission and cure or, at the very least, delayed progression and minimization of secondary disability. The key advantage of clinical staging is that it encourages the balancing of the risks and benefits of treatment within a stepped-care approach. Such a framework has much to offer in terms of guiding treatment selection in the very early stages of mental illness, when evolving mixes of symptoms and comorbidity are the norm, rather than the exception, and current diagnostic tools are of little use.

It has long been recognized that the need for care precedes a formally diagnosable mental illness, and often for significant periods of time (McGorry, 2010). However, because acceptance into our existing mental health services often depends on meeting a certain diagnostic threshold, all too often appropriate care is not available to those living with significant and disabling levels of symptoms and distress who do not yet meet formal criteria for a particular diagnosis. The resulting delay in treatment allows the entrenchment of illness as well as the accumulation of secondary psychosocial disability, both of which may have been averted if a lower threshold for entry into care was set and the opportunity for early and preemptive intervention was available. Determining the threshold at which clinical intervention should be offered is often difficult, particularly in young people, with whom emotional disturbance is common. Although such disturbance often resolves quickly (Patton et al., 2014), this is not always the case for a significant number of young people, who are then at high risk of going on to develop a full-threshold mental illness. Here, the clinical staging model, with its agnostic, rather than diagnostic, approach and emphasis on early preventive intervention comes into its own. This model explicitly acknowledges the need for care in the very early stages of illness, with this being based only on the intensity of symptoms and distress, disturbance in psychosocial functioning, and the persistence of these changes, rather than on specific diagnostic criteria. Adopting such a preemptive approach will require wider acceptance of the value of early intervention, as well as system change to allow the redesign of our existing services and much better resourcing levels, but such an approach has great potential in terms of reducing the human and economic costs associated with poor mental health.

PRODROMES, PREEMPTIVE PSYCHIATRY, AND BROADER ISSUES

The move toward early intervention and a more preemptive psychiatry that has evolved over the last two decades of research into early psychosis raises a number of broader issues for researchers, clinicians, and policymakers alike, particularly when placed within the context of the new insights gained from epidemiological studies into the timing of onset of the major adult-type mental illnesses. We now know that most new cases appear in young people from early adolescence on, with 75 percent of those who experience a mental illness having their first episode by the age of 24 years (Kessler et al., 2005; McGorry, Purcell, Goldstone, & Amminger, 2011). Moreover, mental health concerns are the key health issue for young people, accounting for approximately 50 percent of the burden of disease in this age group. From a preemptive stance, these data indicate that a strong focus on youth mental health—and particularly on early intervention in this age group—offers the best opportunity for reducing the human, social, and economic costs associated with mental illness that we have available to us. Unfortunately, this level of need is not met by our existing services, largely as a result of their historical separation into child and adolescent and adult streams, neither of which are acceptable or appropriate for young people, particularly older adolescents, who are often actively excluded from both service streams. The result of this situation is that young people have the poorest access to mental health care of all age groups across the lifespan, despite their manifest need for appropriate care (McGorry, Goldstone, Parker, Rickwood, & Hickie, 2014), and that this ideal opportunity for preventive, or at least pre-emptive, intervention is lost.

Early intervention is particularly relevant to young people, who tend to present with complex and evolving symptom profiles that may, or may not, evolve into serious mental illnesses. Here, intervening with simple therapies with a strong preventive focus has real potential to prevent the establishment of more severe and enduring illness (McGorry, 2007b; McGorry, Goldstone et al., 2014; McGorry, Purcell, Hickie, & Jorm, 2007). The early psychosis paradigm has provided proof of concept of the value of this approach and has sparked a growing movement advocating for system reform of our mental health services so that they better cater for the needs of our young people, who are so poorly served by the current system. Specific youth mental health services are now beginning to appear that have been designed around the unique clinical, developmental, social, and cultural needs of young people (McGorry et al., 2014). These services offer early intervention with a strong preventive focus in community-based, youth-friendly centers that cater to the broad-spectrum need in this age group, ranging from mild distress to more severe illness. They offer an integrated, multidisciplinary approach to free or low cost treatment in a "one-stop-shop" that also provides access to physical and sexual health care, vocational and educational assistance, and other services commonly used by young people (McGorry, Bates, & Birchwood, 2013; McGorry, Goldstone et al., 2014), which helps to minimize the stigma associated with accessing a mental health service. Their communities have very well accepted such services, with excellent uptake by young people (McGorry, Goldstone et al., 2014; Rickwood, Telford, Parker, Tanti, & McGorry, 2014). Although their value has yet to be formally established, they do appear to be addressing the issues of young peoples' access to mental health care as well as engagement with services, a very positive early outcome (McGorry et al., 2013; Rickwood et al., 2014).

CONCLUSION

The last two decades have seen an enormous growth in our understanding of the psychotic disorders. Research into the early stages of these illnesses has allowed us to build an evidence base to support the value of early intervention with the aim of preventing the onset of illness, or at least minimizing the secondary disability associated with a psychotic illness. This has driven service reforms that have now been adopted world-wide, so that a young person who is at high risk of a psychotic disorder, or experiencing a first episode of illness, can now receive developmentally appropriate, evidence-based care in a specialized service that focuses on maintaining or regaining a normal developmental trajectory and achieving full functional recovery, in the expectation of a good outcome. This is an enormous advance, when just two decades ago preemptive intervention was not considered, and a first psychotic episode was seen as catastrophic, consigning the young person to certain disability.

This move away from the largely palliative treatment approaches that have prevailed until recently has provoked a seismic shift in today's psychiatry toward a more preemptive, personalized medicine, as is already the norm in many areas of physical medicine. Moreover, the success of the early psychosis paradigm, along with our increased awareness of the epidemiology and age of onset of the major mental illnesses, has catalyzed a broader interest in the area of youth mental health more generally, and the enormous public health opportunities that early intervention with a focus on young people's mental health offers.

Much remains to be done for these reforms to bear full fruit. For a truly predictive, personalized medicine able to identify who is at greatest risk of developing a serious mental disorder and the types of interventions that are most appropriate for that person, we need more research into the identification of biomarkers and risk factors for illness. We also need innovative research into the timing, sequence, and structure of therapeutic interventions, and how these might be better targeted to individual needs. Research into systems of care and how these might be optimized is also crucial, along with critical evaluation of new interventions and systems of care as these evolve. Finally, and most importantly, how new knowledge is translated into day-to-day practice is central to any reform process, and how this can be achieved in mental health care is a subject of study in its own right. Much has been achieved within the early psychosis paradigm, and it is now time to build on these advances so that they can be extended to all young people facing the threat of serious mental illness.

REFERENCES

Addington, J., Cornblatt, B. A., Cadenhead, K. S., Cannon, T. D., McGlashan, T. H., Perkins, D.O., . . . Heinssen, R. (2011) At clinical high risk for psychosis: outcome for nonconverters. *American Journal of Psychiatry, 168,* 800–805.

Alvarez-Jimenez, M., Gleeson, J. F., Henry, L. P., Harrigan, S. M., Harris, M. G., Killackey, E., . . . McGorry, P. D. (2012) Road to full recovery: longitudinal relationship between symptomatic remission and psychosocial recovery in first-episode psychosis over 7.5 years. *Psychological Medicine, 42*, 595–606.

American Psychiatric Association. (1997) Practice guideline for the treatment of patients with schizophrenia. *American Journal of Psychiatry, 154*, 1–63.

Amminger, G. P., Schafer, M. R., Papageorgiou, K., Klier, C. M., Cotton, S. M., Harrigan, S. M., . . . Berger, G. E. (2010) Long-chain omega-3 fatty acids for indicated prevention of psychotic disorders: a randomized, placebo-controlled trial. *Archives of General Psychiatry, 67*, 146–154.

Bell, R. Q. (1992) Multiple-risk cohorts and segmenting risk as solutions to the problem of false positives in risk for the major psychoses. *Psychiatry, 55*, 370–381.

Bertelsen, M., Jeppesen, P., Petersen, L., Thorup, A., Ohlenschlaeger, J., le Quach, P., . . . Nordentoft, M. (2008) Five-year follow-up of a randomized multicenter trial of intensive early intervention vs standard treatment for patients with a first episode of psychotic illness: the OPUS trial. *Archives of General Psychiatry, 65*, 762–771.

Crumlish, N., Whitty, P., Clarke, M., Browne, S., Kamali, M., Gervin, M., . . . O'Callaghan, E. (2009) Beyond the critical period: longitudinal study of 8-year outcome in first-episode non-affective psychosis. *British Journal of Psychiatry, 194*, 18–24.

Eaton, W. W., Badawi, M., & Melton, B. (1995) Prodromes and precursors: epidemiologic data for primary prevention of disorders with slow onset. *American Journal of Psychiatry, 152*, 967–972.

Fava, G., & Tossani, E. (2007) Prodromal stage of major depression. *Early Interventional Psychiatry, 1*, 9–18.

Foulds, G. A., & Bedford, A. (1975) Hierarchy of classes of personal illness. *Psychological Medicine, 5*, 181–192.

Fusar-Poli, P., Bonoldi, I., Yung, A. R., & van Os, J. (2012) Predicting psychosis: a meta-analysis of evidence. *Archives of General Psychiatry, 69*, 220–229.

Fusar-Poli, P., Yung, A. R., McGorry, P., & van Os, J. (2014) Lessons learned from the psychosis high-risk state: towards a general staging model of prodromal intervention. *Psychological Medicine, 44*, 17–24.

Hafner, H., Maurer, K., Loffler, W., an der Heiden, W., Hambrecht, H., & Schultze-Lutter, F. (2003) Modeling the early course of schizophrenia. *Schizophrenia Bulletin, 29*, 325–340.

Hafner, H., Maurer, K., Trendler, G., an der Heiden, W., & Schmidt, M. (2005) The early course of schizophrenia and depression. *European Archives of Psychiatry and Clinical Neuroscience, 255*, 167–173.

Harrington, R., & Clark, A. (1998) Prevention and early intervention for depression in adolescence and early adult life. *European Archives of Psychiatry and Clinical Neuroscience, 248*, 32–45.

Hegelstad, W. T., Larsen, T. K., Auestad, B., Evensen, J., Haahr, U., Joa, I., . . . McGlashan, T. (2012) Long-term follow-up of the TIPS early detection in psychosis study: effects on 10-year outcome. *American Journal of Psychiatry, 169*, 374–380.

Henry, L. P., Amminger, G. P., Harris, M. G., Yuen, H. P., Harrigan, S. M., Prosser, A. L., . . . McGorry, P. D. (2010) The EPPIC follow-up study of first-episode psychosis: longer-term clinical and functional outcome 7 years after index admission. *Journal of Clinical Psychiatry, 71*, 716–728.

Hetrick, S. E., Parker, A. G., Hickie, I. B., Purcell, R., Yung, A. R., & McGorry, P. D. (2008) Early identification and intervention in depressive disorders: towards a clinical staging model. *Psychotherapy and Psychosomatics, 77*, 263–270.

Insel, T. R. (2007) The arrival of pre-emptive psychiatry. *Early Interventional Psychiatry, 1*, 5–6.

Kahn, R. S., Fleischhacker, W. W., Boter H, Davidson, M., Vergouwe, Y., Keet, I. P., . . . Grobbee, D.E.(2008) Effectiveness of antipsychotic drugs in first-episode schizophrenia and schizophreniform disorder: an open randomised clinical trial. *Lancet, 371*, 1085–1097.

Kaymaz, N., Drukker, M., Lieb, R., Wittchen, H. U., Werbeloff, N., Weiser, M., . . . van Os, J. (2012) Do subthreshold psychotic experiences predict clinical outcomes in unselected non-help-seeking population-based samples? A systematic review and meta-analysis, enriched with new results. *Psychological Medicine, 42*, 2239–2253.

Kelleher, I., Keeley, H., Corcoran, P., Lynch, F., Fitzpatrick, C., Devlin, N., . . . Cannon, M. (2012) Clinicopathological significance of psychotic experiences in non-psychotic young people: evidence from four population-based studies. *British Journal of Psychiatry, 201*, 26–32.

Kessler, R. C., Berglund, P., Demler, O., Jin, R., Merikangas, K. R., & Walters, E. E. (2005) Lifetime prevalence and age-of-onset distributions of DSM-IV disorders in the National Comorbidity Survey Replication. *Archives of General Psychiatry, 62*, 593–602.

Larsen, T. K., Melle, I., Auestad, B., Haahr, U., Joa, I., Johannessen, J. O., . . . McGlashan, T. (2011) Early detection of psychosis: positive effects on 5-year outcome. *Psychological Medicine, 41*, 1461–1469.

Marshall, M., Lewis, S., Lockwood, A., Drake, R., Jones, P., & Croudace, T. (2005) Association between duration of untreated psychosis and outcome in cohorts of first-episode patients: a systematic review. *Archives of General Psychiatry, 62*, 975–983.

McGorry, P. D. (2007a) Issues for *DSM-V*: clinical staging: a heuristic pathway to valid nosology and safer, more effective treatment in psychiatry. *American Journal of Psychiatry, 164*, 859–860.

McGorry, P. D. (2007b) The specialist youth mental health model: strengthening the weakest link in the public mental health system. *Medical Journal of Australia, 187*, S53–56.

McGorry, P. D. (2010) Risk syndromes, clinical staging and *DSM V*: New diagnostic infrastructure for early intervention in psychiatry. *Schizophrenia Research, 120*, 49–53.

McGorry, P. D. (2013a) Early clinical phenotypes and risk for serious mental disorders in young people: need for care precedes traditional diagnoses in mood and psychotic disorders. *Canadian Journal of Psychiatry, 58*, 19–21.

McGorry, P. D. (2013b) Early clinical phenotypes, clinical staging, and strategic biomarker research: building blocks for personalized psychiatry. *Biological Psychiatry, 74*, 394–395.

McGorry, P., Bates, T., & Birchwood, M. (2013) Designing youth mental health services for the 21st century: examples from Australia, Ireland and the UK. *British Journal of Psychiatry Supplement, 54*, s30–35.

McGorry, P. D., Goldstone, S. D., Parker, A. G., Rickwood, D. J., & Hickie, I. B. (2014) Cultures for mental health care of young people: an Australian blueprint for reform. *Lancet Psychiatry, 1*, 559–568.

McGorry, P., Keshavan, M., Goldstone, S., Amminger, G. P., Allott, K., Berk, M., . . . Hickie, I. B. (2014) Biomarkers and clinical staging in psychiatry. *World Psychiatry*, 13, 211–223.

McGorry, P. D., Nelson, B., Goldstone, S., & Yung, A. R. (2010) Clinical staging: a heuristic and practical strategy for new research and better health and social outcomes for psychotic and related mood disorders. *Canadian Journal of Psychiatry, 55*, 486–497.

McGorry, P. D., Nelson, B., & Goldstone, S. (2012) Providing care to young people with emerging risk of psychosis: Balancing potential risks and benefits. *Clinical Practice, 9*, 669–682.

McGorry, P. D., Purcell, R., Goldstone, S., & Amminger, G. P. (2011) Age of onset and timing of treatment for mental and substance use disorders: implications for preventive intervention strategies and models of care. *Current Opinions in Psychiatry, 24*, 301–306.

McGorry, P. D., Purcell, R., Hickie, I. B., Jorm, A. F. (2007) Investing in youth mental health is a best buy. *Medical Journal of Australia, 187*, S5–S7.

Menezes, N. M., Malla, A. M., Norman, R. M., Archie, S., Roy, P., & Zipursky, R. B. (2009) A multi-site Canadian perspective: examining the functional outcome from first-episode psychosis. *Acta Psychiatrica Scandinavia, 120*, 138–146.

Morgan, C., Lappin, J., Heslin, M., Donohoe, K., Lomas, B., Reininghaus, U., . . . Dazzan, P. (2014) Reappraising the long-term course and outcome of psychotic disorders: the AESOP-10 study. *Psychological Medicine 44*, 2713–2726.

Mrazek, P. J., & Haggerty, R. J. (1994) *Reducing the risks for mental disorder: frontiers for preventive intervention research*. Washington DC: National Academy Press.

Nelson, B., Yuen, H. P., Wood, S. J., Lin, A., Spiliotacopoulos, D., Bruxner, A., . . . Yung, A. R. (2013) Long-term follow-up of a group at ultra high risk ("prodromal") for psychosis: the PACE 400 study. *JAMA Psychiatry, 70*, 793–802.

Norman, R. M., Manchanda, R., Malla, A. K., Windell, D., Harricharan, R., & Northcott, S. (2011) Symptom and functional outcomes for a 5 year early intervention program for psychoses. *Schizophrenia Research, 129*, 111–115.

Patton, G. C., Coffey, C., Romaniuk, H., Mackinnnon, A., Carlin, J. B., Degenhardt, L., . . . Moran, P. (2014) The prognosis of common mental disorders in adolescents: a 14-year prospective cohort study. *Lancet, 383*, 1404–1411.

Perkins, D. O., Gu, H., Boteva, K., & Lieberman, J. (2005) Relationship between duration of untreated psychosis and outcome in first-episode schizophrenia: a critical review and meta-analysis. *American Journal of Psychiatry, 162*, 1785–1804.

Perkins, D. O., Jeffries, C. D., Addington, J., Bearden, C. E., Cadenhead, K. S., Cannon, T. D., . . . Heinssen, R. (2015) Towards a psychosis risk blood diagnostic for persons experiencing high-risk symptoms: preliminary results from the NAPLS project. *Schizophrenia Bulletin, 41*, 419–428.

Pettersson-Yeo, W., Benetti, S., Marquand, A. F., Dell'aqua, F., Williams, S. C., Allen, P., . . . Mechelli, A. (2013) Using genetic, cognitive and multi-modal neuroimaging data to identify ultra-high-risk and first-episode psychosis at the individual level. *Psychological Medicine, 43*, 2547–2562.

Phillips, L. J., Nelson, B., Yuen, H. P., Francey, S. M., Simmons, M., Stanford, C., . . . McGorry, P. D. (2009) Randomized controlled trial of interventions for young people at ultra-high risk of psychosis: study design and baseline characteristics. *Austrlian and New Zealand Journal of Psychiatry, 43*, 818–829.

Rickwood, D. J., Telford, N. R., Parker, A. G., Tanti, C., & McGorry, P. D. (2014) headspace—Australia's innovation in youth mental health: who are the clients and why are they presenting? *Medical Journal of Australia, 200*, 108–111.

Schultze-Lutter, F. (2009) Subjective symptoms of schizophrenia in research and the clinic: the basic symptom concept. *Schizophrenia Bulletin, 35*, 5–8.

Schultze-Lutter, F., Ruhrmann, S., Berning, J., Maier, W., & Klosterkotter, J. (2010) Basic symptoms and ultra-high risk criteria: symptom development in the initial prodromal state. *Schizophrenia Bulletin, 36*, 182–191.

Seeley, J. R., Stice, E., & Rohde, P. (2009) Screening for depression prevention: identifying adolescent girls at high risk for future depression. *Journal of Abnormal Psychology*, 118, 161–170.

Simon, A. E., Borgwardt, S., Riecher-Rossler, A., Velthorst, E., de Haan, L., & Fusar-Poli, P. (2013) Moving beyond transition outcomes: meta-analysis of remission rates in individuals at high clinical risk for psychosis. *Psychiatry Research, 209*, 266–272.

Stochl, J., Khandaker, G. M., Lewis, G., Perez, J., Goodyer, I. M., Zammit, S., . . . Jones, P. B. (2015) Mood, anxiety and psychotic phenomena measure a common psychopathological factor. *Psychological Medicine, 45*, 1483–1493.

Van Der Gaag, M., Smit, F., Bechdolf, A., French, P., Linszen, D. H., Yung, A. R., . . . Cuijpers, P. (2013) Preventing a first episode of psychosis: meta-analysis of randomized controlled prevention trials of 12 month and medium-term follow-ups. *Schizophrenia Research, 149*, 56–62.

van Os, J.. (2013) The dynamics of subthreshold psychopathology: implications for diagnosis and treatment. *American Journal of Psychiatry, 170*, 695–698.

van Os, J., Hanssen, M., Bijl, R. V., & Vollebergh, W. (2001) Prevalence of psychotic disorder and community level of psychotic symptoms: an urban-rural comparison. *Archives of General Psychiatry, 58*, 663–668.

van Os, J. & Linscott, R. J. (2012) Introduction: The extended psychosis phenotype—relationship with schizophrenia and with ultra-high risk status for psychosis. *Schizophrenia Bulletin, 38*, 227–230.

van Rossum, I., Dominguez, M. D., Lieb, R., Wittchen, H.-U., & van Os, J. (2011) Affective dysregulation and reality distortion: a 10-year prospective study of their association and clinical relevance. *Schizophrenia Bulletin, 37*, 561–571.

Varghese, D., Scott, J., Welham, J., Bor, W., Najman, J., O'Callaghan, M., . . . McGrath, J. (2011) Psychotic-like experiences in major depression and anxiety disorders: a population-based survey in young adults. *Schizophrenia Bulletin, 37*, 389–393.

Wigman, J. T., Lin, A., Vollebergh, W. A., et al. (2011) Subclinical psychosis and depression: co-occurring phenomena that do not predict each other over time. *Schizophrenia Research, 130*, 277–281.

Wigman, J. T., van Nierop, M., Vollebergh, W. A., Raaijmakers, Q. A., Nelson, B., . . . Yung, A. R. (2012) Evidence that psychotic symptoms are prevalent in disorders of anxiety and depression, impacting on illness onset, risk, and severity—implications for diagnosis and ultra-high risk research. *Schizophrenia Bulletin, 38,* 247–257.

Woods, S. W., Walsh, B. C., Pearlson, G. D., & McGlashan, T. H. (2006) Glycine treatment of prodromal symptoms. *Schizophrenia Research, 86,* s7–s17.

Yung, A. R., Buckby, J. A., Cotton, S. M., Cosgrave, E. M., Killackey, E. J., Stanford, C., . . . McGorry, P. D. (2006) Psychotic-like experiences in nonpsychotic help-seekers: associations with distress, depression, and disability. *Schizophrenia Bulletin, 32,* 352–359.

Yung, A. R., & McGorry, P. D. (1996a) The initial prodrome in psychosis: descriptive and qualitative aspects. *Australian and New Zealand Journal of Psychiatry, 30,* 587–599.

Yung, A. R., & McGorry, P. D. (1996b) The prodromal phase of first-episode psychosis: past and current conceptualizations. *Schizophrenia Bulletin, 22,* 353–370.

Yung, A. R., Phillips, L. J., McGorry, P. D., McFarlane, C. A., Francey, S., Harrigan, S., . . . Jackson, H. J. (1998) Prediction of psychosis. A step towards indicated prevention of schizophrenia. *British Journal of Psychiatry Supplement, 172,* 14–20.

Yung, A. R, Phillips, L. J., Yuen, H. P., Francey, S. M., McFarlance, C. A., Hallgren, M., & McGorry, P. D. (2003) Psychosis prediction: 12-month follow up of a high-risk ("prodromal") group. *Schizophrenia Research, 60,* 21–32.

Yung, A. R, Phillips, L. J., Yuen, H. P., & McGorry, P. (2004) Risk factors for psychosis in an ultra high-risk group: psychopathology and clinical features. *Schizophrenia Research, 67,* 131–142.

/// 5 /// SCHIZOPHRENIA IN CHILDREN AND ADOLESCENTS

CAROLYN HOWELL, KRISTA BAKER,
and ROBERT FINDLING

INTRODUCTION

Early-onset schizophrenia (EOS) is a diagnosis that may be difficult to make with accuracy for clinicians. The illness often presents with nonspecific symptoms that can mimic other psychiatric illness. This creates not only diagnostic dilemmas, but also treatment challenges. In order to minimize the risk of false positives or false negatives, it is necessary to take a comprehensive cross-sectional assessment as well as a longitudinal history when faced with a patient in whom the diagnosis of youth-onset schizophrenia is being considered. Other key factors that can help in diagnostic decision-making is obtaining a thorough developmental history, identify what the patient's current symptoms are (and where and when they occur), the longitudinal course of these symptoms, and a meticulous family history.

DEFINITION AND EPIDEMIOLOGY

Early onset schizophrenia is defined as onset of illness prior to age 18. A more rare form of the disorder, known as childhood-onset schizophrenia (COS), relates to diagnosis prior to age 13. Investigators have particularly focused on early age of onset because these patients may manifest a more malignant expression of a condition that exists on a continuum across the life cycle. These distinctions are also important given differences in phenomenology and prognosis based on age of onset. Despite these differences, the same criteria are used to diagnose schizophrenia in youth and adults. In fact, in the landmark

Treatment of Early Onset Schizophrenia Study (TEOSS), severity of symptoms in youth was found to be similar to adult populations (Sikich et al., 2008).

In adults, the 12-month prevalence of schizophrenia is about 1 percent in the United States (National Institute of Mental Health [NIMH], 2009). It affects men and women equally, and occurs at similar rates in all ethnic groups around the world (NIMH, 2009). Although the incidence of schizophrenia in males is equal to females in adult onset illness, in youth-onset schizophrenia the rate in males is twice that of females (Stenstrom, Christiansen, Dehlholm-Lambertsen, Nohr-Jensen, & Bilenberg, 2010). This likely relates to later peak onset of illness in males (15–25 years) compared to females (20–29 years) (Castle, 1993; Häfner et al., 1993). The average range of onset for schizophrenia is typically between the ages of 16 and 30, however, the prevalence of onset between ages 13 and 17 is about 4 in 1000 (McGrath, Sukanta, Chant, & Welham, 2008). The prevalence of childhood-onset schizophrenia is very rare. For example, a study completed in North Dakota found a point prevalence of 0.19–0.35 per 10,000 children aged 2–12 (Burd & Kerbeshian, 1987). Given the rarity of childhood onset schizophrenia, it is of paramount importance that clinicians consider a broad differential diagnosis when evaluating a child who is presenting with symptoms that may be present in patients suffering from psychotic illnesses.

EARLY DEVELOPMENTAL FEATURES

There are retrospective studies examining the early childhood development of patients who later develop schizophrenia. As an example, a review of home videos of patients with schizophrenia suggested a higher frequency of abnormal neuromotor development in children who went on to develop schizophrenia compared with their siblings without schizophrenia, (Walker & Lewine, 1990). Specifically, the neuromotor abnormalities found in greater frequency in children who subsequently developed schizophrenia included abnormal hand posturing, choreoathetoid movements of the upper extremities, and associated reactions. An example of an associated reaction is seen when children were told to move the left arm, the right arm would move concurrently. These behaviors were most prominent prior to age four (Walker, 1994).

Fish (1975) described the term *pandysmaturation* (PDM), which is a measure that was proposed as a marker in infancy that would identify those that were genetically vulnerable for developing schizophrenia later in life. By definition, PDM required retarded cranial growth plus delayed and erratic gross and visual motor development. Since Fish, there have been several prospective studies that have evaluated early developmental features of youth that ultimately develop schizophrenia. The majority of these studies were consistent in finding more delayed gross motor skills and visual motor skills in infants that subsequently developed a schizophrenia spectrum disorder later in life (Fish, Marcus, Hans, Auerbach, & Perdue, 1992).

In addition to neuromotor abnormalities, children who go on to develop schizophrenia demonstrate abnormalities in speech and social development. Speech problems include subtle difficulties with receptive and expressive language (Bearden et al., 2000). Problems with social development include solitary play preferences at ages 4–6, decreased social confidence, more anxiety in social situations in early adolescence, and more social maladjustment related to over-reactive behavior (Done, Crow, Johnstone, & Sacker, 1994; Jones, Rogers, Murray, & Marmot, 1994). When taking a thorough history of these children, it is important to pay careful attention to either the presence or absence of delays in motor milestones, difficulties with peer interactions, and anxious predisposition.

PHASES OF ILLNESS (PRODROME/ACTIVE/RESIDUAL)

The phases of schizophrenia include prodrome, active, and residual. For the purposes of this chapter, we will consider some of the phenomenology of the schizophrenia prodrome, as this often occurs during adolescence, and its presence or absence can help confirm or refute a putative diagnosis of schizophrenia. This period represents a heterogeneous group of behaviors prior to onset of frank symptoms. The prodrome may continue for weeks to years without prominent psychotic symptoms.

Historically, the prodrome was thought to be a constellation of symptoms that were evident prior to a frank psychotic state. This has been most commonly conceptualized as a decline in functioning, social withdrawal, changes in mood, amotivation, and subtle psychotic symptoms. Additional symptoms included disturbances in cognition, speech, and energy level (Madaan, Bestha, & Kolli, 2014). There has been a shift in recent conceptualization to attempt to further classify the prodromal period by separating preprodromal or basic symptoms that evolve to a more obvious stage of psychotic illness.

There is no definitive consensus about what the specific identifiable characteristics of a prodrome are; however, most agree that it is most readily recognizable by looking retrospectively after the onset of frank psychotic symptoms have occurred. More recently, there have been increased efforts to characterize the prodrome prospectively in an attempt to intervene early in the course of illness. Other terms have evolved to define this same period to include ultrahigh risk and clinical high-risk state. The components of the high-risk state are attenuated psychotic symptoms (APS), brief limited intermittent psychotic symptoms (BLIPS), and genetic risk and deterioration (GRD) (Correll, Hauser, Auther, & Cornblatt, 2010; Yung et al., 2003).

Early in the course of the prodrome, the individual may exhibit a decline in occupational/academic and interpersonal functioning (Addington & Heinssen, 2012). In addition, they will exhibit more attenuated psychotic symptoms such as unusual thought content, suspicion/paranoia, perceptual abnormalities, grandiosity, and conceptual disorganization (Miller et al., 1999; Phillips, Yung, & McGorry, 2000; Schultze-Lutter et al., 2007). Next is a progression to a more frank state of brief limited intermittent psychosis (BLIPS) characterized by transient psychotic symptoms lasting less than one week (Correlet al., 2010). Researchers have included another group of individuals at high risk for developing schizophrenia, which includes those with a first-degree family member with schizophrenia or schizotypy, and a decline in functioning (Yung et al., 2003) (see Table 5.1).

The predictive power of conversion from a high-risk state to frank psychosis varies substantially with rates estimated between 9 percent and 76 percent depending on the study (Gee & Cannon, 2011). Clinical factors that may increase the risk of conversion from ultrahigh risk to psychotic illness are family history, acuity, and longer duration of attenuated positive symptoms, presence of bizarre thoughts and behaviors, paranoia, decline in global assessment of functioning over the previous year, and use of either

TABLE 5.1 Characteristics of the Prodrome

Pre-Prodromal	High Risk State/Prodromal
Basic Symptoms—changes in emotional responsiveness, mood changes, slowed thinking, inability to divide attention, disturbances of receptive language, decreased ability to discriminate between ideas and perception or fantasy and true memories, unstable ideas of reference, derealization; and visual or acoustic perception disturbances	**Attenuated Psychotic Symptoms**—unusual thought content, suspicion/paranoia, perceptual abnormalities, grandiosity, conceptual disorganization, social isolation and withdrawal, avolition, decreased expression of emotion, and decreased ideational richness **BLIPS**—transient psychotic symptoms that last less than one week before spontaneous resolution. Symptoms may include hallucinations, delusions, and/or disorganized behavior and speech. **GRD**—patients with a first-degree family member with schizophrenia or schizotypy and a decline in functioning (any change in mental state that causes a drop in the global assessment of functioning over the past 12 months).

Schultze-Lutter, et al., 2007; Correll, Hauser, Auther, & Cornblatt, 2010;Yung et al., 2003 cannabis or amphetamines (Madaan et al., 2014). An additional risk factor is childhood history of trauma (Holtzman, Shapiro, Trotman, & Walker, 2012).

The prodrome is an important phase of illness, because it provides an opportunity for early detection and intervention. However, treating individuals at high risk for developing schizophrenia has been a dilemma, and continues to be a subject of debate. As an example, initiating treatment with an antipsychotic may be associated with significant side effects that may make the risk of side effects greater than the benefit, especially given variable conversion rates. Therefore, there is caution against starting antipsychotic treatment at this stage unless there are clear impairing psychotic symptoms that are being targeted with treatment. There is, however, some evidence to suggest that the combination of cognitive behavioral therapy (CBT) and low-dose antipsychotic may delay the progression to a later phase of the prodrome and to a first psychotic episode (Addington & Heinssen, 2012; McGorry et al., 2002).

The prodrome can evolve into the active phase of illness. During this period, frank hallucinations and delusions exist as well as other positive symptoms such as disorganized thought processes and bizarre behavior. Negative symptoms may exist and include flattened or blunted affect, amotivation, anhedonia, and social withdrawal.

The active phase of illness can then transition to the residual phase, which is typically when positive symptoms subside and negative symptoms may persist. However, some people may also be relatively asymptomatic at this time.

PHENOMENOLOGY OF EARLY-ONSET SCHIZOPHRENIA AND DIFFERENTIATION FROM OTHER DISORDERS IN CHILDHOOD

The American Academy of Child and Adolescent Psychiatry (2013) has recently adapted their practice parameters for the diagnosis and treatment of children and adolescents with schizophrenia. The diagnosis in the pediatric population is made using the same criteria as in adults, following the criteria outlined by *Diagnostic and Statistical Manual of Mental Disorders—5th ed. (DSM-5)* (American Psychiatric Association, 2013). Unfortunately, since misdiagnosis is common, this highlights the importance of thoroughly understanding the phenomenology of COS, EOS, and its distinction from other childhood psychiatric illnesses.

Although phenomenologically continuous with its adult counterpart, COS and EOS represent a more severe form of the disorder, with more prominent prepsychotic developmental features, brain abnormalities, and genetic risk factors. In contrast to adult-onset schizophrenia, childhood-onset schizophrenia is more commonly associated with insidious onset, more frequent visual hallucinations, and more inappropriate or blunted affect

(Russell, 1994). Additionally, delusions in children are less complex than in adult schizophrenia and usually take the form of childhood themes (Russell, 1994).

Many children who report hallucinations do not meet criteria for schizophrenia, and many do not have psychotic illnesses. Hallucinations are a fairly common experience, even in the absence of psychopathology (Van Os, Verdoux, Bijil, & Ravelli, 1999). As an example, normative childhood experiences may be confused with psychosis, including overactive imaginations and vivid fantasies. Reports suggestive of psychosis may also stem from an intellectual disability, because hallucinations are reported more frequently in this population. Additionally, anxiety disorder is perhaps the most common category of illness treated in child psychiatry, and children may have nonpsychotic perceptual disturbances in this context. Often, the content of hallucinations involves anxious themes. It is not uncommon for anxious prepubertal children to report illusions and other perceptual disturbances mostly at night when anxiety is at its peak.

Post-traumatic stress disorder is another anxiety spectrum illness in which hallucinations may present as a part of the phenomenology. Visual hallucinations must be differentiated from internal reexperiencing of symptoms, such as flashbacks. Mistreated youth are particularly vulnerable to report such symptoms, which may represent dissociation and/or anxiety, including intrusive thoughts/worries, derealization, or depersonalization. Similarly, when a patient has symptoms consistent with obsessive- compulsive disorder and describes hallucinations, this must be differentiated from unwanted intrusive images that are distressing, and, therefore, more aptly considered obsessions.

Affective psychoses (especially bipolar disorder) can present with a variety of mood and psychotic symptoms. Severe mania in teenagers often presents with florid psychosis, including hallucinations, delusions, and thought disorder. Psychotic depression may present with mood congruent or incongruent hallucinations or delusions. Alternatively, symptoms of schizophrenia, such as negative symptoms, may be confused with a depressive disorder. The overlap in symptoms increases the likelihood of misdiagnosis. Longitudinal reassessment is the key to ensuring diagnostic accuracy.

Autism is a neurodevelopmental disorder that is difficult to distinguish from childhood onset schizophrenia. In Bleuler's historical description of schizophrenia, autism is described of one of the "four A's" and relates to social withdrawal or preferring to live in a fantasy world rather than interacting appropriately with the social world. Autism spectrum disorders (ASD) are distinguished from schizophrenia by the absence of psychotic symptoms, and by the predominance of the characteristic deviant language patterns, aberrant social relatedness, and/or repetitive behaviors. The earlier age of onset and the absence of a normal period of development also differentiate autism from schizophrenia. The premorbid abnormalities for children with schizophrenia also tend to be less pervasive and severe than those with autism. Additionally, children with schizophrenia often have premorbid and/or comorbid problems with social oddities and aloofness, which may be confused with ASD. Once psychotic symptoms become apparent, the diagnosis of schizophrenia takes precedence. These symptoms that antecede psychosis are likely nonspecific markers of disrupted brain development, and may also reflect potential shared etiologic mechanisms that are common to both syndromes. Table 5.2 describes the essential similarities and differences when comparing EOS with other forms of mental illness in children and adolescents.

When interviewing a child, it is critical to frame questions in a developmentally appropriate context, while skillfully exploring the subtle differences that are critical to differentiating the complex phenomenology. As stated in the recent revision to AACAP (2013) parameters, "The mere fact that a child responds affirmatively to questions regarding hallucinations or delusions does not *ipso facto* mean they are psychotic. Psychotic symptoms occur in the context of an illness, and psychotic illnesses are rare in youth, especially in children younger than age 12 years" (p. 980). True psychotic symptoms are generally confusing to the individual and are experienced as distressing external phenomena

TABLE 5.2 Examples of Differential Diagnoses

Illness	Similarities to Early Onset Schizophrenia	Differences from Early Onset Schizophrenia
OCD	Intrusive thoughts and images that may be confused with hallucinations. Patient may have poor insight into obsessions and, therefore, symptoms may seem more upsetting.	Obsessive thoughts and compulsive behaviors are not true hallucinations and are distressing. Delusional beliefs may not be distressing.
PTSD	Flashbacks and nightmares may be confused with hallucinations. Patients may also experience hallucinations of the voice of the perpetrator or in other ways related to trauma	Intrusive thoughts, nightmares, and flashbacks associated with PTSD are internal experiences that are differentiated from externally located hallucinations.
Affective Psychosis	Hallucinations and paranoid/persecutory delusions can exist	Hallucinations and delusions in affective psychosis exist only in the context of mood symptoms.
ASD	Early disturbances in speech and language, possible cognitive deficits, motor skill deficits, abnormalities in play and social deficits. Echolalia can exist with both illnesses.	Early developmental signs and symptoms are evident as early as 18 months in ASD (earlier than schizophrenia) and are often more severe. Psychotic symptoms are not evident in ASD.

beyond their control. Highly descriptive, detailed, organized, and/or situation-specific reports are less likely to represent true psychosis. Overt signs of the illness should be evident on the mental status exam and in descriptions of the child's behavior. Without overt evidence of psychosis, the validity of symptom reports suggestive of schizophrenia in children needs to be carefully scrutinized.

IMAGING

Further support for the neurodevelopmental hypothesis of schizophrenia became available with the advent of brain imaging studies in the 1970s. Existing literature provides evidence to support similar neuroanatomical findings in adult-onset and early-onset schizophrenia. Neuroimaging (most often MRI data) findings common to both include enlarged lateral ventricles compared with healthy controls, as well as reduced grey matter volumes in the cortex, hippocampal-amygdala region, and parahippocampal gyrus (Lewis, 1997; Shenton, Dickey, Frumin, & McCarley, 2001; Sporn et al., 2003). A main difference between early-onset and childhood-onset neuroanatomical findings is the progression of gray matter volume reduction. As an example, Sporn and colleagues (2003) discovered that children with COS displayed exaggerated gray matter losses involving not only the frontal, parietal regions, but also the temporal lobes. Losses tend to originate in the parietal lobe and spread anteriorly over time. The rate of grey matter loss leveled off in early adulthood. Neuroimaging data also reveal abnormalities in cortical folding in both adult and early-onset populations (Cachia et al., 2008, Penttila et al., 2008) Follow-up longitudinal studies show that cortical thinning in COS may plateau in early adulthood when it becomes similar to the adult regional pattern (Greenstein et al., 2006, Sporn et al., 2003).

COGNITION

Multiple areas of basic neurocognition are impaired in EOS. Specific cognitive deficits in early onset schizophrenia include general cognitive ability, processing speed, working memory, attention, visuospatial skills, executive control, verbal fluency, verbal learning/memory, and visual memory (Nieto & Castellanos, 2011). Cognitive dysfunction is an early indicator of illness and is evident even in the prodromal phase. It is believed that the majority of cognitive dysfunction and decline occurs prior to onset of first episode. (Kahn & Keefe, 2013).

Decline in cognitive function in youth and adults, regardless of the age of onset, seems to occur between the ages of 7 and 18 years and is even more pronounced in those individuals with EOS (Frangou, 2013). A meta-analysis by Rajji, Ismail, and Mulsant (2009) examined age of onset and cognition in schizophrenia and found that the severity of the cognitive deficit was correlated to the time of onset. EOS patients, when compared to adult first-episode schizophrenia patients, tested lower on arithmetic, executive function, IQ, psychomotor speed of processing, and verbal memory. (Rajji et al., 2009).

A study evaluating the effects of treatment with antipsychotics on cognition in youth with schizophrenia demonstrated only modest improvement in cognitive abilities (Frazier et al., 2012). Cognitive deficits may be predictors of overall functional ability (Green, 1996), which highlights the need for future studies focusing on treatments that can improve aspects of cognition. One such example is cognitive remediation, which capitalizes on the concept of brain plasticity. Given the evidence in the adult literature, studies evaluating the efficacy of cognitive remediation therapy in early onset schizophrenia may be a promising future direction.

PSYCHOPHARMACOLOGICAL TREATMENT

Antipsychotics have existed since the 1950s, beginning with the introduction of chlorpromazine. This and other first-generation antipsychotics have been widely used in adult and pediatric populations. However, they have a liability of causing extrapyramidal symptoms (EPS) by virtue of their antagonism of the D2 receptor. The second-generation antipsychotics are distinguished from first generation by their reduced propensity to cause EPS. There are several second-generation antipsychotics that are approved by the US Food and Drug Administration (FDA) for use in pediatric schizophrenia (see Table 5.3).

Second-generation or atypical antipsychotic agents are considered the first line treatment for schizophrenia spectrum disorders in youth. According to AACAP (2013) parameters, it is recommended that these agents be used in conjunction with psychotherapeutic interventions. There have been several randomized controlled trials examining antipsychotic agents for EOS. Older studies support the use of loxapine (Pool, Bloom, Mielke, Roniger, & Gallant, 1976) and haloperidol (Spencer, Kafantaris, Padron-Gayol,

TABLE 5.3 Atypical Antipsychotics Approved by the FDA for Use in Youth

Atypical Antipsychotic	Ages for Approved Use in Schizophrenia
Aripiprazole	Adolescents 13–17
Olanzapine	Adolescents 13–17
Paliperidone	Adolescents 12–17
Quetiapine	Adolescents 13–17
Risperidone	Adolescents 13–17

Rosenberg, & Campbell, 1992). For adolescents with EOS, industry-sponsored randomized, placebo-controlled trials in adolescents with schizophrenia support the efficacy of risperidone (Haas et al., 2009); aripiprazole (Findling et al., 2008); olanzapine (Kryzhanovskaya et al., 2009) quetiapine (Findling et al., 2013) and paliperidone (Singh et al., 2011).

The Treatment of Early Onset Schizophrenia Spectrum Disorders Study (TEOSS) compared olanzapine, risperidone, and molindone for youth with early-onset schizophrenia spectrum disorders, using a randomized double-blind design. Fewer than 50 percent of participants (n = 119) responded over eight weeks of acute treatment (Sikich et al., 2008). There were no significant differences found among the treatment groups in response rates or the magnitude of symptom reduction. Patients receiving olanzapine gained significantly more weight than participants in the other two treatment arms. There were no statistically significant differences in mean EPS ratings among groups with the exception of higher rates of akathisia in the molindone group.

Safety and effectiveness data addressing the use of antipsychotic medications for EOS remain limited, and for the most part reflect short-term use. Comparative trials are generally lacking. The choice of which agent to use first is typically based on FDA approval status, side-effect profile, patient and family preference, clinician familiarity, and cost. Individual responses to different antipsychotics are variable, and if insufficient effects are evident after a six-week trial using adequate dosages, a different antipsychotic agent should be tried. Table 5.4 shows selected randomized controlled trials evaluating safety and efficacy with atypical antipsychotics in youth with schizophrenia. Most compare an antipsychotic to placebo, or are head-to-head trials comparing two antipsychotics. The exception is a study by Haas and colleagues (2009), where very low dose risperidone (0.15mg–0.6 mg) was compared to risperidone at higher doses (1.5mg–6 mg). A theme that emerges from the collective studies is that placebo can have a positive effect on symptoms, but most antipsychotics are more efficacious than placebo, moderate to higher doses may be more effective than very low doses, but higher doses are associated with greater side effects.

Metabolic side effects to antipsychotics are a substantial concern, and can hugely impact morbidity and mortality. Consensus guidelines developed for monitoring for metabolic syndrome include obesity, hyperlipidemia, hyperglycemia, and hypertension, all of which contribute to cardiovascular disease. AACAP (2013) has more specific recommendations for pediatric patients, and suggest following up on metabolic parameters (including fasting glucose and lipid profile) every six months, with more frequent monitoring as clinically indicated.

TABLE 5.4 Selected studies of antipsychotics in adolescent schizophrenia

Treatment Arm	Author, year	Number	Age Range	Duration	Efficacy Assessments	Outcome
Clozapine versus haloperidol	Kumra et al. 1996	21	6–18	6 weeks	BPRS, Bunney-Hamburg Psychosis Rating Scale, CGAS, BPRS-C, SAPS, SANS	Clozapine was superior to haloperidol in all measures of psychosis
Clozapine versus olanzapine	Shaw et al., 2006	25	7–16	8 weeks	CGI, SANS, BPRS	Both groups showed improvement. Clozapine group had greater improvements in negative symptoms
Clozapine versus "high dose olanzapine (up to 30 mg/day)	Kumra et al., 2008	39	10–18	12 weeks	BPRS, CGI	2/3 of clozapine group had a 30 percent reduction in BPRS and 1/3 of olanzapine group had a 30 percent reduction in BPRS.
Aripiprazole versus placebo	Findling et al., 2008	302	13–17	6 weeks	PANSS	Significant reduction in PANSS positive symptom score displaying improvement in negative symptoms.
Olanzapine versus placebo	Kryzhanovskaya et al., 2008	107	13–17	6 weeks	BPRS-C, CGI, PANSS, OAS	Clinical improvements found for olanzapine but significant side effects were noted.
Risperidone versus placebo	Haas et al., 2009	160	13–17	6 weeks	PANSS, CGI, CGAS	Both treatment groups improved significantly
Risperidone 1.5–6.0 mg/day versus 0.15–0.6 mg/day	Haas, et al., 2009	257	13–17	8	PANSS, CGI	Patients in regimen 1.5-6 mg/day group showed greater improvement.

(*continued*)

TABLE 5.4 (Continued)

Treatment Arm	Author, year	Number	Age Range	Duration	Efficacy Assessments	Outcome
Paliperidone (1 of 3 weight based fixed doses) versus placebo	Singh et al., 2011	201	12–17	6	PANSS, CGI, CGAS	Clinical improvement in medium dosed group.
Quetiapine versus placebo	Findling et al., 2012	220	13–17	6 weeks	PANSS, CGI	Clinical improvement in quetiapine group.
Ziprasidone versus placebo	Findling et al., 2013	276	13–17	6 weeks	PANSS, CGI, BPRS, KID-SCID	Failed to separate from placebo

Excerpts of chart from Madaan, Dvir, & Wilson, 2008.

PANSS: Positive and Negative Symptom Scale.

CGAS: Children's Global Assessment Scale.

CGI: Clinical Global Impression.

SANS: Scale for the Assessment of Negative Symptoms.

SAPS: Scale for the Asssessment of Positive Symptoms.

BPRS: Brief Psychotic Rating Scale.

OAS: Overt Aggression Scale.

In addition to metabolic side effects, movement side effects are also a potential for concern. This is particularly relevant to youth, as they may be more prone to develop extrapyramidal symptoms as a result of being treated with antipsychotics. In particular, younger male patients are more at risk for developing acute dystonias (Keepers & Casey, 1987). A good rule to follow when prescribing antipsychotics to children and adolescents is to follow evidence-based dosing schemas. For antipsychotics approved by the FDA for use in adolescents, specific FDA dosing guidelines should be followed.

There are long-acting injectable antipsychotics available for use. AACAP (2013) parameter guidelines indicate that the use of depot antipsychotics should only be considered in adolescents with schizophrenia with documented chronic psychotic symptoms and a history of poor medication adherence. There is a lack of studies evaluating safety and efficacy of long-acting injectable antipsychotic medication in the pediatric population. AACAP also recommends that ongoing medication therapy should be provided to most youth with schizophrenia to improve functioning and prevent relapse.

PSYCHOSOCIAL TREATMENTS

Psychopharmacology is considered a first line of treatment for schizophrenia; however, there are side effects such as EPS and metabolic syndrome that can be associated with its use (Chien, Leung, Yeung, & Wong, 2013). Adherence can also substantially complicate effectiveness of medication. Therefore, psychosocial interventions are often seen as adjunct treatments to psychopharmacology that can address adherence as well as target overall functioning and quality of life. When adherence is optimal, medication targets the positive and, to a lesser degree, negative symptoms of schizophrenia. However, psychosocial interventions are often necessary to target more comprehensively the overall functional outcomes for people with schizophrenia. A significant portion of individuals continue to experience ongoing distress from auditory hallucinations, delusions, cognitive decline, and interruption of social and academic functioning despite pharmacological interventions (Rector & Beck, 2001). There are myriad psychosocial interventions available that address these areas; however, the intervention should optimally be tailored to the person's cognitive ability, life circumstances, and personal goals. The following psychosocial interventions are the most commonly used/cited. It is important to note that there is a relative lack of literature assessing efficacy and side effects of psychotherapeutic interventions in youth with schizophrenia compared to adults. Additionally, adaptations may be necessary when working with youth under the age of 13.

Cognitive Behavioral Therapy (CBT) is grounded in the context of a strong therapeutic alliance, supportive relationship, and maintaining a collaborative process between the client and provider throughout therapy. The underpinning of CBT is that erroneous cognitive processing and misinformation (termed cognitive distortions) contribute to the development of hallucinations and delusions. Once hallucinations and delusions are formed, they are maintained the same way that ordinary beliefs are maintained: supporting evidence is garnered and refuting evidence is dismissed (Rector & Beck, 2001). Clients are urged to identify psychosocial goals and work with the clinician to identify cognitive distortions that maintain symptoms and prevent goal attainment.

Additionally, in CBT, there is an emphasis on normalizing symptoms and teaching patients that hearing voices can occur for a number of reasons in people not diagnosed with schizophrenia, such as sleep deprivation, extreme isolation, and various medical illness. In addition, perceptual disturbances are particularly common in the pediatric population and can occur in the context of normal development (i.e., children externalizing blame for disruptive or inappropriate behaviors), anxiety disorders, autism spectrum disorders (Sikich, 2013), and intellectual disabilities (Chaudhury, 2010). The goal of normalizing these experiences is that it aids in reducing stress for the individual and assists with a less stigmatizing view of oneself. Patients are encouraged to learn and utilize coping strategies to reduce the frequency and distress of the symptoms that are impeding their ability to meet their life goals. CBT does not aim to eliminate persistent symptoms but, rather, to provide people with the ability to cope with the symptoms that are blocking their functional improvement.

The fundamental focus of family therapy is psychoeducational in nature. The main components to be addressed are education regarding schizophrenia as an illness, including knowledge of symptom presentation and treatment options including medication. This form of therapy is aimed at teaching family members and caregivers communication and problem-solving skills with a goal of lowering the emotional climate of the household, if problematic. Households with high expressed emotion or hostile communication styles are associated with higher relapse rates (Chien et al., 2013). Families/caregivers need to have reasonable expectations of the child's performance or functional ability while continuing to encourage growth and developmentally appropriate autonomy. Family therapy is also known to be effective when delivered in a multifamily therapy context, where an additional aspect of treatment is providing mutual support to one another (McFarlane, 2002).

Social-skills therapy (SST) aims to reduce the impact that schizophrenia invariably causes in psychosocial functioning. Social-skills therapy can be delivered in individual or group setting, often allowing for role play to practice emotion recognition, initiating and maintaining conversations, appropriate social skills development in school or work environment, and generalizing techniques for application in the real-world setting (Chien et al., 2013). The content of these programs can vary and should be specific to the deficits that each individual experiences.

Cognitive remediation approaches are typically utilized with older adolescents and adults. The goals of this approach are to target cognitive ability including memory, attention, processing, and executive functioning, as well as social cognition. The goal can either be restoration of these abilities or strategies aimed at compensation for functional impairments (Patterson & Leeuwenkamp, 2008). Interventions can be delivered in paper and pencil format, but are more commonly delivered in computer games/assessments, and in a group format. Cognitive remediation has been shown to enhance areas of basic neurocognition and social cognition early in the course of illness. However, an area of future focus is the generalizability of tasks learned to everyday life.

CONCLUSION

Patients typically present with symptoms consistent with schizophrenia between the ages of 15 and 30. Although onset prior to age 13 (COS) is extremely rare and generally has a poorer prognosis compared to its adult counterpart, onset during adolescence is relatively common and also associated with a poorer prognosis. Diagnosing schizophrenia in youth has significant challenges due to its often insidious onset and symptom overlap with other childhood/adolescent mental illnesses. Neuroimaging data have revealed similar brain abnormalities in youth and adult onset schizophrenia, with subtle differences specific to childhood onset schizophrenia. Cognitive deficits are reported in the literature for pediatric and adult populations; however, studies indicate that the deficits tend to occur earlier and be more pronounced in youth with schizophrenia. Treatments for EOS include antipsychotic medications as well as various psychosocial and behavioral interventions. However, more studies are needed to further evaluate the efficacy and safety of these interventions.

REFERENCES

Addington, J., & Heinssen, R. (2012). Prediction and prevention of psychosis in youth at clinicalhigh risk. *Annual Review of Clinical Psychology, 8*, 269–289.

American Academy of Child and Adolescent Psychiatry. (2013). *Practice parameter for the assessment and treatment of children and adolescents with schizophrenia.* Retrieved from http://www.aacap.org/App_Themes/AACAP/docs/practice_parameters/Schizophrenia_Sept13.pdf

American Psychiatric Association (2013). *Diagnostic and statistical manual of mental disorders* (5th ed.). Arlington, VA: American Psychiatric Publishing.

Bearden, C. E., Rosso, I. M., Hollister, J. M., Sanchez, L. E., Hadley, T., & Cannon, T. D. (2000). A prospective cohort study of childhood behavioral deviance and language abnormalities as predictors of adult schizophrenia. *Schizophrenia Bulletin, 26*(2), 395–410.

Burd, L., & Kerbeshian, J. (1987). A North Dakota prevalence study of schizophrenia presenting in childhood. *Journal of the American Academy of Child and Adolescent Psychiatry, 26*(3), 347–350.

Cachia, A., Paillere-Martinot, M. L., Galinowski, A., Januel, D., de Beaurepaire, R., Bellivier, F., . . . Martinot, J. L. (2008). Cortical folding abnormalities in schizophrenia patients with resistant auditory hallucinations. *Neuroimage, 39*(3), 927–935.

Castle, D. J. (1993). Rate of schizophrenia among males and females. *British Journal of Psychiatry, 150*(9), 1431–1432.

Chaudhury, S. (2010). Hallucinations: Clinical aspects and management. *Industrial Psychiatry Journal, 19*(1), 5–12.

Chien, W. T., Leung, S. F., Yeung, F. K., & Wong, W. K. (2013). Current approaches to treatments for schizophrenia spectrum disorders, part II: Psychosocial interventions and patient-focused perspectives in psychiatric care. *Neuropsychiatric Disease and Treatment, 9*, 1463–1481.

Correll, C. U., Hauser, M., Auther, A. M., Cornblatt, B. A. (2010). Research in people with psychosis risk syndrome: a review of the current evidence and future directions. *Journal of Child Psychology and Psychiatry, 51* (4), 390–431

Done, D. J., Crow, T. J., Johnstone, E. C., & Sacker, A. (1994) Childhood antecedents of schizophrenia and affective illnesses: social adjustment at ages 7 and 11. *British Medical Journal, 309*, 699–703.

Findling, R. L. McKenna, K., Earley, W. R., Stankowski, J., & Pathak, S. (2012). Efficacy and safety of quetiapine in adolescents with schizophrenia investigated in a 6-week, double-blind, placebo-controlled trial. *Journal of Child and Adolescent Psychopharmacology, 22*(5), 327–342.

Findling, R. L., Robb, A., Nyilas, M., Forbes, R. A., Na Jin, M. S., Ivanova, S., & Carson, W. H. (2008). A multiple-center, randomized, double-blind, placebo-controlled study of oral aripiprazole for treatment of adolescents with schizophrenia. *American Journal of Psychiatry, 165*(11), 1432–1441.

Findling, R. L., Pathak, S., Earley, W., Liu, S., & Delbello, M. (2013). Safety, tolerability, and efficacy of quetiapine in youth with schizophrenia or bipolar disorder: A 26-week, open-label, continuation study. *Journal of Child and Adolescent Psychopharmacology, 23*(7), 490–501.

Fish, B. (1975). Biologic antecedents of psychosis in children. In Freedman, D. X. (Ed.), *Biology of the major psychoses: A comparative analysis* (49–80). New York, NY: Raven.

Fish, B., Marcus, J., Hans, S., Auerbach, J., & Perdue, S. (1992) Infants at risk for schizophrenia: Sequelae of a genetic neurointegrative defect. *Archives of General Psychiatry, 49*, 221–235.

Frangou, S. (2013). Neurocognition in early-onset schizophrenia. *Child Adolescent Psychiatry Clinics of North America, 22*(4), 715–726

Frazier, J. A., Giuliano, A. J., Johnson, J. L., Yakutis, L., Youngstrom, E. A., Breiger, D., . . . Hooper, S. R. (2012). Neurocognitive outcomes in the treatment of early-onset schizophrenia spectrum disorders study. Journal of the American Academy of Child and Adolescent Psychiatry, *51*(5), 496–505.

Gee, D. G., & Cannon, T. D. (2011). Prediction of conversion to psychosis: Review and future directions. *Revista Brasileira de Psiquiatria, 33*(Suppl. 2), S129–S142.

Green, M. F. (1996). What are the functional consequences of neurocognitive deficits in schizophrenia? *American Journal of Psychiatry, 153*(3), 321–330.

Greenstein, D., Lerch, J., Shaw, P., Clasen, L., Giedd, J., Gochman, P., . . .Gogtay, N. (2006). Childhood onset schizophrenia: cortical brain abnormalities as young adults. *Journal of Child Psychology and Psychiatry, 47*(10), 1003–1012.

Haas, M., Eerdekens, M., Kushner, S., Singer, J., Augustyns, I., Quiroz, J., . . . Kusumakar, V. (2009). Efficacy, safety and tolerability of two risperidone dosing regimens in adolescent schizophrenia: Double-blind study. *The British Journal of Psychiatry, 194*, 158–164.

Häfner, H., an der Heiden, W., Hambrecht, M., Riecher-Rossler, A., Maurer, K., Loffler, W., & Fatkenheuer, B. (1993). A chapter in systematic schizophrenia research—the search for causal explanations for sex differences in age of onset. *Der Nervenarzt, 64*(11), 706–716.

Holtzman, C. W., Shapiro, D. I., Trotman, H. D., & Walker, E. F. (2012). Stress and the prodromal phase of psychosis. *Current Pharmaceutical Design, 18*(4), 527–533.

Jones, P., Rodgers, B., Murray, R., & Marmot, M. (1994). Child development risk factors for adult schizophrenia in the British 1946 birth cohort. *Lancet, 344*, 1398–1402.

Kahn, R. S., & Keefe, R. S. (2013). Schizophrenia is a cognitive illness: Time for a change in focus. *JAMA Psychiatry*. *70*(10), 1107–1112.

Keepers, G. A., Casey, D. E. (1987). Prediction of neuroleptic-induced dystonia. *Journal of Clinical Psychopharmacology, 7*(5), 342–345.

Kryzhanovskaya, L., Schulz, S. C., McDougle, C., Frazier J., Dittman, R., Robertson-Plouch, C., . . . Tohen, M. (2009). Olanzapine versus placebo in adolescents with schizophrenia: A 6-week randomized, double-blind, placebo-controlled trial. *Journal of Academy of Child & Adolescent Psychiatry, 48*(1), 60–70.

Kumra, S., Frazier, J. A., Jacobsen, L. K., McKenna, K., Gordon, C. T., Lenane, M. C., . . . Rapoport, J. L. (1996). Childhood-onset schizophrenia. A double-blind clozapine-haloperidol comparison. *Archives of General Psychiatry, 53*(12), 1090–1097.

Kumra, S., Kranzler, H., Gerbino-Rosen, G., Kester, H. M., DeThomas, C., Cullen, K., . . . Kane, J. M. (2008). Clozapine versus "high-dose" olanzapine in refractory early-onset schizophrenia: an open-label extension study. *Journal of Child Adolescent Psyhcophamacology, 18*(4) 307–316.

Lewis, D. A. (1997). Development of the prefrontal cortex during adolescence: insights into vulnerable neural circuits in schizophrenia. *Neuropsychopharmacology, 16*(6), 385–398.

Madaan, V., Bestha, D. P., & Kolli, V. (2014). Schizophrenia prodome: An optimal approach. *Current Psychiatry, 13*(3), 16–20, 29–30.

Madaan, V., Dvir, Y., & Wilson, D. R. (2008). Child and adolescent schizophrenia: pharmacological approaches. *Pharmacotherapy, 9*(12), 2053–2068.

McFarlane, W. (2002). *Multifamily groups in the treatment of severe psychiatric disorders*. New York, NY: Guilford Press.

McGorry, P. D., Yung, A. R., Phillips, L. J., Yuen, H. P., Francey, S., Cosgrave, E. M., & Jackson, H. (2002). Randomized controlled trial of interventions designed to reduce the risk of progression to first-episode psychosis in a clinical sample with subthreshold symptoms. *Archives of General Psychiatry, 59*(10), 921–928.

McGrath, J., Sukanta, S., Chant, D., & Welham, J. (2008). Schizophrenia: A concise overview of incidence, prevalence, and mortality. *American Journal of Epidemiology, 30*(1), 67–76.

Miller, T. J., McGlashan, T. H., Woods, S. W., Stein, K., Driesen, N., Corcoran, C. M., . . . Davidson, L. (1999). Symptom assessment in schizophrenic prodromal states. *Psychiatric Quarterly, 70*(4), 273–287.

Nieto, R., & Castellanos, F. (2011). A meta-analysis of neuropsychological functioning in patients with early onset schizophrenia and pediatric bipolar disorder. *Journal of Clinical Child & Adolescent Psychology, 40*(2) 266–280.

National Institutes of Mental Health (2009). *Schizophrenia: What is schizophrenia*. Retrieved from http://www.nimh.nih.gov/health/publications/schizophrenia/index.shtml

Patterson, T. L., & Leeuwenkamp, O. R. (2008). Adjunctive psychosocial therapies for the treatment of schizophrenia. *Schizophrenia Research, 100*(1–3), 108–119.

Penttila, J., Paillere-Martinot, J. L., Mangin, J. F., Burke, L. Corrigall, R., Frangou, S., & Cachia, A., (2008). Global and temporal cortical folding in patients with early-onset schizophrenia. *Journal of the American Academy of Child and Adolescent Psychiatry, 47*(10), 1125–1132.

Phillips, L. J., Yung, A. R., & McGorry, P. D. (2000). Identification of young people at risk of psychosis: Validation of personal assessment and crisis evaluation clinic intake criteria. *The Australian and New Zealand Journal of Psychiatry, 34*(Suppl.), S164–S169.

Pool, D., Bloom W., Mielke, D. H., Roniger, J. J., & Gallant, D. M. (1976). A controlled evaluation of loxitane in seventy-five adolescent schizophrenia patients. *Current Therapeutic Research, Clinical and Experimental, 19*(1), 99–104.

Rajji, T. K., Ismail, Z., & Mulsant, B. (2009). Age at onset and cognition in schizophrenia: Meta-analysis. *The British Journal of Psychiatry, 195*, 286–293.

Rector, N. A., & Beck, A. T. (2001). Cognitive behavioral therapy for schizophrenia: An empirical review. *The Journal of Nervous and Mental Disease, 189*(5), 278–287.

Russell, A. T. (1994). The clinical presentation of childhood-onset schizophrenia. *Schizophrenia Bulletin,* 2(4), 631–646.

Schultze-Lutter, F., Ruhrmann, S., Picker, H., von Reventlow, H. G., Brockhaus-Dumke, A., & Klosterkötter, J. (2007). Basic symptoms in early psychotic and depressive disorders. *British Journal of Psychiatry, 51,* 31–37.

Shaw, P., Sporn, A., Gogtay, N., Overman, G. P., Greenstein, D., Gochman, P., . . . Rapoport, J. L. (2006). Childhood-onset schizophrenia: a double-blind, randomized clozapine-olanzapine comparison. *Archives of General Psychiatry, 63*(7), 721–730.

Shenton, M. E., Dickey, C. C., Frumin, M., & McCarley, R. W. (2001). A review of MRI findings in schizophrenia. *Schizophrenia Research, 49*(1–2), 1–52.

Sikich, L. (2013). Diagnosis and evaluation of hallucinations and other psychotic symptoms in children and adolescents. *Child and Adolescent Psychiatric Clinics of North America,* 22(4), 655–673.

Sikich, L., Frazier, J. A., McClellan, J., Findling, R. L., Vitiello, B., Ritz, L., . . . Lieberman, J. A. (2008). Double-blind comparison of first- and second-generation antipsychotics in early-onset schizophrenia and schizo-affective disorder: Findings from the treatment of early-onset schizophrenia spectrum disorders (TEOSS) study. *The American Journal of Psychiatry, 165*(11), 1420–1431.

Singh, J., Robb, A., Vijapurkar, U., Nuamah, I., & Hough, D. (2011). A randomized, Double blind study of paliperidone extended release in treatment of acute schizophrenia in adolescents. *Biological Psychiatry, 70*(12) 1179–1187.

Spencer, E. K., Kafantaris, V., Padron-Gayol, M. V., Rosenberg, C. R., & Campbell, M. (1992). Haloperidol in schizophrenic children: Early findings from a study in progress. *Psychopharmacology Bulletin, 28*(2), 183–186.

Sporn, A. L., Greenstein, D. K., Gogtay, N., Jeffries, N. O., Lenane, M., Gochman, P., . . . Rapoport, J. L. (2003). Progressive brain volume loss during adolescence in childhood-onset schizophrenia. *American Journal of Psychiatry, 160*(12), 2181–2189.

Stenstrom, A. D., Christiansen, E., Dehlholm-Lambertsen, B., Nohr-Jensen, P., & Bilenberg, N. (2010). Rising incidence rates of schizophrenia among children and adolescents *Ugeskr Laeger, 172*(31), 2131–2135.

van Os, J., Verdoux, H. R., Bijl, R., Ravelli, A. (1999). Psychosis as an extreme of continuous variation in dimensions of psychopathology (1999). In H. Häfner, W. Gattaz (Eds.), *Search for the Causes of Schizophrenia,* (vol. 4, pp. 59–79). Berlin: Springer.

Walker, E. F. (1994) Developmentally moderated expressions of the neuropathology underlying schizophrenia. *Schizophrenia Bulletin, 20,* 453–480.

Walker, E., & Lewine, R. J. (1990). Prediction of adult-onset schizophrenia from childhood home movies of the patients. *The American Journal of Psychiatry, 147*(8), 1052–1056.

Yung, A. R., Phillips, L. J.,Yuen, H. P., Francey, S. M., McFarlane, C. A., Hallgren, M., McGorry, P. D. (2003). Psychosis prediction: 12-month follow up of a high-risk ("prodromal") group. *Schizophrenia Research, 60,* 21–32.

/// 6 /// PSYCHOTICISM DUE TO PERSONALITY DISORDERS OR STRESS-RELATED PHENOMENA

JONATHAN HOMANS
and KATHARINE J. NELSON

INTRODUCTION

The realm of mental health evaluation and treatment entails a high degree of subtlety and nuance. The issues faced by patients, families, providers and health care systems are not black and white. The *Diagnostic and Statistical Manual (DSM), International Classification of Disease (ICD),* and all other categorical paradigms of diagnosis are built upon separating phenomena based on symptoms and time-course. This framework is then superimposed onto an individual's presentation in an attempt to make sense of the illness. These are our best attempts at simplifying myriad presentations of human suffering into workable pieces; but, although we strive to design diagnoses which represent reality, often these diagnoses do an incomplete job of representing reality itself. The symptoms of a diagnosis are one level closer to the reality of an individual's experience than is a diagnosis. Single symptoms, however, are present in multiple different patterns of illness. There are no diagnoses in the *DSM* that are made based on a single symptom. This idea is important to clinical care, because diagnosis drives the treatment plan. Thus, utmost precision in arriving at a diagnostic formulation that reflects reality as much as possible is critical to doing well by your patients.

Psychotic symptoms are not exclusive to the diagnosis of schizophrenia, nor are they contained entirely within the broader category of primary psychotic disorders (schizophrenia, schizoaffective disorder, bipolar disorder, or major depressive disorder with psychotic features). Trauma-associated symptoms, dissociative disorders, borderline and paranoid personality disorder, grief, delirium, or psychologically mediated phenomena need to be considered when developing a psychiatric differential for psychotic symptoms. There are exotic and captivating qualities to psychotic symptoms that catch people's attention, raise hackles, and attract morbid fascination. Auditory hallucinations are certainly more commanding of our attention than a patient reporting *decreased energy*. Because these symptoms command such fascination and attention, it is important to recognize that psychotic symptoms are not confirmative of a specific diagnosis, similar to the idea that the symptom of *decreased energy* may be associated with a variety of disorders and does not necessarily imply major depression.

This chapter is devoted to understanding these "other" psychiatric diagnoses that are associated with psychotic symptoms. There has been much clinical and academic work done to clearly understand the boundaries of disorders like bipolar disorder and schizophrenia in relationship to stress-related psychotic phenomena found in disorders like post-traumatic stress disorder (PTSD) or borderline personality disorder (BPD). This chapter seeks to describe and understand these areas of overlap and ambiguity regarding psychotic symptoms. We begin by exploring hallucinations in healthy populations and move on to discussing hallucinations and negative symptom clusters found in PTSD and BPD.

HALLUCINATIONS ARE PART OF THE NORMAL HUMAN EXPERIENCE

There have been several cross-sectional studies examining hallucinations that occur in healthy individuals. Choong, Hunter, and Woodruff (2007) catalogued numerous cross-sectional studies in a variety of populations, including college students in psychology classes and nursing students, and found the presence of at least brief auditory hallucinations in 30–84 percent of participants. It is important to note that these experiences largely consisted of hearing one's name shouted out in a crowd or hearing one's own thoughts spoken aloud.

There are other situations that commonly result in more pronounced hallucinations. Carlsson and Nilsson (2007) reported that 49 percent of bereaved spouses experienced some form of hallucinations following the death of their loved one. "It was common to hear footsteps of the deceased or hear the deceased shout the spouse's name from an adjacent room. " Four percent of the bereaved spouses in this study reported having spoken with their loved one and 13 percent actually saw the deceased loved one. These types of hallucinations appear to be nonpathologic and part of the normal human experience. It is important to note that these hallucinations in normal populations have some qualities that are commonly associated with primary psychotic disorders. As is suggested by the bereavement study, placing an individual under more psychological stress increases the likelihood of hallucinatory experiences.

HALLUCINATIONS ARE A COMMON OUTCOME OF TRAUMA REGARDLESS OF DIAGNOSIS

Trauma, particularly in childhood, is a common and horrific occurrence with profound ramifications later in life. Read and Argyle (1999) looked at 100 consecutive admissions to an inpatient psychiatry unit and interviewed the inpatients to understand their exposure to trauma and evaluate for current psychotic symptoms. Twenty-two percent of the patients reported physical or sexual abuse, and of those reporting abuse, 77 percent reported one psychotic symptom (50 percent hallucinations, 45 percent delusions) and 27 percent had some form of thought disorder. Of these individuals, only 4 met full criteria for schizophrenia. This evidence suggests the mere fact of having a history of trauma places people at a significant risk for developing psychotic symptoms in adulthood, regardless of diagnosis.

People who experience sexual or physical abuse in childhood and seek mental health treatment as an adult are very likely to develop psychotic symptoms and the majority of these do not meet criteria for schizophrenia. In an outpatient sample of 200 patients, Read, Agar, Argyle, and Aderhold (2003) found that 52 percent of those who suffered childhood sexual abuse reported auditory hallucinations. Childhood sexual and physical abuse and adult sexual abuse were significantly related to hearing voices comment on their surroundings and voices commanding patients to harm or kill themselves. Conceptually, sexual or physical abuse in a child has the potential to be so psychologically damaging that it can dislodge the anchors of reality. Studies such as these strongly suggest that hallucinations can be a consequence of severe trauma, but hallucinations are not considered part of the most common trauma-related diagnosis, post-traumatic stress disorder (PTSD). Further complicating the situation is that certain presentations of PTSD share symptoms with schizophrenia.

POST-TRAUMATIC STRESS DISORDER

Post-traumatic stress disorder is an evolving diagnostic entity that represents a significant deviation in mood and functioning following a traumatic event. Our societal interest in PTSD has largely been driven by major wars, beginning with WWI. Wartime experiences have led to the classic presentation of intrusive memories, flashbacks, nightmares, hypervigilance, and marked physiologic response (elevated blood pressure and heart rate, elevated breathing rate) (American Psychiatric Association, 2013; DSM-5). There has been increasing research and awareness of other post-trauma symptoms including those that feature predominantly negative symptoms including dissociation, avoidance of reminders, negative cognitions, persistent and exaggerated negative beliefs, markedly diminished interest in activities, detachment from others and persistent inability to experience positive emotions. These negative symptoms can have significant overlap with psychotic diagnoses.

The spectrum of PTSD includes presentations that are easily confused with psychotic diagnosis. Trauma is not "one-size-fits-all," and it is difficult to argue that a single traumatic event, such as a car crash, should be placed in the same category as serial rape by a family member throughout childhood. The classic PTSD symptoms noted in the previous paragraph apply less well to victims of severe and repeated trauma early in life. In an attempt to better describe this group, the diagnostic entity of *complex PTSD* has been proposed by Pelcovitz et al. (1997). At times, complex PTSD can superficially mimic schizophrenia—particularly in patients who are affectively restricted, guarded, and suspicious of others due to inability to trust and fear of victimization. Dissociation may mimic either florid hallucinations or disorganization, especially during the process of inpatient hospitalization when patients may be retraumatized or experience repeated episodes of dissociation without refuge. Therefore, people who have survived severe child abuse have significant rates of both psychotic symptoms and symptoms easily mislabeled as psychotic, as described earlier.

Identification of past trauma is an important aspect of assessment for all mental health professionals. It is beyond the scope of this chapter to provide a complete approach to this topic; however, a few basic principles should be observed. In order for patients to feel comfortable discussing theses sensitive and at times exquisitely painful topics, a trusting relationship with the practitioner needs to be developed. Clear explanation of confidentiality and an investment in time and expressed interest in the patient are important aspects to make space for disclosure of this type of sensitive information. It is also important not to dig for a history of trauma, because this can result in stress, confusion, and may affect historical memory. The most important strategy is to remain open-minded and patient, especially in cases in which large periods of a patient's childhood are not remembered, and to allow for an evolving diagnostic formulation.

BORDERLINE PERSONALITY DISORDER

Since its inception, the relationship between borderline personality disorder (BPD) and psychotic symptoms has been extensively debated. This is a critically important clinical question, because the treatment algorithms for BPD and psychotic disorders are very different. In order to navigate this clinical issue, we will provide a framework for understanding BPD as well as discuss areas of overlap between symptoms of primary psychotic disorders and BPD.

The term *personality disorder* refers to diagnostic criteria that attempt to describe individuals with rigid personality characteristics, believed to be stable over time, present across multiple situations, and resulting in functional impairment. Classically, personality disorders were conceptualized as treatment resistant and relatively fixed; however, this understanding has changed over time, especially in the case of BPD, which has now been demonstrated to respond to treatment and carries a more favorable prognosis than previously believed (Gunderson, 2009).

Borderline personality disorder is best understood as a developmental disorder manifesting as chronic mood dysregulation impacting interpersonal relationships, self-image, and social and occupational attainment, and it is associated with nonsuicidal self-injury and suicidal behavior. This results in chronic emotional dysregulation and interpersonal dysfunction, which can include psychotic features in times of extreme stress (American Psychiatric Association, 2013).

When BPD was first described by early psychiatrists, it was described as *pseudoneurotic schizophrenia*. Some features of the disorder appeared to be similar to depression and anxiety, whereas other features looked more like schizophrenia or psychotic illness.

> *Some psychiatrists concede that the clinical and psychodynamic structure of these cases differs from the neuroses—although retaining a great deal of resemblance to the neurotic disturbances—and call them "borderline cases." Again, others are struck by the similarity of mental changes and personality structure to schizophrenia and will diagnose them as schizophrenics.* (Hoch & Polatin, 1949)

Despite the clear differences in the prototypes of schizophrenia and borderline personality disorder, there are areas in which these diagnoses overlap and can create diagnostic dilemmas. Psychotic symptoms are widely acknowledged as part of the symptom cluster that makes up BPD. In 1987, the American Psychiatric Association's *Diagnostic and Statistical Manual* criteria for BPD included "transient, stress-related paranoid ideation or severe dissociative symptoms." These criteria are retained in *DSM-5*.

There has been a large amount of mental and scientific resources devoted to defining how much psychosis can be present in BPD before one is classified under a primary psychotic diagnosis. In one of the largest prospective studies of BPD, Zanarini, Frankenburg, Wedig, and Fitzmaurice (2013) examined the natural course of BPD over several decades. This study recruited 290 patients from inpatient services who met stringent criteria for BPD and "had no history or current symptoms of schizophrenia, schizoaffective disorder, bipolar I disorder, or an organic condition that could cause serious psychiatric symptoms." (p. 672) Despite rigorous exclusion of primary psychotic disorders, psychotic symptoms were common. At the baseline assessment, 51.7 percent had paranoia, 61.7 percent had ideas of reference. Hallucinations and delusions were also common reaching 48.6 percent and 41.0 percent respectively, although these hallucinations were circumscribed, short-lived, and nonbizarre. More severe psychotic symptoms (generalized, bizarre or persistent delusions or hallucinations) were less common but still occurred in 3.5 percent (delusions) and 2.1 percent (hallucinations) of the baseline sample. These percentages fluctuated over the course of the follow-up reaching 4.8 percent for delusions and 4.1 percent for hallucinations at maximum during the study. This study demonstrates that psychotic symptoms occur in a significant proportion of patients with BPD even when the sample is rigorously vetted, a practice not routinely followed in clinical practice.

An obstacle to understanding the complete picture of the literature in this area lies in the definitions and exclusion criteria for a majority of clinical trials. Most studies examining BPD, patients with prominent psychotic symptoms are excluded and in studies looking at schizophrenia, patients with BPD are excluded. Several smaller studies have looked specifically at psychotic symptoms in community patients with BPD where this type of comorbidity was not excluded. Three studies totaling 98 patients meeting criteria for BPD yielded rates of psychosis ranging from 21.2 to 84.6 percent (Chopra & Beatson, 1986; Kingdon et al., 2010; Pope, Jonas, Hudson, Cohen, & Tohen, 1985). In a larger study of 113 patients with BPD, Coid et al. (2009) found that 8.8 percent tested positive on a psychosis screen. What is clear is that psychotic symptoms are an important part of BPD, but the extent and severity of this remains unclear. Later in this chapter we will discuss qualitative aspects of these symptoms.

TRAUMA IS A COMMON RISK FACTOR FOR BPD, PTSD, AND SCHIZOPHRENIA

As discussed previously, traumatic experiences, particularly during childhood and adolescence, can have a profound impact on development and psychiatric symptoms in adults. Understanding a history of trauma is fundamental in understanding one's patients and accurately explaining their current symptoms. Despite this importance, the identification of trauma alone does not exclude or confirm diagnoses. Although PTSD requires a history of trauma, trauma also remains a major risk factor for psychotic disorders and BPD. This results in three ways in which accurate diagnosis may be confounded:

1. *Trauma is not considered and, therefore, an accurate diagnosis of PTSD is missed.*
2. *The clinician mistakenly believes trauma (particularly sexual trauma) is required to develop BPD.* Although abuse and neglect is present in the childhood narratives of some cases of BPD, we must avoid narrowly extrapolating these components to all cases. In numerous studies examining the association of BPD and childhood trauma, researchers have found a significant, but not universal association. Golier and colleagues (2003) looked at the relationship between abuse in childhood and adolescence, personality disorders and abuse and assaults in adulthood. Of those with BPD, 52.8 percent experienced physical abuse/assault, 29.2 percent experienced sexual abuse/assault, and 40.3 percent experienced crime during their childhood/adolescence. Although these percentages are quite high compared with the general populations, they are not completely correlated. Also in this study, 25 percent of the adults meeting criteria for BPD also met criteria for PTSD.
3. *The identification of significant trauma mistakenly leads to a diagnosis of PTSD or BPD and the diagnosis of schizophrenia is missed.* Antecedent trauma is actually a major risk factor for the development of schizophrenia. Swett, Surrey, and Cohen (1990) interviewed 125 men meeting criteria for schizophrenia in an outpatient clinic. In this sample there were high rates of childhood trauma including physical abuse (48 percent), sexual abuse (7 percent), and both (8 percent). Statistical analysis demonstrated a significant association between trauma before age of 18 and psychoticism, somatization, depression, anxiety, and global severity scales of the SCL-90 R.

Another study directly compared patients with schizophrenia versus patients with BPD, for differences in rates of childhood trauma and psychotic symptoms and found significantly higher rates in BPD of severe emotional (92 versus 42 percent), and sexual abuse (67 versus 20 percent). It is important to note that although there is a statistical difference between these groups, rates of abuse remain high in those meeting criteria for schizophrenia. There were no statistical differences between the rates of physical abuse, or emotional or physical neglect. (Kingdon et al., 2010)

Larger studies examining associations between adverse childhood experiences and development of psychosis find similar trends. Varese and colleagues (2012) conducted a meta-analysis of 41 articles, including 18 case control studies (2,048 psychotic patients and 1,856 nonpsychotic controls) and found that trauma was associated with increased risk of psychosis (2.78 odds ratio 2.34–3.31)—comparable across case control, prospective cohort and population-based cross-sectional studies. All types of abuse were correlated with increased risk of developing schizophrenia including sexual abuse, physical abuse, emotional abuse, bullying, and neglect. Interestingly, only abuse types that involved an abuser targeting a victim (i.e., bullying or sexual abuse) resulted in significant associations; whereas, more random sources of trauma (death of a parent) were not significantly associated with psychosis. In order to illustrate the magnitude of the association, the authors went on to state that if one assumes causality between traumatic events and later development of psychosis, if the trauma were prevented this would result in a 33 percent reduction in the rate of schizophrenia.

SYMPTOM OVERLAP AND COMORBIDITY IN SCHIZOPHRENIA, PTSD, AND BPD

Given that trauma is a common risk factor for these three disorders, it could be expected that there is some amount of diagnostic overlap, *but to what degree*? This question is actually much more difficult to answer. This difficulty is largely due to problematic approaches to study design. For instance, a large-scale epidemiological study by Stinson and colleagues (2008) presented psychiatric diagnostic data on a community sample that included over 34,000 individuals. Despite gathering comorbidity data between BPD and a variety of diagnoses including substance use, mood, anxiety, personality, and bipolar disorders, the study did not assess for the presence of primary psychotic disorders, such as schizophrenia. This is an unfortunate trend that results in only small studies gathering the amount of diagnostic detail necessary to determine rates of comorbidity between BPD and schizophrenia. Coid and colleagues (2006) found high rates of comorbidity between psychosis and BPD by demonstrating that a cluster B diagnoses (BPD, histrionic personality disorder, antisocial personality disorder or narcissistic personality disorder) were 7 times more likely to also have a psychotic disorder compared with controls ($P<0.01$). Kindgon and colleagues (2010) found a comorbidity rate of BPD and schizophrenia of 35.6 percent among an outpatient sample. These estimates are likely influenced by their sample size, but do underscore that comorbidity between BPD and other disorders can and does occur. Figure 6.1 provides an estimate of overlap based on the aforementioned samples.

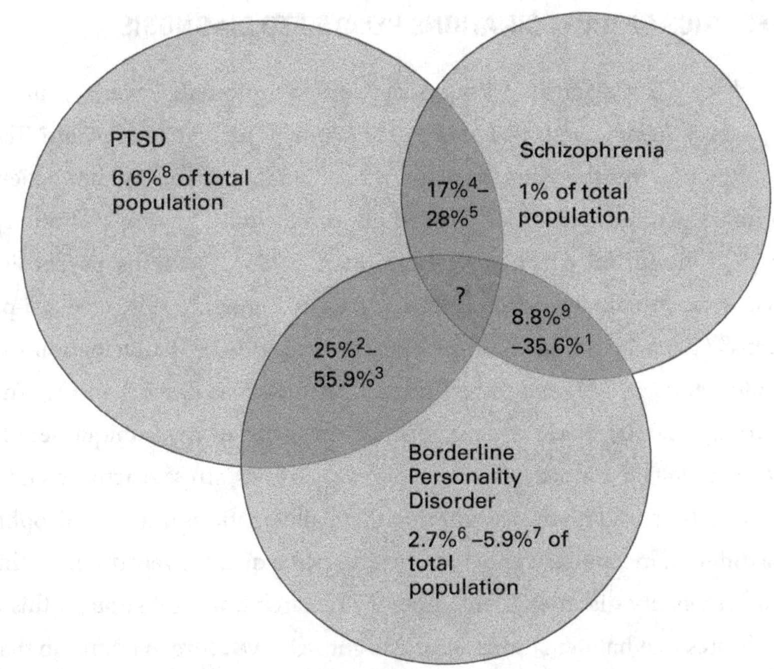

FIGURE 6.1 Rates of PTSD, Schizophrenia, and BPD diagnostic comorbidity.
1: Kingdon, Ashcroft, Bhandari, Gleeson, Warikoo, Symons, ... Mehta, 2010. 2: Golier, Yehuda, Bierer, Mitropoulou, New, Schmeidler, ... Siver, L., 2003. 3: Zanarini, Frankenburg, Dubo, Sickel, Trikha, Levin, & Reynolds,. 19984: Fan, Henderson, Nguyen, Cather, Freudenreich, Evins, ... Goff, 2008. 5: Mueser, Goodman, Trumbetta, Rosenberg, Osher, Vidaver, ... Foy, 1998. 6: Tomko, Trull, Wood, & Sher, 2013. 7: Grant, Chou, Goldstein, Huang, Stinson, F., Saha, T., ... Ruan, 2008. 8: Pagura, Stein, Bolton, Cox, Grant, & Sareen, 2010. 9: Coid, Yang, Tyrer, Roberts, & Ullrich, 2006.

Post-traumatic stress disorder has significant overlap with both BPD and schizophrenia. Zanarini and colleagues (1998) examined overlap between BPD and PTSD and found that 55.9 percent of BPD patients also met criteria for PTSD. Zlotnick, Franklin, and Zimmerman (2002) considered whether comorbidity between BPD and PTSD was associated with more severe clinical severity, but no significant association was found. PTSD rates in schizophrenia are significant. Estimates of prevalence of PTSD in schizophrenia range from 17–28 percent (Fan et al., 2008; Mueser et al., 1998). The clinical ramifications of PTSD and schizophrenia comorbidity were studied by Fan and colleagues (2008) who found that individuals with PTSD and schizophrenia had decreased attention, working memory, executive function, and quality-of-life ratings compared to those with only schizophrenia. This indicates that identification of PTSD in schizophrenia has important functional and prognostic implications.

CHARACTERISTICS OF HALLUCINATIONS RELATED TO DIAGNOSIS

With the lack of clear diagnostic boundaries and symptomatic overlap, *are there any reliable methods of dividing patients based on the nature of psychotic symptoms*? There have been many attempts over the years to categorize hallucinations that are not believed to be part of a primary psychotic disorder. Coined phrases include: "micropsychotic episodes" (Soloff, 1979), "hysterical psychosis" (Lotterman, 1985), "factious psychosis" (Pope et al.,1985), "pseudohallucinations" (Heins, Gray, & Tennant, 1990), "quasi-psychotic hallucinations" (Zanarini, Gunderson, & Frankenburg, 1990), "hallucination-like symptoms" (Skodol et al., 2002), and "stress-related psychosis" (Glaser, Van Os, Thewissen, & Myin-Germeys, 2010). Each of these terms comes with its own unique set of qualitative criteria including location, explanation, bizarre qualities, stress reactivity, and so forth. These terms are also based on the assumption that hallucinations due to schizophrenia are caused by a different mechanism and, therefore, must be qualitatively different than those caused by a personality disorder. Contemporary research does not support this assumption, and indicates that hallucinations across diagnoses have more in common than not.

There have been several studies comparing hallucinations between people with mental health diagnosis and those who do not meet criteria for any diagnosis. Daalman and colleagues (2011) attempted to study qualitative differences in patients with psychosis and people who reported hearing voices, but did not meet criteria for mental illness. Through a detailed interview process, the researchers assessed a large range of qualitative features including frequency, duration, location, loudness, explanation of origin, emotional valence, controllability, number of voices, total distress, age of onset, personification, voices speaking in third person (Table 6.1). There were surprisingly few significant differences between the two groups. Location (inside or outside of the body), loudness, number of voices, and personification (if the voices were recognized as acquaintances) did not differ between psychotic and nonpsychotic individuals. Several qualitative features were statistically different, but not different enough to provide any diagnostic utility. These included explanation of origin, controllability, age of onset, and voices speaking in the third person. The only measures that appear to be diagnostically useful were frequency, duration, distress, and emotional valence. What emerges from this data is that, for diagnostic purposes, the most important feature of hallucinations is how much dysfunction and distress these symptoms cause the patient. Those with psychotic diagnoses experience hallucinations for a majority of the time and they caused significant annoyance, distress and dysfunction.

A similar study looking at fMRI differences between psychotic and nonpsychotic voice hearers showed no statistical differences in patterns of brain activation between

TABLE 6.1 Qualitative differences in patients with psychoses versus participants who experience auditory hallucinations but do not meet criteria for mental illness (healthy voice hearers)

	Psychotic patients	**Healthy voice hearers**
Frequency:	Every hour	Every three days
Duration:	40 minutes	2–3 minutes
Emotional valence:	Seldom unpleasant	Majority of voices unpleasant and/or annoying
Distress:	Almost no discomfort or disruption to daily life	Moderate to severe distress and disruption of daily life

Daalman, Boks, Diederen, Weijer, Blom, Kahn, & Sommer, 2011

these two groups (Dierderen et al., 2012). They go on to say that there was no detectable difference in the brain networks implicated by the results of this study.

Kingdon and colleagues (2010) studied a group of 111 individuals who met criteria for either BPD or schizophrenia. This is a rare study that allowed for comorbidity between BPD and schizophrenia and, thus, is helpful in extrapolating to real-world clinical samples. Samples were not identical, and those meeting criteria for schizophrenia were more likely to be older, male, and inpatient than those with BPD. Paranoia was more common in those with only schizophrenia (61 percent) and both diagnoses (65 percent), than in BPD alone (29 percent, $p< 0.009$). Hallucinations were also common in this clinical sample including 50 percent of BPD participants, 60 percent of schizophrenia participants and 90 percent of those meeting criteria for both disorders. Qualitative analyses between these groups found no significant differences in the frequency, duration, location, belief about origin, intensity of distress, disruption of life, or controllability. Participants with BPD did show significantly higher amount and degree of negative content and amount of distress than the schizophrenia or the comorbid group. Another study (Hepworth, Ashcroft, & Kingdon, 2013), which used the same study population but a more in-depth analysis of hallucinations, found that those who met criteria for BPD had significantly greater emotional resistance (attempts to ignore or suppress) the voices, and those with schizophrenia alone reported significantly more emotional engagement (positive emotional responses to voices, such as reassurance).

These findings have been replicated in a third study by Slotema and colleagues (2012) who undertook a phenomenological study of hallucinations in females with BPD and >1 auditory hallucinations per month, schizophrenia, and healthy controls who also reported auditory hallucinations > 1 per month. They found similar significant qualitative differences between healthy voice hearers and those with pathology for frequency, duration, degree of negative content, and disruption of life. Only disruption to life was significantly higher in the schizophrenia group as compared with the BPD group. What these studies reinforce is that there is little in the *quality* of hallucinatory experiences that is exclusively found in psychotic disorders. The differences that *are* important are more simple—*How does this affect the patient in front of me*? If hallucinations are an almost constant problem that is causing distress and dysfunction, then they are more likely to be due to a psychotic disorder, such as schizophrenia.

CONCLUSION

Although this discussion provides little in the way of clear advice, hopefully it underscores the complexity of this frequent diagnostic dilemma. Simple rules that allow for accurate separation of symptoms into a single diagnosis do not exist. Diagnostic comorbidity and common underlying risk factors occur frequently. What is most important is understanding the overall diagnostic presentation and patient narrative, rather than focusing one's attention too far in a single direction by adhering to one symptom or piece of history. Psychotic symptoms need to be interpreted in the entire context of a patient's presentation. The most important aspect to take into account when considering the role of psychotic symptoms in diagnostic formulation is the impact on the patient. Fully understanding a patient's experience is more important than applying a label.

CASE ILLUSTRATIONS

Case 1:

A 42-year-old woman, Carla, is hospitalized several times over the past two decades. She lives alone with her five cats and has not been able to keep her job as a grocery clerk. She is supported through social security disability. She has completed one year of community college, but discontinued due to mental health symptoms. She has had a series of romantic relationships with men, but has never been married. She has been assigned to a treatment team through her county services (which includes a psychiatrist, nurse, and social worker). The illness episodes requiring hospitalization vary in character. Some of her hospitalizations have been related to extreme paranoia where she feels like her neighbors have implanted listening devices in her home. Often, these symptoms occur in the context of decreasing or stopping her antipsychotic medication. Based on these symptoms, she carries the diagnosis of paranoid schizophrenia. However, Carla also struggles with long-standing history of alcoholism and ongoing suicidality, identity disturbance, affective instability with prominent depression, and impulsive behavior not influenced by delusions or hallucinations. Several of her hospitalizations have been in the context of conflict with her father. During these episodes, she uses alcohol after arguing with her father and presents to the emergency room intoxicated and experiencing guilt, sadness, and suicidal thoughts and urges. The case of Carla illustrates an individual struggling with comorbid schizophrenia and BPD. Precision in identifying her presenting issues is necessary to determine the proper intervention and treatment plan. In some cases, increase or re-initiation of her antipsychotic medication is the primary intervention; at other times, chemical dependency support and other psychotherapeutic interventions to address guilt and shame are required to promote recovery and stabilization.

Case 2:

David is a 56-year-old divorced homeless male. He has been homeless since age 39 when his wife declined to allow him to live in their home due to his chemical use and frequent conflict. He is a former laborer, but has not been employed in several years. He has no source of support, other than general assistance or food stamps through his county's social services. His wife was concerned that his anger was impacting the children. David has struggled with alcohol and cocaine addiction since he was a teenager. He is hospitalized for urges to jump off a bridge or walk in front of traffic. He states he is no longer able to live in this "cruel world." He described his childhood as very painful. He was taken from his family at age 3 and situated in a series of foster-care placements. He was sexually abused by male family members in at least two of the foster placements. During periods of heavy alcohol use, he hears the voice of his abusers saying "you're no good" or "you should just kill yourself." He does not typically experience these hallucinations when he is feeling well. He demonstrates aspects of PTSD, including flashbacks and avoidance of distressing thoughts or memories. He often feels "paranoid" about his safety while living on the streets, as he has frequently been the victim of robbery. He uses alcohol and cocaine to "numb the pain." He does not demonstrate negative symptoms of schizophrenia. Trials of antipsychotic medication have been helpful for sleep, but have not changed the frequency or character of the hallucinations or his fears. His diagnostic presentation most closely aligns with post-traumatic stress disorder, chemical dependency, and extreme psychosocial stress. Although he is experiencing auditory hallucinations, during an extended psychiatric evaluation he does not reveal symptoms that meet criteria for schizophrenia. His hallucinations and suicide urges appear to be related to the impact of early childhood trauma, ongoing stress, and chemical use. David's fearfulness is less likely related to delusional paranoia and more likely legitimate fear due to the high risk of continued victimization.

Case 3:

Donovan is a 26-year-old single male. He completed 3.5 years of an undergraduate degree but did not obtain enough credits to graduate due to his frustrations with the college administration and professors he felt were singling him out by grading his assignments more critically compared to his peers. He identifies as gay and has had a series of brief, intense romantic relationships, which are usually ended by his partner at the time. He experiences significant sadness and anger following these break-ups, wondering why he has been repeatedly abandoned. He describes himself as alienated from his family, stating they have never really understood him. During times of sadness and shame following interpersonal conflict, he contemplates suicide and by researching methods for suicide online. He does not use drugs or alcohol, as he does not enjoy the feeling of being "out of control." He has several versions of a suicide note saved in a computer file. He uses safety pins to repeatedly pierce his earlobes and the webs of skin between his fingers. On at least three occasions following rejection, he has experienced extreme distress and anger, manifesting as feeling like he is hovering above his body, sees flashes of light, believes that everyone in his residence hall unit could read his thoughts, heard the voice of his father repeatedly telling him he'll "never be good enough" and punched the wall damaging the sheetrock. These episodes lasted less than two hours. Although he experienced these transient stress-related psychotic phenomena, his diagnostic picture is most consistent with BPD, rather than schizophrenia.

REFERENCES

American Psychiatric Association. (2013). *Diagnostic and statistical manual of mental disorders* (5th ed.). Washington, DC: Author.

Carlsson, M. & Nilsson, I. (2007). Bereaved spouses' adjustment after the patients' death in palliative care. *Palliative & Supportive Care, 5*, 397–404.

Choong, C., Hunter, M., & Woodruff, P. (2007). Auditory hallucinations in those populations that do not suffer from schizophrenia. *Current Psychiatry Reports, 9*, 206–212.

Chopra, H. & Beatson, J. (1986). Psychotic Symptoms in Borderline Personality Disorder. *American Journal of Psychiatry, 143*, 1605–1607.

Coid, J., Yang, M., Bebbington, P., Moran, P., Brugha, T., Jenkins, R., . . .Ullrich, S. (2009). Borderline personality disorder: health service use and social functioning among a national household population. *Psychological Medicine, 39*, 1721–1731.

Coid, J., Yang, M., Tyrer, P., Roberts, A., & Ullrich, S. (2006). Prevalence and correlates of personality disorder in Great Britain. *British Journal of Psychiatry, 188*, 423–431.

Daalman, K., Boks, M., Diederen, K., Weijer, A., Blom, J., Kahn, R., & Sommer, I. (2011). The Same or Different? A Phenomenological Comparison of Auditory Verbal Hallucinations in Healthy and Psychotic Individuals. *Journal of Clinical Psychiatry*, 72(3), 320–325.

Dierderen, K., Daalman, K., Weijer, A., Neggers, S., Gastel, W., Blom, J., . . . Sommer, I. (2012). Auditory Hallucinations Elicit Similar Brain Activation in Psychotic and Nonpsychotic Individuals. *Schizophrenia Bulletin*, *38*(5), 1074–1082.

Fan, X., Henderson, D., Nguyen, D., Cather, C., Freudenreich, O., Evins, A., . . . Goff, D. (2008). Posttraumatic stress disorder, cognitive function and quality of life in patients with schizophrenia. *Psychiatric Research*, *159*(1–2) 140–146.

Glaser, J., Van Os, J., Thewissen, V., & Myin-Germeys, I. (2010). Psychotic reactivity in borderline personality disorder. *Acta Psychiatrica Scandinavica*, *121*, 125–134.

Golier, J., Yehuda, R., Bierer, L., Mitropoulou, V., New, A., Schmeidler, J., . . . Siver, L. (2003). The relationship of borderline personality disorder to posttraumatic stress disorder and traumatic event. *American Journal of Psychiatry*, *160*, 2018–2024.

Gunderson, J. (2009). Borderline personality disorder: ontogeny of a diagnosis. *American Journal of Psychiatry*, *166*, 530–539.

Heins, T., Gray, A., & Tennant, M. (1990). Persisting hallucinations following childhood sexual abuse. *Australian and New Zealand Journal of Psychiatry*, *24*, 561–565.

Hepworth, C., Ashcroft, K., & Kingdon, D. (2013). Auditory hallucinations: a comparison of beliefs about voices in individuals with schizophrenia and borderline personality disorder. *Clinical Psychology & Psychotherapy*, *20*, 239–45.

Hoch, P. & Polatin, P. (1949). Pseudoneurotic forms of schizophrenia. *Psychiatric Quarterly*, *23*(2), 248–276.

Kingdon, D., Ashcroft, K., Bhandari, B., Gleeson, S., Warikoo, N., Symons, M., . . . Mehta, R. (2010). Schizophrenia and borderline personality disorder: similarities and differences in the experience of auditory hallucinations, paranoia, and childhood trauma. *The Journal of Nervous and Mental Disease*, *198*, 399–403.

Lotterman, A. (1985). Prolonged psychotic states in borderline personality disorder. *Psychiatric Quarterly*, *57*, 33–46.

Mueser, K., Goodman, L., Trumbetta, S., Rosenberg, S., Osher, F., Vidaver, R., . . . Foy, D. (1998). Trauma and Posttraumatic Stress Disorder in Severe Mental Illness. *Journal of Consulting and Clinical Psychology*, *66*, 493–499.

Pagura, J., Stein, M., Bolton, J., Cox, B., Grant, B., & Sareen, J. (2010). Comorbidity of borderline personality disorder and posttraumatic stress disorder in the U.S. population. *Journal of Psychiatric Research*, *44*(16), 1190–1198.

Pelcovitz, D., van der Kolk, B., Roth, S., Mandel, F., Kaplan, S., & Resick, P. (1997). Development and criteria set and a structured interview for disorders of extreme stress (SIDES). *Journal of Traumatic Stress*, *10*, 3–16.

Pope, H., Jonas, J., Hudson, J., Cohen, B., & Tohen, M. (1985). An empirical study of psychosis in borderline personality disorder. *American Journal of Psychiatry*, *142*, 1285–1290.

Read, J. & Argyle, N. (1999). Hallucinations, delusions, and thought disorder among adult psychiatric inpatients with a history of child abuse. *Psychiatric Services*, *50*(11), 1467–1472.

Read, J., Agar, K., Argyle, N., & Aderhold, V. (2003). Sexual and physical abuse during childhood and adulthood as predictors of hallucinations, delusions and thought disorder. *Psychology and Psychotherapy: Theory, Research and Practice*, *76*, 1–22.

Skodol, A., Gunderson, J., Pfohl, B., Widiger, T., Livesley, J., & Siever, L. (2002). The borderline diagnosis I: Psychopathology, comorbidity, and personality structure. *Biological Psychiatry*, *51*, 936–950.

Slotema, C., Daalman, K., Blom, J., Diederen, K., Hoek, H., & Sommer, I. (2012). Auditory verbal hallucinations in patients with borderline personality disorder are similar to those in schizophrenia. *Psychological Medicine*, *42*, 1873–1878.

Stinson, F., Dawson, D., Goldstein, R., Chou, S., Huang, B., Smith, . . . Grant, B. (2008). Prevalence, correlates, disability, and comorbidity of DSM-IV borderline personality disorder: results from the Wave 2

National Epidemiologic Survey on Alcohol and Related Conditions. *Journal of Clinical Psychiatry, 69*(4), 533–545.

Soloff, P. (1979). Physical restraint and the nonpsychotic patient: clinical and legal perspectives. *Journal of Clinical Psychiatry, 40*(7), 302–305.

Swett, C., Surrey, J., & Cohen, C. (1990). Sexual and physical abuse histories and psychiatric symptoms among male psychiatric outpatients. *The American Journal of Psychiatry, 147*, 632–636.

Tomko, R., Trull, T., Wood, P., & Sher, K. (2013). Characteristics of borderline personality disorder in a community sample: Comorbidity, treatment utilization, and general functioning. *Journal of Personality Disorders, 28*(5), 1–17.

Varese, F., Smeets, F., Drukker, M., Lieverse, R., Lataster, T., Viechtbauer W., . . . Bentall, R. (2012). Childhood adversities increase the risk of psychosis: A meta-analysis of patient-control, prospective- and cross-sectional cohort studies. *Schizophrenia Bulletin, 38*(4), 661–671.

Zanarini, M., Gunderson, J., & Frankenburg, F. (1990). Cognitive features of borderline personality disorder. *American Journal of Psychiatry, 147*, 57–63.

Zanarini, M., Frankenburg, F., Dubo, E., Sickel, A., Trikha, A., Levin, A., & Reynolds, V. (1998). Axis I comorbidity of borderline personality disorder. *American Journal of Psychiatry, 155*, 1733–1739.

Zanarini, M., Frankenburg, F., Wedig, M., & Fitzmaurice, G. (2013). Cognitive experiences reported by patients with borderline personality disorder and Axis II comparison subjects: A 16-year prospective follow-up study. *American Journal of Psychiatry, 170*(6), 671–679.

Zlotnick, C., Franklin, C., & Zimmerman, M., (2002). Is comorbidity of posttraumatic stress disorder and borderline personality disorder related to greater pathology and impairment? *American Journal of Psychiatry, 159*, 1940–1943.

/// 7 /// COGNITIVE PROCESSES IN SCHIZOPHRENIA

NAOMI T. TABAK and MICHAEL F. GREEN

INTRODUCTION AND HISTORICAL CONTEXT

When most people think of schizophrenia, they tend to think of the positive symptoms of the disorder: the generally distressing auditory hallucinations and delusions that have shaped the common notion of schizophrenia. However, understanding cognitive functioning in schizophrenia may provide a richer picture of the disorder. Although the study of cognition in schizophrenia has expanded greatly in the past 20 years, the topic has been a focus for much longer. In fact, Emil Kraepelin, who famously differentiated between schizophrenia (dementia praecox) and bipolar disorder also documented attentional processing abnormalities in schizophrenia in the early 1900s (Kraepelin, 1971). Eugen Bleuler, who coined the term *schizophrenia*, not only noted these cognitive abnormalities, but also considered them to be central to the illness. He believed that cognitive deficits, which he labeled as fundamental symptoms, were more stable and primary features of the disorder than the accessory (positive) symptoms (Bleuler, 1950). Although we now know that Bleuler's instincts were correct, this early distinction was counterintuitive, and the field largely forgot about it for much of the twentieth century.

With the rise of experimental psychology starting in the 1950s, researchers began to utilize more objective methods to understand the nature of schizophrenia. During this post–World War II era, integrative and translational research projects emerged and refocused interest in cognition. Joseph Zubin and his contemporaries started to examine event-related potentials (ERPs) in combination with cognitive tasks (Sutton, Braren, Zubin, & John, 1965), beginning a line of research that continues today. Other researchers turned to studies of reaction time (Cancro, Sutton, Kerr, & Serman, 1971), and modeling attention and information processing (Braff, 1993; Nuechterlein & Dawson, 1984) to determine how these processes differed from the prevailing models of normal cognitive functioning.

By the end of the twentieth century, the interest in studying cognition in schizophrenia was strong and further propelled by several key findings. First, the advent of neuroimaging methodologies led to clear conclusions that the brains of schizophrenia patients showed structural and functional differences compared to people without the disorder. Patients had enlarged ventricles, indicating reduced brain tissue relative to cerebral spinal fluid, and failed to activate their frontal lobes during cognitive tasks in the same way as control participants (Andreasen et al., 1992; Weinberger, Torrey, Neophytides, & Wyatt, 1979). Second, as it became clear that cognitive functioning was compromised in schizophrenia, initial efforts started to improve cognition. Early cognitive remediation studies utilized a variety of methods to test whether performance deficits could be modified (Green, Satz, Ganzell, & Vaclav, 1992; van der Gaag, Kern, van den Bosch, & Liberman, 2002). Although limited, these early investigations demonstrated that cognitive deficits are not fixed; they can be improved with appropriate treatment. And researchers began to realize that improving these deficits might have a profound impact on community functioning in schizophrenia.

This brief historical review sets the stage for our discussion of the current state of research on cognitive functioning in schizophrenia. We will begin with an overview of known cognitive deficits in schizophrenia, including types and range of deficits. We will make a sharp differentiation between nonsocial and social cognition and will spend time reviewing both domains. We will then discuss developing approaches for treating cognitive and social cognitive deficits in schizophrenia. In this chapter, we cannot do justice to the complexity and richness of the major trends and topics in the vast literature on cognitive functioning in schizophrenia. Entering the search terms *cognition and schizophrenia* into PubMed yields nearly 10,000 abstracts. In the last two years alone, there have been at least 700 papers published per year on this topic. Hence, this chapter can only serve as a snapshot of our current knowledge.

COGNITION IN SCHIZOPHRENIA

Cognition broadly refers to the mental acts or processes involved in perceiving, learning, remembering, and using knowledge. The types of cognition that are most commonly studied in schizophrenia include: (a) perception, (b) attention, (c) memory, (d) processing speed, and (e) reasoning and problem solving. We now know that cognitive deficits are a core feature of schizophrenia; that is, they are not by-products of psychotic symptoms or medication effects. Evidence for this comes from several lines of research, which have shown that cognitive deficits are present before the onset of psychotic symptoms and other clinical features (Cornblatt, Lenzenweger, Dworkin, & Erlenmeyer-Kimling, 1992), are not strongly related to clinical symptom severity (Bilder et al., 2000), and are relatively stable across changes in clinical state and medication status (Finkelstein, Cannon, Gur, Gur, & Moberg, 1997). In addition, these deficits are detectable (in attenuated form) in first-degree relatives of patients (Cannon et al., 1994), indicating a genetic contribution. In this section, we briefly review some of the findings on known cognitive deficits in schizophrenia, drawing largely from review papers and meta-analyses.

Perception. Current models of cognitive impairment in schizophrenia are influenced by evidence for distributed brain dysfunction in the disorder, with impairments in basic perceptual processing (bottom-up) as well as higher-order processing (top-down). Studies of perception in schizophrenia utilize behavioral, neurophysiological (event-related potentials, ERP), and functional magnetic resonance imaging (fMRI) methodologies to understand responses to visual and auditory stimuli. For example, mismatch negativity (MMN) is a common ERP paradigm that has been used extensively in schizophrenia research. MMN is a preattentive ERP component that reflects an automatic process of detecting an "oddball" stimulus that differs in some way (e.g., pitch or duration) from other "standard" stimuli. On this task and similar paradigms, research has demonstrated that patients with schizophrenia demonstrate deficits in early stages of auditory and visual processing and these deficits have downstream consequences for subsequent processes that rely on clear and intact auditory and visual information. For example, deficits in pitch processing lead to impairments in higher-level tasks, such as auditory emotion recognition, whereas basic deficits in the visual system lead to impairments in recognizing faces (Javitt, 2009). As we will discuss later, there is also evidence for a path linking these early processing deficits to real-world functional outcomes in schizophrenia.

Attention. Many components of attention are impaired in schizophrenia. *Selective attention* can be assessed with the Stroop task, which also measures speed of processing and cognitive control. In this task, participants read words (names of colors) that are printed in colored ink. The print color (e.g., red) is either congruent (red) or incongruent (green) with the word being read. Participants must, therefore, focus on only one aspect of the stimulus and inhibit task-irrelevant responses. Most people are slower on incongruent trials of the Stroop task. However, schizophrenia patients consistently demonstrate disproportionate difficulty inhibiting overlearned responses on the Stroop, as reflected by longer response times and decreased accuracy compared to healthy control participants (Westerhausen, Kompus, & Hugdahl, 2011). *Sustained attention* or vigilance has also been widely studied in schizophrenia with many versions of the Continuous Performance Test

(CPT). Generally, the CPT requires participants to monitor a series of rapidly displayed numbers or letters and to respond (by pressing a button) every time they see a target event (e.g., letter X) or target sequence (A followed by an X). Participants must avoid responding to nontargets. Schizophrenia patients consistently demonstrate difficulties in distinguishing between targets and nontargets on this type of task (Nuechterlein, 1991). In daily life, impairments in attention/vigilance may manifest as difficulty reading a book or paying attention to the plot of a movie.

Memory. Meta-analytic studies have demonstrated wide-ranging memory deficits in schizophrenia. *Verbal and spatial episodic memory* involves remembering previously learned information (facts, ideas, stories, or events). This neurocognitive domain is among the most impaired in schizophrenia and may be largely accounted for by impairments in the learning or encoding stage (Cirillo & Seidman, 2003). Because of this type of impairment, patients may have difficulty remembering where they left their house keys (spatial) or which items to pick up at the grocery store (verbal). *Working memory* refers to the ability to temporarily store and manipulate information and is assessed through a variety of neuropsychological tests that ask participants to remember verbal (e.g., a list of digits) or visuospatial information (e.g., objects). In everyday life, this may translate into problems remembering a phone number or address that someone else has just provided verbally. Although working memory deficits are traitlike features of schizophrenia that exist regardless of task modality and length of the delay period, some evidence suggests that deficits in visuospatial working memory may be more robust than verbal working memory deficits (Lee & Park, 2005). Patients tend to perform better during recognition tasks and when retrieval cues are provided during recall. Finally, unlike the situation with dementia, patients with schizophrenia do not have a deficit in memory retention, and do not show rapid forgetting (Paulsen et al., 1995).

Processing Speed. Processing speed refers to how quickly an individual can execute a sequence of different cognitive operations. It is often measured with digit symbol coding tasks, in which participants look at a key that links digits with symbols and then uses the key to quickly code a series of digits with their corresponding symbols. Although this is a rather low-level task, many higher-order cognitive processes rely on the ability to be mentally quick and accurate. It has been argued that this domain of cognition yields the largest level of impairments in schizophrenia. Although age and duration of illness may influence processing speed, other clinical moderators (e.g., medication status, symptom severity, and education) do not seem to account for this robust deficit (Dickinson, Ramsey, & Gold, 2007). *Fluency* is another component of processing speed that is commonly studied in schizophrenia. It is typically assessed by asking participants to name as many words as possible beginning with a specific letter (phonemic fluency) or in a specific category (semantic fluency). Patients with schizophrenia demonstrate deficits in both phonemic and semantic fluency, with some evidence for larger disturbances in semantic fluency (Henry & Crawford, 2005). Slow processing speed may be especially impaired in certain work tasks in which people are expected to quickly and accurately use a computer, cash register, or other type of device.

Reasoning and Problem Solving. Reasoning and problem solving include a number of executive functioning skills. The Wisconsin Card Sorting Task, which has been well studied in schizophrenia, requires participants to sort cards based on an abstract rule that changes over the course of the task. Participants must learn the new rule and flexibly shift their responses to continue answering correctly. There are also nonverbal tests of reasoning and problem solving that require patients to perform mazes, complete a sequence of visual patterns, or construct a visual pattern using blocks. These tasks require relatively high-level skills, as they involve the integration of lower-level processes (e.g. perception, processing speed) with strategic planning and decision making. Despite the involvement of other processes, reasoning is a separable cognitive factor that is reliably impaired and associated with long-term outcome in schizophrenia (Nuechterlein et al., 2004; Reed, Harrow, Herbener, & Martin, 2002). Good reasoning and problem solving are integral to many aspects of daily life, as demands are constantly changing. For example, figuring out how to get to an appointment on time when the bus schedule has changed requires an individual to flexibly adapt and find novel solutions.

Areas of preserved functioning. Because schizophrenia patients demonstrate impairments in most cognitive domains in a neuropsychological battery, there is a view that they have generalized cognitive deficits that affects all aspects of cognition. However, several areas of preserved performance have been identified, suggesting that the impairment is not entirely generalized. For example, patients are relatively intact in some aspects of attention (attentional selection for working memory storage and speed of attention shifting), procedural memory, and early components of visual processing (Gold, Hahn, Strauss, & Waltz, 2009; Green, Horan, & Sugar, 2013). We are still learning about the nature and scope of these intact cognitive processing domains in schizophrenia, and further research utilizing cognitive neuroscience methods will continue to shed light on their nature and significance.

SOCIAL COGNITION IN SCHIZOPHRENIA

Although nonsocial cognition in schizophrenia has a very long history, the study of social cognition in schizophrenia is relatively recent. This historical oversight is surprising since we have known from the earliest clinical conceptualizations that patients with schizophrenia have difficulty interpreting and responding to social information. The recent surge in interest has overlapped with the expansion of social cognitive neuroscience and the emerging understanding about the neural bases for social processing. As social cognitive scientists have developed novel fMRI approaches to probe these processes in healthy participants, exciting translational opportunities have arisen for clinical researchers. This neuroscientific research has shown that, in both healthy samples and in patients, the processing of nonsocial and social stimuli is supported by partially independent neural systems (van Overwalle, 2009).

Simply put, social cognition refers to the mental operations underlying social interactions (Green et al., 2008), including perceiving emotions and interpreting and generating responses to people in our social environment. The most commonly studied social cognitive domains in schizophrenia include: (a) emotional processing, (b) social perception, (c) attributional bias, and (d) mental state attribution. Schizophrenia patients demonstrate impairments on at least three of these domains, with large effects for emotional processing, social perception, and mental state attribution (Savla, Vella, Armstrong, Penn, & Twamley, 2013). Like other cognitive deficits, social cognitive impairments represent a core feature of schizophrenia in that they are present early in the illness, are stable over time, are not accounted for by symptom severity, and are present in first-degree relatives of patients (Penn, Corrigan, Bentall, Racenstein, & Newman, 1997).

Emotional processing. This domain of social cognition includes a number of skills related to the ability to perceive and use emotional information to facilitate adaptive functioning. Emotion perception, which involves identifying or discriminating between emotions displayed in still photographs, auditory stimuli, or videos, has been the most extensively studied social cognitive process in schizophrenia. Patients are consistently and significantly impaired on this ability, with large effect sizes for patient versus control differences (Kohler, Walker, Martin, Healey, & Moberg, 2010). Although other aspects of emotional processing have been studied less extensively, evidence suggests that patients demonstrate deficits in their ability to understand, manage, and regulate their emotional responses (Eack et al., 2010).

Social perception. Social perception is the ability to make inferences about social situations from contextual information and social cues (e.g., facial expressions, vocal intonations, and communicative gestures). This ability is generally assessed by watching videotaped vignettes that display an interaction between several actors. The participant must then make inferences about complex or ambiguous social situations. Patients with schizophrenia have difficulty utilizing available contextual information when perceiving social stimuli (Penn, Ritchie, Francis, Combs, & Martin, 2002).

Attributional Style. Attributional style refers to how individuals characteristically explain the causes of positive and negative events. There are typically three attributional styles that are studied in psychological research: external personal attributions (attributing causes to other people), external situational attributions (attributing causes to the situation), and internal attributions (attributing causes to oneself). Schizophrenia patients who have paranoid beliefs or persecutory delusions often utilize external personal attributions for negative events, in that they jump to conclusions about others' intentions and assume (often in the absence of clear evidence) that others are out to get them or trying to hurt them (Bentall, Corcoran, Howard, Blackwood, & Kinderman, 2001; Garety & Freeman, 1999).

Mental State Attribution. Mental state attribution (also called mentalizing or theory of mind) is the ability to understand the mental states of other people. It includes the ability to understand false beliefs, intentions, humor, deception, and indirect speech (hints, metaphor, sarcasm, and irony). Many of the methods used to study mental state attribution have been adapted from developmental research on healthy children and those with autism spectrum disorders. Some mental state attribution tasks assess one's ability to understand irony, hints, metaphors, and the idea that another person can hold a false belief (e.g., believing an object is hidden somewhere when it is, in fact, hidden elsewhere), whereas other tasks test the ability to infer another's intentions from information provided in a short story. On a wide range of paradigms, schizophrenia patients demonstrate deficits with large effect sizes in mental state attribution (Bora, Yucel, & Pantelis, 2009; Sprong, Schothorst, Vos, Hox, & van Engeland, 2007).

FUNCTIONAL CORRELATES OF COGNITIVE IMPAIRMENT

Over time, treatments for schizophrenia have shifted their focus from solely alleviating psychotic symptoms to also considering integration of patients into their communities. This shift has been influenced by the recovery movement, which emphasizes improving recovery through pursuit of personally meaningful goals and aspirations. In addition, accumulating evidence has confirmed that treating psychotic symptoms does not automatically translate into improved community functioning. We now know that cognitive factors, including social cognition, are key determinants of both functional capacity and real-world functioning. Whereas real-world functioning is measured by one's actual level of functional attainment in different life domains (e.g., work, independent living, social relationships), functional capacity refers to patients' ability to perform daily activities under simulated conditions. Functional capacity is measured in the lab with role-play exercises that mimic real-world activities, but performance on these tasks does not always map onto patients' real-world performance.

Deficits in memory, attention, reasoning, problem solving, and processing speed are strongly related to both real-world functioning and functional capacity, in cross-sectional and longitudinal studies (Green, Kern, Braff, & Mintz, 2000; Green, Kern, & Heaton, 2004). In fact, these relationships tend to be stronger than relationships between psychotic symptoms and functional outcome. Although composite measures of neurocognition account for a substantial amount of the variance in functional outcome (Green, Kern, et al., 2004), more recent research has focused on identifying the intervening steps between cognitive ability and daily living.

As might be expected, social cognition is one of these intervening variables. Not only are impairments in social cognition reliably associated with functional outcome in schizophrenia (Couture, Penn, & Roberts, 2006; Green et al., 2008), but numerous studies have shown that social cognition mediates the association between nonsocial neurocognition and functional outcome (Schmidt, Mueller, & Roder, 2011). Understanding others' emotional states and being able to use this information to function adaptively in society is critical for community integration. A meta-analysis of neurocognition, social cognition, and functional outcome in 52 studies found relatively strong associations across studies for the relationship between outcome and key social cognitive domains (emotional processing, social perception, and mental state attribution). In fact, social cognition was more strongly associated with community functioning than neurocognition across studies (Fett et al., 2011).

Other factors that contribute to functional outcome in schizophrenia include dysfunctional attitudes and negative symptoms. According to Beck and colleagues, people with schizophrenia repeatedly encounter discouraging and aversive life experiences, largely resulting from their cognitive impairments. Over time, these experiences contribute to dysfunctional beliefs, including defeatist beliefs about one's ability to successfully perform tasks. In turn, these defeatist beliefs lead to decreased motivation and interest in these tasks. Clinically, this lack of motivation and interest is seen as negative symptoms (Beck & Rector, 2005). There is emerging support for this connection between cognition, beliefs, and negative symptoms. For example, a study from our group demonstrated that there is a single path linking early cognitive impairments in visual perception through social cognition, defeatist beliefs, motivational negative symptoms, and functional outcome (Green, Hellemann, Horan, Lee, & Wynn, 2012). This single pathway model suggests that successful community functioning relies both on patients' cognitive and social cognitive abilities, as well as their beliefs and motivation to apply these abilities to real-world challenges.

INTERVENTIONS FOR COGNITIVE IMPAIRMENTS

The realization that cognitive deficits are key determinants of functional outcome in schizophrenia created an increased enthusiasm for developing pharmacological and behavioral treatments that target cognitive functioning. However, there was a lack of consensus regarding which cognitive domains should be targeted and there was no standardized assessment battery to evaluate the efficacy of new treatments. In 2002, the National Institute of Mental Health (NIMH) sponsored the Measurements and Treatment Research to Improve Cognition in Schizophrenia (MATRICS) initiative. Two main objectives of this initiative was deciding on the key domains of cognition in schizophrenia that are relevant to treatment studies, and developing a consensus cognitive battery for clinical trials (Green, Nuechterlein, et al., 2004). The MATRICS Initiative helped to coordinate and stimulate research on cognitive enhancement in schizophrenia. Although MATRICS was initially conceived for pharmacological interventions, the resulting assessment battery, the MATRICS Consensus Cognitive Battery (MCCB) is utilized in many trials of nonpharmacological treatments as well. The MCCB assesses seven domains of cognition that are reliably impaired in schizophrenia: attention/vigilance, speed of processing, working memory, verbal learning, visual learning, reasoning and problem solving, and social cognition.

Pharmacological interventions. The development of antipsychotic medications has led to a substantial reduction in psychotic symptoms for many people with schizophrenia. Although these medications demonstrate clinical efficacy, unfortunately they have done little to change the overall rates of recovery and community functioning for people with the disorder (World Health Organization, 2001). This lack of success is likely because antipsychotic medications do not provide cognitive benefits. When atypical antipsychotic medications were first introduced, there were high expectations for cognitive benefits. However, data from large-scale trials soon demonstrated that there were few differences between first and second-generation medications in terms of their cognitive effects (Marder, 2006). Because of these disappointing results, researchers are exploring the possibilities of novel pharmacological agents for treating cognitive deficits. Modafinil, GABA-based agents, alpha 7 nicotinic, and glutamatergic drugs have all been suggested as potential compounds (Citrome, 2014; Harvey & Bowie, 2012). Although there are several promising leads, no cognition-enhancing drugs for schizophrenia are approved at this time. Hence, psychosocial interventions aimed at cognitive remediation and social cognitive skills training show greater potential at the moment for improving cognition and outcomes in patients with schizophrenia.

Cognitive remediation. Cognitive remediation interventions were initially developed for neurological patients but are increasingly being used to treat cognitive deficits in schizophrenia and other conditions. This family of interventions includes programs that teach strategies to improve cognition, as well as compensatory strategies to reduce the problems associated with cognitive impairments. In addition, neuroplasticity-based approaches, which target early perceptual processing and working memory operations through intensive practice, have been developed and tested in schizophrenia (Fisher, Holland, Merzenich, & Vinogradov, 2009). Many of these approaches are computer assisted and involve repetitive practice of drills that target attention, memory, and executive functioning. There are many advantages to computer-assisted cognitive remediation, including the opportunity for unlimited repetition of training tasks, exposure to multimedia stimulations (which is believed to foster neural plasticity), automatic adjustment of difficulty levels, various forms of reinforcement, and objective recording of participants' task performance (Grynszpan et al., 2011). Computer-assisted cognitive remediation yields a medium effect size for improving general cognition and small effect sizes for improvements on specific cognitive measures in schizophrenia. Further, combining this approach with social group therapies seems to be especially useful in boosting social cognitive skills (Grynszpan et al., 2011). A meta-analysis of 40 studies that included multiple cognitive remediation approaches similarly documented small to moderate improvement in cognitive performance across a variety of program and patient conditions. In addition, this review found that cognitive remediation can improve functional outcomes, especially when combined with psychiatric rehabilitation programs (Wykes, Huddy, Cellard, McGurk, & Czobor, 2011).

Social cognitive skills training. Several research groups have now developed interventions for improving social cognition in schizophrenia. Two well-validated training programs (Horan, Kern, Green, & Penn, 2008; Penn, Roberts, Combs, & Sterne, 2007) include training on emotional processing, social perception, attributional style, and theory of mind. These interventions, which combine psychoeducation, repetitive skill practice, strategy games, role-plays, and homework exercises, are delivered in group format over 12–24 weeks. There are also more targeted interventions, which focus on one specific domain of social cognition (e.g., emotion perception or mental state attribution). Results from a meta-analysis suggested that social cognition training programs produce moderate to large improvements on measures of facial affect recognition and smaller, but significant, effects on mental state attribution. In the same meta-analysis, social cognition training was associated with moderate to large improvements on observer-rated measures of functioning in both inpatients and outpatients (Kurtz et al., 2012).

CONCLUSION

In the past, schizophrenia was viewed as a life-long struggle with a poor prognosis. Currently, it is viewed as a serious condition, but with reasons to be hopeful. One of the reasons for this more optimistic stance about the illness is that the field is starting to understand the factors that determine recovery, not simply reduce symptoms. Cognition is clearly one of these factors.

Current research on cognition in schizophrenia spans many areas of investigation, some of which were discussed in this chapter, and many of which were not. We focused on the definition of the domains, their relationships to daily functioning, and the emerging role of interventions for cognition. We also emphasized the increasing role of cognition for processing social information (i.e. social cognition).

In many instances, research into cognition in schizophrenia follows closely in time developments in neuroscience. Hence, as developments in biological and brain science (e.g., markers of infection and inflammation, optogenetics, genomic risk factors, epigenetics, pluripotent stem cells, advanced neuroimaging paradigms, etc.) are used in schizophrenia, implications for the cognition of schizophrenia soon follow. Indeed one of the advantages of cognition compared with other features of schizophrenia is that it can be directly tied to known brain circuits, as well as to daily functioning. Cognition is central to the disorder. From the perspective of history, phenomenology, and neuroscience, the examination of cognition of schizophrenia is not separable from the study of schizophrenia itself.

REFERENCES

Andreasen, N. C., Rezai, K., Alliger, R., Swayze, V. W., Flaum, M., Kirchner, P., . . . O'Leary, D. S. (1992). Hypofrontality in neuroleptic-naive patients and in patients with chronic schizophrenia. Assessment with xenon 133 single-photon emission computed tomography and the Tower of London. *Archives of General Psychiatry, 49*(12), 943–958. Retrieved from http://www.ncbi.nlm.nih.gov/pubmed/1360199

Beck, A. T., & Rector, N. A. (2005). Cognitive approaches to schizophrenia: theory and therapy. *Annual Review of Clinical Psychology, 1*, 577–606. doi:10.1146/annurev.clinpsy.1.102803.144205

Bentall, R. P., Corcoran, R., Howard, R., Blackwood, N., & Kinderman, P. (2001). Persecutory delusions: A review and theoretical integration. *Clinical Psychology Review, 21*(8), 1143–1192. doi:10.1016/S0272-7358(01)00106-4

Bilder, R. M., Goldman, R. S., Robinson, D., Reiter, G., Bell, L., Bates, J. A., . . . Lieberman, J. A. (2000). Neuropsychology of first-episode schizophrenia: initial characterization and clinical correlates. *American Journal of Psychiatry, 157*(4), 549–559. Retrieved from http://www.ncbi.nlm.nih.gov/pubmed/10739413

Bleuler, E. (1950). *Dementia praecox or the group of schizophrenias*. New York, NY: International Universities Press.

Bora, E., Yucel, M., & Pantelis, C. (2009). Theory of mind impairment in schizophrenia: meta-analysis. *Schizophrenia Research, 109*(1–3), 1–9. doi:10.1016/j.schres.2008.12.020

Braff, D. L. (1993). Information processing and attention dysfunctions in schizophrenia. *Schizophrenia Bulletin, 19*(2), 233–59. Retrieved from http://www.ncbi.nlm.nih.gov/pubmed/8322034

Cancro, R., Sutton, S., Kerr, J., & Serman, A. A. (1971). Reaction time and prognosis in acute schizophrenia. *Journal of Nervous and Mental Disease, 153*, 351–359.

Cannon, T. D., Zorrilla, L. E., Shtasel, D., Gur, R. E., Gur, R. C., Marco, E. J., . . . Price, R. A. (1994). Neuropsychological functioning in siblings discordant for schizophrenia and healthy volunteers. *Archives of General Psychiatry, 51*(8), 651–661. Retrieved from http://www.ncbi.nlm.nih.gov/pubmed/8042914

Cirillo, M. A., & Seidman, L. J. (2003). Verbal declarative memory dysfunction in schizophrenia : From clinical assessment to genetics and brain mechanisms, *Neuropsychology Review, 13*(2), 43–77.

Citrome, L. (2014). Unmet needs in the treatment of schizophrenia: new targets to help different symptom domains. *Journal of Clinical Psychiatry, 75*, Supp 1, 21–26.

Cornblatt, B. A., Lenzenweger, M. F., Dworkin, R. H., & Erlenmeyer-Kimling, L. (1992). Childhood attentional dysfunctions predict social deficits in unaffected adults at risk for schizophrenia. *The British Journal of Psychiatry. Supplement, 18*, 59–64. Retrieved from http://www.ncbi.nlm.nih.gov/pubmed/1389043

Couture, S. M., Penn, D. L., & Roberts, D. L. (2006). The functional significance of social cognition in schizophrenia: a review. *Schizophrenia Bulletin, 32*(Suppl 1), S44–S63. doi:10.1093/schbul/sbl029

Dickinson, D., Ramsey, M. E., & Gold, J. M. (2007). Overlooking the obvious: a meta-analytic comparison of digit symbol coding tasks and other cognitive measures in schizophrenia. *Archives of General Psychiatry, 64*(5), 532–542.

Eack, S. M., Greeno, C. G., Pogue-Geile, M. F., Newhill, C. E., Hogarty, G. E., & Keshavan, M. S. (2010). Assessing social-cognitive deficits in schizophrenia with the Mayer-Salovey-Caruso Emotional Intelligence Test. *Schizophrenia Bulletin, 36*(2), 370–380. doi:10.1093/schbul/sbn091

Fett, A.-K. J., Viechtbauer, W., Dominguez, M.-G., Penn, D. L., van Os, J., & Krabbendam, L. (2011). The relationship between neurocognition and social cognition with functional outcomes in schizophrenia: a meta-analysis. *Neuroscience and Biobehavioral Reviews, 35*(3), 573–88. doi:10.1016/j.neubiorev.2010.07.001

Finkelstein, J. R. J., Cannon, T. D., Gur, R. E., Gur, R. C., & Moberg, P. (1997). Attentional dysfunctions in neuroleptic-naive and neuroleptic-withdrawn schizophrenic patients and their siblings. *Journal of Abnormal Psychology, 106*(2), 203–212.

Fisher, M., Holland, C., Merzenich, M. M., & Vinogradov, S. (2009). Using neuroplasticity-based auditory training to improve verbal memory in schizophrenia. *The American Journal of Psychiatry, 166*(7), 805–811. doi:10.1176/appi.ajp.2009.08050757

Garety, P. A., & Freeman, D. (1999). Cognitive approaches to delusions : A critical review of theories and evidence. *British Journal of Clinical Psychology, 38*, 113–154.

Gold, J. M., Hahn, B., Strauss, G. P., & Waltz, J. A. (2009). Turning it upside down: Areas of preserved cognitive function in schizophrenia. *Neuropsychology Review, 19*(3), 294–311. doi:10.1007/s11065-009-9098-x.TURNING

Green, M. F., Hellemann, G., Horan, W. P., Lee, J., & Wynn, J. K. (2012). From perception to functional outcome in schizophrenia: modeling the role of ability and motivation. *Archives of General Psychiatry, 69*(12), 1216–1224. doi:10.1001/archgenpsychiatry.2012.652

Green, M. F., Horan, W. P., & Sugar, C. a. (2013). Has the generalized deficit become the generalized criticism? *Schizophrenia Bulletin, 39*(2), 257–262. doi:10.1093/schbul/sbs146

Green, M. F., Kern, R. S., Braff, D. L., & Mintz, J. (2000). Neurocognitive deficits and functional outcome in schizophrenia: Are we measuring the "right stuff"? *Schizophrenia Bulletin, 26*(1), 119–136.

Green, M. F., Kern, R. S., & Heaton, R. K. (2004). Longitudinal studies of cognition and functional outcome in schizophrenia: implications for MATRICS. *Schizophrenia Research, 72*(1), 41–51. doi:10.1016/j.schres.2004.09.009

Green, M. F., Nuechterlein, K. H., Gold, J. M., Barch, D. M., Cohen, J., Essock, S., . . . Marder, S. R. (2004). Approaching a consensus cognitive battery for clinical trials in schizophrenia: The NIMH-MATRICS conference to select cognitive domains and test criteria. *Biological Psychiatry, 56*(5), 301–307. doi:10.1016/j.biopsych.2004.06.023

Green, M. F., Penn, D. L., Bentall, R., Carpenter, W. T., Gaebel, W., Gur, R. C., . . . Heinssen, R. (2008). Social cognition in schizophrenia: an NIMH workshop on definitions, assessment, and research opportunities. *Schizophrenia Bulletin, 34*(6), 1211–1220. doi:10.1093/schbul/sbm145

Green, M. F., Satz, P., Ganzell, S., & Vaclav, J. F. (1992). Wisconsin Card Sorting Test performance in schizophrenia: remediation of a stubborn deficit. *The American Journal of Psychiatry, 149*(1), 62–67. Retrieved from http://www.ncbi.nlm.nih.gov/pubmed/1728187

Grynszpan, O., Perbal, S., Pelissolo, A., Fossati, P., Jouvent, R., Dubal, S., & Perez-Diaz, F. (2011). Efficacy and specificity of computer-assisted cognitive remediation in schizophrenia: a meta-analytical study. *Psychological Medicine, 41*(1), 163–173. doi:10.1017/S0033291710000607

Harvey, P. D., & Bowie, C. R. (2012). Cognitive enhancement in schizophrenia: Pharmacological and cognitive remediation approaches. *Psychiatric Clinics of North America, 35*(3), 683–698. doi:10.1016/j.psc.2012.06.008.Cognitive

Henry, J. D., & Crawford, J. R. (2005). A meta-analytic review of verbal fluency deficits in schizophrenia relative to other neurocognitive deficits. *Cognitive Neuropsychiatry, 10*(1), 1–33. doi:10.1080/13546800344000309

Horan, W. P., Kern, R. S., Green, M. F., & Penn, D. L. (2008). Social Cognition Training for Individuals with Schizophrenia: Emerging Evidence. *American Journal of Psychiatric Rehabilitation, 11*(3), 205–252. doi:10.1080/15487760801963652

Javitt, D. C. (2009). When doors of perception close: bottom-up models of disrupted cognition in schizophrenia. *Annual Review of Clinical Psychology, 5*, 249–275. doi:10.1146/annurev.clinpsy.032408.153502

Kohler, C. G., Walker, J. B., Martin, E. a, Healey, K. M., & Moberg, P. J. (2010). Facial emotion perception in schizophrenia: a meta-analytic review. *Schizophrenia Bulletin, 36*(5), 1009–1019. doi:10.1093/schbul/sbn192

Kraepelin, E. (1971). *Dementia praecox and paraphrenia*. Huntington, NY: Robert E. Krieger Publishing.

Kurtz, M. M. and Richardson, C. L. (2012). Social cognitive training for schizophrenia: a meta-analytic investigation of controlled research. *Schizophrenia Bulletin 38*(5),1092–1104.

Lee, J., & Park, S. (2005). Working memory impairments in schizophrenia: a meta-analysis. *Journal of Abnormal Psychology, 114*(4), 599–611. doi:10.1037/0021-843X.114.4.599

Marder, S. R. (2006). Drug initiatives to improve cognitive function. *Journal of Clinical Psychiatry, 67*(Suppl 9), 31–35.

Nuechterlein, K. H. (1991). Vigilance in schizophrenia and related disorders. In S. Steinhauer, J. Gruzelier, & J. Zubin (Eds.), *Handbook of schizophrenia. neuropsychology, psychophysiology and information processing* (vol. 5, pp. 397–433). Amsterdam: Elsevier Science.

Nuechterlein, K. H., Barch, D. M., Gold, J. M., Goldberg, T. E., Green, M. F., & Heaton, R. K. (2004). Identification of separable cognitive factors in schizophrenia. *Schizophrenia Research, 72*(1), 29–39. doi:10.1016/j.schres.2004.09.007

Nuechterlein, K. H., & Dawson, M. E. (1984). Information processing and attentional functioning in the developmental course of schizophrenic disorders. *Schizophrenia Bulletin, 10*(2), 160–203. Retrieved from http://www.ncbi.nlm.nih.gov/pubmed/6729409

Paulsen, J. S., Heaton, R. K., Sadek, J. R., Perry, W., Delis, D. C., Braff, D., . . . Jeste, D. V. (1995). The nature of learning and memory impairments in schizophrenia. *Journal of the International Neuropsychological Society, 1*(1), 88–99. Retrieved from http://www.ncbi.nlm.nih.gov/pubmed/9375213

Penn, D. L., Corrigan, P. W., Bentall, R. P., Racenstein, J. M., & Newman, L. (1997). Social cognition in schizophrenia. *Psychological Bulletin, 121*(1), 114–132.

Penn, D. L., Ritchie, M., Francis, J., Combs, D., & Martin, J. (2002). Social perception in schizophrenia: the role of context. *Psychiatry Research, 109*(2), 149–159. Retrieved from http://www.ncbi.nlm.nih.gov/pubmed/11927140

Penn, D. L., Roberts, D. L., Combs, D., & Sterne, A. (2007). The development of the social cognition and interaction training program for schizophrenia spectrum disorders. *Psychiatric Services, 58*(4), 449–451.

Reed, R. A., Harrow, M., Herbener, E. S., & Martin, E. M. (2002). Executive function in schizophrenia: Is it linked to psychosis and poor life functioning? *Journal of Nervous and Mental Disease, 190*(11), 725–732.

Savla, G. N., Vella, L., Armstrong, C. C., Penn, D. L., & Twamley, E. W. (2013). Deficits in domains of social cognition in schizophrenia: a meta-analysis of the empirical evidence. *Schizophrenia Bulletin, 39*(5), 979–992. doi:10.1093/schbul/sbs080

Schmidt, S. J., Mueller, D. R., & Roder, V. (2011). Social cognition as a mediator variable between neurocognition and functional outcome in schizophrenia: empirical review and new results by structural equation modeling. *Schizophrenia Bulletin, 37*(Suppl 2), S41–54. doi:10.1093/schbul/sbr079

Sprong, M., Schothorst, P., Vos, E., Hox, J., & van Engeland, H. (2007). Theory of mind in schizophrenia: meta-analysis. *The British Journal of Psychiatry : The Journal of Mental Science, 191*, 5–13. doi:10.1192/bjp.bp.107.035899

Sutton, S., Braren, M., Zubin, J., & John, E. R. (1965). Evoked-potential correlates of stimulus uncertainty. *Science, 150*(3700), 1187–1188. Retrieved from http://www.ncbi.nlm.nih.gov/pubmed/5852977

Van der Gaag, M., Kern, R. S., van den Bosch, R. J., & Liberman, R. P. (2002). A controlled trial of cognitive remediation in schizophrenia. *Schizophrenia Bulletin, 28*(1), 167–176. Retrieved from http://www.ncbi.nlm.nih.gov/pubmed/12047016

Van Overwalle, F. (2009). Social cognition and the brain: a meta-analysis. *Human Brain Mapping, 30*(3), 829–858.

Weinberger, D. R., Torrey, E. F., Neophytides, A. N., & Wyatt, R. J. (1979). Lateral cerebral ventricular enlargement in chronic schizophrenia. *Archives of General Psychiatry, 36*(7), 735–739.

Westerhausen, R., Kompus, K., & Hugdahl, K. (2011). Impaired cognitive inhibition in schizophrenia: a meta-analysis of the Stroop interference effect. *Schizophrenia Research, 133*(1–3), 172–181. doi:10.1016/j.schres.2011.08.025

World Health Organization. (2001). *World Health Report 2001, Mental Health: New* Understanding, N*ew Hope*. Geneva, Switzerland: World Health Organization.

Wykes, T., Huddy, V., Cellard, C., McGurk, S. R., & Czobor, P. (2011). A meta-analysis of cognitive remediation for schizophrenia: methodology and effect sizes. *The American Journal of Psychiatry, 168*(5), 472–485. doi:10.1176/appi.ajp.2010.10060855

PART II

PATHOPHYSIOLOGY AND FUTURE OUTLOOK

/// 8 /// GENETICS OF SCHIZOPHRENIA

AMANDA B. ZHEUTLIN, REBECCA FORTGANG, and TYRONE D. CANNON

INTRODUCTION

Although it has been known for several decades that genetic factors play a major role in the etiology of schizophrenia, it has been only recently that the field has had the tools to probe the genetic architecture of the syndrome. As these tools have been applied to increasingly large samples of cases and controls to reveal DNA variations that occur more frequently among those with schizophrenia, one overriding conclusion has been reached: there is a humbling degree of complexity in the genetic foundations of schizophrenia. Risk for the disorder is now understood to be conferred by thousands of common single nucleotide variants, each of very small effect, as well as by thousands of larger mutations, each quite rare and of putatively larger effect (Purcell et al., 2014; Schizophrenia Working Group of the Psychiatric Genomics, 2014). This degree of genetic complexity is perhaps not surprising in view of the substantial heterogeneity in symptomology, course, treatment response, and other clinical features of the syndrome (Cannon & Keller, 2006; Tan, Callicott, & Weinberger, 2008; Walton et al., 2013). Although many of the variants detected in genome-wide association studies implicate disruptions in certain biological pathways, including synaptic plasticity and immune function (Ohi et al., 2014; Schizophrenia Working Group of the Psychiatric Genomics, 2014), which are emphasized in current models of schizophrenia pathophysiology (Cannon, Kaprio, Lonnqvist, Huttunen, & Koskenvuo, 1998; Pogue-Geile & Yokley, 2010), only a tiny fraction of the risk-increasing variants have thus far been conclusively identified.

The goal of this chapter is to provide an overview of recent advances in the genetics of schizophrenia. We first consider the question of the magnitude of genetic involvement and the range of syndromes likely to share genetic influences in common with this syndrome.

These issues are addressed from the perspective of genetic epidemiology, focusing primarily on studies of twins and nuclear families. We then turn to the molecular genetic basis of schizophrenia, highlighting findings of recent genome-wide association studies and discussing several challenges that the complexity of this syndrome raises for elucidating the full host of liability-conferring mutations. It is important to recognize that genes do not code for schizophrenia or any of its symptoms directly, but rather, indirectly, by impacting a number of biological signaling cascades and neural systems, which can be conceptualized as representing intermediate phenotypes or endophenotypes for schizophrenia (Cannon & Keller, 2006; Greenwood, Light, Swerdlow, Radant, & Braff, 2012; Tan et al., 2008; Toulopoulou et al., 2007). Apart from increasing sample sizes to facilitate mapping more variants associated with risk for schizophrenia, the next great challenge is revealing the links between risk-conferring mutations and disruptions in the brain systems underlying the expression of schizophrenia. These efforts will help to realize the promise of genetics to a personalized medicine approach in psychiatry: developing intervention targets based on knowledge of the mechanisms of abnormal gene action in particular cases.

HERITABILITY: HOW "GENETIC" IS SCHIZOPHRENIA?

Heritability refers to the proportion of observed variance in a phenotype that is attributable to genetic influences. Schizophrenia's heritability has been estimated at about 80–85 percent in studies of monozygotic (MZ) and dizygotic (DZ) twins (Cannon et al., 1998; Cardno & Gottesman, 2000). MZ twin pairs share 100 percent of their genetic code, and DZ twin pairs on average share 50 percent—or approximately the same amount as any two siblings (Plomin, DeFries, & McClearn, 2008). In principle, the heritable component of a trait could be further subdivided into the component that is attributable to additive genetic influences and the component that is attributable to nonadditive or dominance genetic influences. Additive genetic variance emerges from the sum of allelic effects across multiple genes. Nonadditive genetic variance emerges in the presence of interactions between alleles, either at the same locus (dominance effects) or different loci (epistatic effects). In twin modeling studies of schizophrenia, only additive genetic influences have been detected statistically. However, it is highly likely that twin studies to date have been too small to detect a measurable nonadditive component to heritability in the context of a robust additive component, leaving open the possibility that gene-gene interaction effects account for some share of the 80–85 percent heritability.

The remaining 15–20 percent of variance in schizophrenia is attributable to nongenetic factors. This nongenetic, or environmental, component could, in principle, be further subdivided into the part due to shared, or common, environmental influences and the part due to individual-specific environmental influences. Shared environmental influences include factors such as socioeconomic status and geographic location that hold for all members of a family (and equally so for members of twin pairs, whether MZ or DZ; Plomin, 2011). Twin modeling studies have not detected a measurable influence of shared family factors on risk for schizophrenia, though a small shared environmental component has been detected in some studies of nuclear families that include other types of kinships including half-siblings and adoptees (Lichtenstein et al., 2009). This means that the 15-20 percent of variance in schizophrenia due to non-genetic factors is primarily attributable to environmental effects specific to individuals. Such factors could include differential exposures to environmental pathogens (including drug abuse), head injuries, etc. Nevertheless, it is important to keep in mind that for the most part, environmental risk factors for schizophrenia are thought to be illness promoting only in the presence of predisposing genotypes (as in gene by environment interactions, denoted $g \times e$). The proportion of variance in schizophrenia attributable to $g \times e$ effects is not known. Such effects are currently grouped together (i.e., confounded) with the estimate for genetic effects in the case of $g \times e$ for shared environmental influences and with the estimate for nongenetic effects in the case of $g \times e$ for individual-specific environmental influences. Importantly, pre- and perinatal complications, such as maternal infection and fetal oxygen deprivation, which are among the most robust environmental risk factors for schizophrenia, probably contribute in a gene-dependent manner (Cannon et al., 2002; Mittal, Ellman, & Cannon, 2008). The higher heritability estimates for schizophrenia observed in twin studies (80–85 percent) than in some recent studies of nuclear families (65–70 percent) also suggests that environmental influences more likely be shared by co-twins in the same pregnancy (and in particular by MZ twins who are monochorionic) than by children from separate pregnancies, are major contributors to risk.

Genetic epidemiological methods have also been used to discern whether schizophrenia shares genetic risk factors in common with other psychiatric syndromes. Schizophrenia and bipolar disorder, while classically conceptualized as distinct syndromes according to Kraepelin, actually share a very high level of genetic overlap—on the order of 50–65 percent (Craddock, O'Donovan, & Owen, 2006; Lichtenstein et al., 2009; Purcell et al., 2009). Schizoaffective disorder has been found to also show high genetic correlations with both schizophrenia and bipolar disorder. Schizophrenia and bipolar disorder have both shared and syndrome-specific genetic inputs, but genetic contributions to schizoaffective disorder have been shown to entirely overlap with schizophrenia and bipolar disorder (Cardno, Rijsdijk, Sham, Murray, & McGuffin, 2014).

MOLECULAR GENETICS: WHAT GENES INCREASE RISK FOR SCHIZOPHRENIA?

Molecular genetic data—genetic information at the resolution of individual base pairs—has opened the field to investigate questions that could not be addressed by classic heritability studies. Heritability modeling can explain *how much* variance in incidence of schizophrenia is genetic, but not *what* genetic variants contribute. Molecular genetic studies are poised to uncover specific genetic variants that influence phenotypes. Any heritable phenotype in principle could be investigated, though molecular genetic techniques have mostly been leveraged to uncover variants increasing risk for syndromal or disease status. Exceptions to this include large-scale investigations of genetic influences on height (Yang et al., 2010) and IQ (Davies et al., 2011).

Some illnesses are genetically simple. Huntington's disease (HD) is caused by a mutation in a single gene, *huntingtin,* making it a Mendelian disorder. Mendelian disorders manifest in the presence of one copy of the disease-related variant. Assuming the individual lives through the period of risk for onset of disease, presence of the mutation is always associated with disease expression (100 percent sensitivity); absence is always associated with a lack of expression (100 percent specificity). Unlike HD, psychiatric illnesses are genetically complex. The current estimate of the number of independent single nucleotide polymorphisms (SNPs)—individual base-pair mutations—that contribute to schizophrenia is around 8,400 (Purcell et al., 2009; Schizophrenia Working Group of the Psychiatric Genomics, 2014). Each of these variants has a very small effect on risk for schizophrenia. Because of this, one would need many such variants to manifest schizophrenia as a phenotype. However, it is unknown how many such variants or in what configuration is required for schizophrenia. Furthermore, none of these variants may be specific to schizophrenia. Thus, ascertaining the genetic architecture of schizophrenia has introduced a variety of hurdles not initially anticipated by psychiatric geneticists.

Molecular genetic methods can classify and investigate genetic information in a variety of ways, including by type of mutation (e.g., deletion, duplication, translocation), frequency of mutation (i.e., common versus rare mutations), structural component (i.e., affecting promoter, exon, intron, etc.), gene, gene network (i.e., sets of genes that are functionally related), and chromosome, among many others (Heck et al., 2014; Hou & Zhao, 2013; Lee et al., 2012; Ohi et al., 2014; Purcell et al., 2014; Schork et al., 2013). These are some of the classifications psychiatric geneticists are currently using to organize the massive amount of genetic information available to discern how genetic variation might map onto neural function and behavior to promote or protect against disease.

Recent work on the genetics of schizophrenia has revealed the importance of both common and rare genetic variants (Lee et al., 2012; Purcell et al., 2014; Stefansson et al., 2014; Szatkiewicz et al., 2014), enrichment of disease-promoting variants in the coding regions of genes (Schork et al., 2013), and specific involvement of a variety of genes associated with glutamate (Ayalew et al., 2012; Ohi et al., 2014) and GABA function (Wang, Liu, & Aragam, 2010), calcium and sodium channel expression (Cross-Disorder Group of the Psychiatric Genomics, 2013; Dickinson et al., 2014; Hertzberg, Katsel, Roussos, Haroutunian, & Domany, 2015; Ripke et al., 2013), immune function (Schizophrenia Working Group of the Psychiatric Genomics, 2014), and many other pathways hypothesized to be involved in the pathophysiology of schizophrenia.

MISSING HERITABILITY

Many of the first genetic disorders studied were Mendelian in nature, or much less genetically complex than mental illnesses such as schizophrenia (Diehl & Kendler, 1989). Huntington's disease is a good example, as is Alzheimer's disease, for which genotype at a locus in the gene APOE predicts 10–20 percent of the variance in prevalence (Bookheimer & Burggren, 2009). As recently as several decades ago, psychiatric geneticists were in pursuit of "the" schizophrenia gene or "schizogene," hoping that the genetic basis of schizophrenia would be analogous to that of Alzheimer's, which is also highly heritable, but non-Mendelian. Several mutations identified in pedigrees of families with high prevalence of schizophrenia seemed promising candidates for such a "schizogene," but ultimately each of these mutations had only modest effects in larger samples (e.g., DISC1; Sullivan, 2013). Such large mutations were present only in a small number of schizophrenia patients and had low specificity (i.e., also occurred in nonaffected family members), and different rare (but low penetrance) mutations were identified in different pedigrees (Stefansson et al., 2014; Szatkiewicz et al., 2014).

With the advent of genome sequencing came the opportunity to search more systematically for these disease-conferring variants. Genome-wide association studies (GWAS), the first of which investigated age-related macular degeneration (Klein et al., 2005), are designed to look for differences in allele frequencies as a function of a phenotype of interest, usually case status (i.e., patient versus nonpatient). These studies employ large samples of unrelated individuals, testing for an association between the phenotype and each of 500,000 to 2 million SNPs.

Originally, this type of study was expected to reveal all the genes that contributed to schizophrenia in relatively short order. However, even as sample sizes began growing from hundreds to thousands to tens of thousands of participants, often only a few genetic variants would meet the stringent significance thresholds required when conducting millions of statistical tests (Purcell et al., 2009; Ripke et al., 2013). Collectively, the identified pool of genome-wide significant variants accounted for less than 4 percent of the variance in case status—much less than the 65–80 percent heritability estimates from family and twin studies. This became known as the problem of "missing heritability."

COMMON VARIANT, COMMON DISEASE

There are billions of base pairs in the human genome. These are primarily composed of sequences held constant across all humans. A very small portion of this code varies between individuals and an even smaller percentage represents chunks of DNA or individual base pairs that vary commonly (i.e., the rare allele occurs in 1 percent or more of the population). These regions, and the polymorphisms in them, are "common variants" and are so-called because a substantial portion of a population (2 percent–50 percent, typically) carries a mutation at this genomic location. Common genetic variation is much easier to assess than rare variation, by virtue of its frequency in the population, but for the same reason typically has much smaller effects on phenotypes.

Several theories have emerged with possible explanations for the elusiveness of schizophrenia-related genes. One of the best developed is the common variant, common disease model (Reich & Lander, 2001). This model asserts that common genetic variation may contribute to psychopathology in addition to large, deleterious mutations, which are by virtue of their higher phenotypic impact, almost always rare at a population level. If thousands of common variants influence schizophrenia status, each contributing a very small increase in risk, this may explain the relatively low recurrence risk for schizophrenia (10 percent in offspring with one affected parent), while still accounting for the high heritability estimates (Cannon & Keller, 2006). As such, the CV/CD model posits that individual risk alleles for a psychiatric illness are distributed broadly in the general population. In this model, while any particular schizophrenia-related variant occurs at a high rate among unaffected individuals, those with and without the clinical phenotype differ in the aggregation of such risk variants, with affected individuals at the relative extreme of the underlying aggregated continuum of risk variants (Cannon & Keller, 2006).

Under this hypothesis—that common variants have small effect sizes, but together contribute substantial genetic risk for schizophrenia—two parallel lines of research emerged. The first was a push to increase sample size and thus increase statistical power to detect small effects. Over the last decade, the sample sizes in schizophrenia GWAS have grown from hundreds of individuals to close to 150,000 (Mah et al., 2006; Purcell et al., 2009; Ripke et al., 2013; Schizophrenia Working Group of the Psychiatric Genomics, 2014). The larger studies have had, as predicted, more success in identifying significant genetic variants associated with schizophrenia. As compared with early studies, which returned few significant hits, the largest study to date identified 108 genomic regions (Mah et al., 2006; Schizophrenia Working Group of the Psychiatric Genomics, 2014). However, even these 108 regions together only account for less than 4 percent of the variance in disease status.

Another line of research opted instead to lower the stringent p-value thresholds enforced by standard statistical rules. Purcell et al. (2009) suggested that many variants, even in extremely large samples, will still fail to cross the significance thresholds but will meet more nominal significance thresholds. He aggregated across thousands of nominally significant SNPs—most of which did not meet standard GWAS significance thresholds—to create a single, polygenic score approximating genetic risk for schizophrenia more broadly. These polygenic scores accounted for far more of the variance in disease status than any individual SNP and provided substantial evidence for the contribution of common variants to risk for schizophrenia (Purcell et al., 2009).

OTHER GENETIC RISK FACTORS

Most common variants contributing to risk for schizophrenia have yet to be identified at genome-wide levels of significance (i.e., $p < 10^{-8}$). However, even if we had already mapped all the common risk variants, it is likely that much of the genetic variance would remain unexplained (Purcell et al., 2009). This portion, which has been estimated to be 30–50 percent of the variance in disease status, is due instead to rare mutations and epistatic effects (i.e., gene-gene interactions) (Schizophrenia Working Group of the Psychiatric Genomics, 2014).

The most frequently investigated form of rare mutation in schizophrenia is copy-number variation. Copy number variants (CNVs) are portions of the genome that are either duplicated or deleted. When these mutations occur in coding regions of the DNA, they can result in highly deleterious changes in function. One example is Down syndrome, which is caused by an additional copy of chromosome 21 and leads to profound intellectual disability. CNVs associated with schizophrenia are typically not as severe, though it is much harder to make general claims about the penetrance of rare variants, since very few individuals will have CNVs of the same length in the same genomic location and since most CNVs probably operate to increase risk against a non-zero background of common risk variants (Purcell et al., 2014; Stefansson et al., 2014; Szatkiewicz et al., 2014).

Additionally, risk-associated genes almost certainly do not increase risk strictly in an additive, linear way. Genes interact biologically—the exact patterns and systems of these interactions remain current avenues of inquiry. As such, their effects on phenotypic outcomes should be expected to interact statistically. Several examples of gene–gene interactions increasing risk for schizophrenia have been offered (e.g., Andreasen et al., 2012; Kang et al., 2011; Nicodemus et al., 2010), though this aspect of the field is still in its infancy.

Together, common variants, rare mutations, and epistatic effects between genes contribute to the substantial genetic component of schizophrenia. Environmental effects, along with gene–environment interactions also contribute to risk for schizophrenia. Although some risk-associating variants have been identified, the vast majority of the contributing genes remain to be uncovered. Advances in bioinformatics are expected to aid substantially in gene-finding efforts, and an improvement in phenotypic definition may also improve results.

ENDOPHENOTYPES: HOW DO GENES INCREASE RISK FOR SCHIZOPHRENIA?

Nearly all efforts to uncover the genetic factors relevant in schizophrenia, as well as all other psychiatric illnesses, have relied on case-control comparisons. Such studies by design can only detect genetic variants that tend to be present in cases and absent from controls. Thus, their success relies on two assumptions: (1) that all cases will have similar genetic profiles, and (2) that individuals without schizophrenia will lack disease-related genetic variation. However, clinicians have long known that there is a great deal of heterogeneity within schizophrenia patients, which is almost certainly reflected at the gene level. Additionally, more recent work characterizing first-degree relatives of patients, as well as individuals with subsyndromal levels of psychotic symptoms, suggests genetic variants for schizophrenia are actually distributed among the general (nonaffected) population, as predicted by the CV/CD model (Cannon & Keller, 2006; Tan et al., 2008).

Gottesman and Shields (1972) suggested that schizophrenia, as defined at the syndromal level, may not be the optimal level at which to seek associations with genetics. Instead, they proposed an approach adapted from insect biology: the "endophenotype." In the insect literature, the term had been used to denote characteristics of grasshoppers that were not obvious and external (termed exophenotypes) but rather were microscopic or internal, requiring specialized measurement to discern. These endophenotypes were thought to explain behavioral variation in grasshoppers that could not be explained by exophenotypes. The authors used this term in the context of schizophrenia to refer to phenotypes associated with schizophrenia but that are not the disorder themselves, such as eye-movement abnormalities. These traits, more narrowly defined than the syndrome, were expected to involve fewer genes and, therefore, in a sense to be more proximal to the genetics of schizophrenia than the end state of the disorder itself. In other words, these traits were thought to be intermediate between the disease-promoting genetic variations and clinical syndrome (Gottesman & Gould, 2003).

Since the initial conceptualization of psychiatric endophenotypes, other terms are used to denote highly similar constructs, including intermediate phenotypes (Meyer-Lindenberg & Weinberger, 2006), biomarkers, subclinical traits, and vulnerability markers. Additionally, several components of the endophenotype concept have shifted since the term was initially applied in 1972. The notion that they cannot be directly observed but must be measured using specialized instruments is no longer central to their definition, as the field of endophenotypes has expanded to include self-reported, neuropsychological, and cognitive traits, along with neural and endocrinological markers.

The assumption that endophenotypes are less complex genetically than clinical syndromes has also not proven true. Some argue that endophenotypes are just as difficult to pin down genetically as disorders are, and the effect sizes of genetic loci on endophenotypes are no greater than on psychiatric disorders themselves (Flint & Munafò, 2007; Iacono, Vaidyanathan, Vrieze, & Malone, 2014). However, further refining of a particular endophenotype may aid in reducing complexity at the genetic level. Additionally, the endophenotype approach remains a fruitful way to identify elements of disorders that represent shared genetic variance with the disorder outcome. It also identifies traits that, if associated with the disorder, do not only emerge symptomatically ("clinical phenotypes") but also are present earlier in life, so can be used as potential markers of liability prior to onset. These traits, in some cases, can also be more readily investigated in animal models.

WATERSHED ANALOGY OF ENDOPHENOTYPES

A useful way of conceptualizing the biological components of a complex phenotype such as schizophrenia is to imagine the clinical syndrome as the ultimate body of water in a watershed, the culmination of many distinct tributaries, streams, and rivers—endophenotypes at different levels of function—which flow into it (Cannon & Keller, 2006). In this analogy, thousands of genes individually contribute to hundreds of cell-signaling mechanisms (e.g., synaptic density in the prefrontal cortex), which underlie specific neural systems (e.g., working memory circuits) that, in turn, map onto primary clinical symptoms (e.g., cognitive deficits). Symptoms aggregate to form clinical syndromes like schizophrenia. Based on this framework, disruptions in any of these systems alone may not be enough to result in expression of the clinical syndrome, but the cumulative effects of many disruptions could. Thus, schizophrenia may be a collection of abnormal biological processes that impinge on an ultimate clinical phenotype. As such, examining each process individually may be more tractable than trying to connect thousands of genes to a complex set of symptoms, like schizophrenia, without any mechanisms in between (Cannon & Keller, 2006; Tan et al., 2008). Herein lies the most salient advantage of endophenotypes.

Endophenotypes include quantitative, heritable, phenotypic measures related to the disorder that varies dimensionally across the general population. If these phenotypes lie between the clinical syndrome and genes promoting the disease, they should be heritable (i.e., have some genetic basis) and be related to the development of the disease, rather than a secondary result of having the illness. Although mental disorders are currently defined categorically (an individual either does or does not have an illness), it is highly unlikely that the biological processes underlying these disorders are discrete (e.g., memory performance, synaptic density, receptor protein expression, etc., are all continuously varying phenomena). As such, endophenotypes should represent variation across the population. Additionally, there should be many endophenotypes for one complex disorder. Whereas early conceptualizations required that endophenotypes be specific to a single disorder, more recent findings demonstrate high rates of overlap in the genetic contribution to different disorders. This indicates instead that related disorders should share common endophenotypes (e.g., schizophrenia and bipolar disorder have substantial genetic and phenotypic overlap, so a subset of endophenotypes for one should be present in the other).

Many potential schizophrenia endophenotypes have been offered. Some of the first-identified endophenotypes included deficits in sustained attention deficit, working memory, and smooth-pursuit eye movement (Calkins, Curtis, Iacono, & Grove, 2004; Holzman, Proctor, & Hughes, 1973). One of the most reliable endophenotypes in schizophrenia—and most profound areas of cognitive impairment—is episodic memory (Greenwood et al., 2013; van Erp et al., 2008). Several other potential cognitive endophenotypes have been proposed, as well, including processing speed, set shifting, sequencing, verbal learning, spatial memory, general cognitive ability, and others (see Ohi et al., 2014; Snitz, MacDonald, & Carter, 2006 for a review).

A plethora of neural abnormalities, both gross and specific, have been reported in schizophrenia, including gray matter abnormalities in many brain regions (Mathew et al., 2014; Turner et al., 2012), reduced white matter integrity (Wheeler & Voineskos, 2014), and consistent findings of ventricular enlargement (Cannon et al., 1992). Specific aberrations in the prefrontal cortex, both structurally and functionally, have also been identified as endophenotypes, including structural abnormalities in polar and dorsolateral prefrontal regions (Cannon et al., 2002) and altered functional activity in the prefrontal cortex during performance of a working-memory and executive function tasks (Callicott et al., 2003; Owens et al., 2012).

Other endophenotypes have been proposed, including sensory processing and event related potential measures such as prepulse inhibition and P300 and P50 waves (Bramon et al., 2005; Bramon, Rabe-Hesketh, Sham, Murray, & Frangou, 2004), as well as traits such as coping style (Fortgang, Hultman, & Cannon, 2015) and impulsivity (Fortgang, Hultman, & Cannon). Locating endophenotypes will not only help us understand the nature of liability, but also will help with consistent detection and diagnosis of schizophrenia-spectrum disorders. Perhaps most importantly, it also represents the possibility of prevention of psychosis (Stone et al. 2005).

LIABILITY-THRESHOLD MODEL OF PSYCHIATRIC ILLNESS

If endophenotypes that underpin psychiatric illness vary dimensionally across the population, risk factors for those disorders should also be distributed in this manner. The relationship between aggregate risk and phenotypic severity (i.e., degree of a particular phenotype such as negative affect) represents the liability-threshold model (Cannon & Keller, 2006; Lee & Wray, 2013). Here, we would expect individuals who meet criteria for schizophrenia to fall on the extreme ends of the distributions of many related phenotypes, reflecting aggregation of risk at the tail end of the integrated distribution. However, individuals with varying degrees of risk, like relatives of patients who share genetic risk factors, or individuals with subclinical symptoms, should fall higher on both risk and phenotypic severity relative to the population mean.

Consistent with this prediction, nonill siblings of patients with schizophrenia show moderate impairment—less than patients, but more than controls—on endophenotype measures (Tan et al., 2008). Siblings show similar phenotypic profiles neurocognitively, as well as neurologically, to patients with schizophrenia, though the impairments are attenuated in severity (e.g., Callicott et al., 2003; Iacono et al., 2014; van Scheltinga, Bakker, van Haren, Derks, Buizer-Voskamp, Boos, et al., 2013). Unaffected monozygotic twins also show more similarity to patients than dizygotic twins on endophenotype measures, further confirming the genetic component to the phenotypic overlap (van Erp et al., 2008). Finally, individuals that report subclinical symptoms or have related diagnoses (e.g., schizotypal personality disorder) show similar phenotypic and genetic profiles (Hazlett et al., 2015). These patterns support the view that genes confer risk for schizophrenia via these dimensional endophenotypes, thus giving advantage to testing those phenomena directly in searching for causal gene variants linked to schizophrenia.

LINKING GENES TO ENDOPHENOTYPES TO SCHIZOPHRENIA

Many approaches have been used to link genes associated with schizophrenia to endophenotypes for schizophrenia. Consistent with the endophenotype approach, shared variance between schizophrenia and its neurocognitive endophenotypes is partially (up to 92 percent) accounted for by shared genetic variance (Toulopoulou et al., 2007). Similarly, candidate genes for schizophrenia identified through linkage studies, genome-wide association studies, and animal models of psychosis have been associated with many endophenotypes for schizophrenia, including measures of executive function, memory, prepulse inhibition, and others (Greenwood et al., 2012).

More widespread molecular genetic approaches have also been employed. Polygenic scores that approximate aggregate genetic risk for schizophrenia have been associated with symptoms of schizophrenia (Derks et al., 2012; Fanous et al., 2012), as well as other schizophrenia-related endophenotypes, including IQ (McIntosh et al., 2013; van Scheltinga, Bakker, van Haren, Derks, Buizer-Voskamp, Cahn, et al., 2013), structural MRI measures (van Scheltinga, Bakker, van Haren, Derks, Buizer-Voskamp, Boos, et al., 2013; Whalley et al., 2013), and working memory blood-oxygen-level-dependent (BOLD) activation (Walton et al., 2013). In these studies, higher genetic risk for schizophrenia is associated with lower performance or less robust neurophysiology. Finally, a few recent studies have identified sets of genes related to endophenotypes for schizophrenia, including general cognitive ability (Lencz et al., 2014), working memory (Heck et al., 2014), auditory verbal memory (Zheutlin et al.), and impulsivity (unpublished data), that also relate to schizophrenia case status. These represent the first attempts to use endophenotypes themselves to find schizophrenia-related genes, rather than using previously identified schizophrenia risk genes to predict variance on an endophenotype measure.

Future work testing for molecular evidence of shared etiology between putative endophenotypes and schizophrenia are poised to make substantial advances in our understanding of the genetics of the disorder. Comprehensive knowledge of those variants that predict a particular trait in the general population, as well as in patient samples, could offer insight into the genetic architecture of complex diseases like schizophrenia and help to identify specific genetic susceptibility for symptom clusters (e.g., gene pathways conferring risk for a particular cognitive impairment).

CONCLUSION

Although it has long been known that schizophrenia is highly genetic (Kallmann & Rypins, 1938), only recently have psychiatric geneticists started to identify genes that confer risk for illness, a process that has only just begun. Alongside work uncovering abnormalities at parallel levels of analysis including cellular signaling, neural circuit connectivity, and cognitive processes, gene-finding efforts in schizophrenia may help uncover the key neurobiological mechanisms disrupted in schizophrenia.

Heritability models using twin and family designs have quantified the genetic component of schizophrenia and discerned substantial genetic overlap with other psychiatric illnesses, along with many cognitive processes (Cannon et al., 1998; Craddock et al., 2006; Lichtenstein et al., 2009; Purcell et al., 2009; Toulopoulou et al., 2007). Molecular genetic techniques have uncovered the complexity of the genetic architecture of risk for schizophrenia, identifying over 100 impacted genes, with estimates of thousands more yet to be found (Purcell et al., 2009; Ripke et al., 2013; Schizophrenia Working Group of the Psychiatric Genomics, 2014). Of those, roughly half are likely to be common variants, each of very small effect, while the rest will be rare variants of larger impact. More advanced methods of parsing genetic information have identified systems of genes that are likely involved including those related to glutamate signaling, synaptic plasticity, and immune function, among other processes. Further advances in modeling complicated genetic effects will likely impact our understanding of schizophrenia genetics in the future.

Endophenotypes, which help bridge the biological gap between genes and behavior, will likely also advance understanding of the pathophysiology of schizophrenia. Burgeoning evidence of the dimensionality of clinical symptomology and those risk factors that underlie illness suggests that investigating biologically proximate aspects of disease (e.g., cognitive processes, abnormalities in brain maturation) will aid in uncovering disease-related mechanisms and risk factors. Already, many examples of the genetic overlap between risk for schizophrenia and related cognitive and neural measures have been reported (e.g., Callicott et al., 2003; Walton et al., 2013; Whalley et al., 2013). By ascertaining the mechanisms underlying impaired processes in schizophrenia, including the multitude of cognitive deficits, trouble with motivation, affect, and effort, as well as those systems related to the development of psychosis, it is the hope of the field that we can advance early detection and prevention, as well as develop new, more targeted treatments.

REFERENCES

Andreasen, N. C., Wilcox, M. A., Ho, B. C., Epping, E., Ziebell, S., Zeien, E., . . . Wassink, T. (2012). Statistical epistasis and progressive brain change in schizophrenia: an approach for examining the relationships between multiple genes. *Molecular Psychiatry, 17*(11), 1093–1102. doi: 10.1038/mp.2011.108

Ayalew, M., Le-Niculescu, H., Levey, D. F., Jain, N., Changala, B., Patel, S. D., . . . Niculescu, A. B. (2012). Convergent functional genomics of schizophrenia: from comprehensive understanding to genetic risk prediction. *Molecular Psychiatry, 17*(9), 887–905. doi: 10.1038/mp.2012.37

Bookheimer, S., & Burggren, A. (2009). APOE-4 genotype and neurophysiological vulnerability to Alzheimer's and cognitive aging. *Annual Review of Clinical Psychology, 5*, 343–362. doi: 10.1146/annurev.clinpsy.032408.153625

Bramon, E., McDonald, C., Croft, R. J., Landau, S., Filbey, F., Gruzelier, J. H., . . . Murray, R. M. (2005). Is the P300 wave an endophenotype for schizophrenia? A meta-analysis and a family study. *Neuroimage, 27*(4), 960–968.

Bramon, E., Rabe-Hesketh, S., Sham, P., Murray, R. M., & Frangou, S. (2004). Meta-analysis of the P300 and P50 waveforms in schizophrenia. *Schizophrenia Research, 70*(2), 315–329.

Calkins, M. E., Curtis, C. E., Iacono, W. G., & Grove, W. M. (2004). Antisaccade performance is impaired in medically and psychiatrically healthy biological relatives of schizophrenia patients. *Schizophrenia Research, 71*(1), 167–178.

Callicott, J. H., Mattay, V. S., Verchinski, B. A., Marenco, S., Egan, M. F., & Weinberger, D. R. (2003). Complexity of prefrontal cortical dysfunction in schizophrenia: more than up or down. *American Journal of Psychiatry, 160*(12), 2209–2215.

Cannon, T. D., Kaprio, J., Lonnqvist, J., Huttunen, M., & Koskenvuo, M. (1998). The genetic epidemiology of schizophrenia in a Finnish twin cohort. A population-based modeling study. *Archives of General Psychiatry, 55*(1), 67–74.

Cannon, T. D., & Keller, M. C. (2006). Endophenotypes in the genetic analyses of mental disorders. *Annual Review of Clinical Psychology, 2*, 267–290. doi: 10.1146/annurev.clinpsy.2.022305.095232

Cannon, T. D., Raine, A., Herman, T. M., Mednick, S. A., Schulsinger, F., & Moore, M. (1992). Third ventricle enlargement and lower heart rate levels in a high-risk sample. *Psychophysiology, 29*(3), 294–301.

Cannon, T. D., Thompson, P. M., van Erp, T. G., Toga, A. W., Poutanen, V.-P., Huttunen, M., . . . Khaledy, M. (2002). Cortex mapping reveals regionally specific patterns of genetic and disease-specific gray-matter deficits in twins discordant for schizophrenia. *Proceedings of the National Academy of Sciences, 99*(5), 3228–3233.

Cannon, T. D., van Erp, T. G., Rosso, I. M., Huttunen, M., Lonnqvist, J., Pirkola, T., . . . Standertskjold-Nordenstam, C. G. (2002). Fetal hypoxia and structural brain abnormalities in schizophrenic patients, their siblings, and controls. *Archives of Genetic Psychiatry, 59*(1), 35–41.

Cardno, A. G., & Gottesman, I. I. (2000). Twin studies of schizophrenia: from bow-and-arrow concordances to star wars Mx and functional genomics. *American Journal of Medical Genetics, 97*(1), 12–17.

Cardno, A. G., Rijsdijk, F. V., Sham, P. C., Murray, R. M., & McGuffin, P. (2014). A twin study of genetic relationships between psychotic symptoms.

Craddock, N., O'Donovan, M. C., & Owen, M. J. (2006). Genes for schizophrenia and bipolar disorder? Implications for psychiatric nosology. *Schizophrenia Bulletin, 32*(1), 9–16. doi: 10.1093/schbul/sbj033

Cross-Disorder Group of the Psychiatric Genomics, C. (2013). Identification of risk loci with shared effects on five major psychiatric disorders: a genome-wide analysis. *Lancet, 381*(9875), 1371–1379. doi: 10.1016/S0140-6736(12)62129-1

Davies, G., Tenesa, A., Payton, A., Yang, J., Harris, S. E., Liewald, D., . . . Deary, I. J. (2011). Genome-wide association studies establish that human intelligence is highly heritable and polygenic. *Molecular Psychiatry, 16*(10), 996–1005. doi: 10.1038/mp.2011.85

Derks, E. M., Vorstman, J. A. S., Ripke, S., Kahn, R. S., Ophoff, R. A., & Con, S. P. G. (2012). Investigation of the genetic association between quantitative measures of psychosis and schizophrenia: A polygenic risk score analysis. *Plos One, 7*(6). doi: ARTN e37852. doi 10.1371/journal.pone.0037852

Dickinson, D., Straub, R. E., Trampush, J. W., Gao, Y., Feng, N., Xie, B., . . . Weinberger, D. R. (2014). Differential effects of common variants in SCN2A on general cognitive ability, brain physiology, and messenger RNA expression in schizophrenia cases and control individuals. *JAMA Psychiatry, 71*(6), 647–656. doi: 10.1001/jamapsychiatry.2014.157

Diehl, S. R., & Kendler, K. S. (1989). Strategies for linkage studies of schizophrenia: pedigrees, DNA markers, and statistical analyses. *Schizophrenia Bulletin, 15*(3), 403–419.

Fanous, A. H., Zhou, B. Y., Aggen, S. H., Bergen, S. E., Amdur, R. L., Duan, J. B., . . . Genome-Wide, S. P. (2012). Genome-wide association study of clinical dimensions of schizophrenia: Polygenic effect on disorganized symptoms. *American Journal of Psychiatry, 169*(12), 1309–1317. doi: 10.1176/Appi.Ajp.2012.12020218

Flint, J., & Munafò, M. R. (2007). The endophenotype concept in psychiatric genetics. *Psychological medicine, 37*(2), 163–180.

Fortgang, R., Hultman, C. M., & Cannon, T. Dissecting impulsivity as an endophenotype in schizophrenia, bipolar disorder, and depression using the discordant co-twin design. *Unpublished manuscript.*

Fortgang, R., Hultman, C. M., & Cannon, T. (2015). Coping Styles in Twins Discordant for Schizophrenia, Bipolar Disorder and Depression. *Under Review.*

Gottesman, I. I., & Gould, T. D. (2003). The endophenotype concept in psychiatry: etymology and strategic intentions. *American Journal of Psychiatry, 160*(4), 636–645.

Gottesman, I. I., & Shields, J. (1972). Schizophrenia and genetics: A twin study vantage point.

Greenwood, T. A., Light, G. A., Swerdlow, N. R., Radant, A. D., & Braff, D. L. (2012). Association Analysis of 94 Candidate Genes and Schizophrenia-Related Endophenotypes. *Plos One, 7*(1). doi: ARTN e29630. doi 10.1371/journal.pone.0029630

Greenwood, T. A., Swerdlow, N. R., Gur, R. E., Cadenhead, K. S., Calkins, M. E., Dobie, D. J., . . . Braff, D. L. (2013). Genome-wide linkage analyses of 12 endophenotypes for schizophrenia from the consortium on the genetics of schizophrenia. *American Journal of Psychiatry, 170*(5), 521–532. doi: 10.1176/Appi.Ajp.2012.12020186

Hazlett, E. A., Rothstein, E. G., Ferreira, R., Silverman, J. M., Siever, L. J., & Olincy, A. (2015). Sensory gating disturbances in the spectrum: Similarities and differences in schizotypal personality disorder and schizophrenia. *Schizophrenia Research, 161*(2–3), 283–290. doi: 10.1016/j.schres.2014.11.020

Heck, A., Fastenrath, M., Ackermann, S., Auschra, B., Bickel, H., Coynel, D., . . . Papassotiropoulos, A. (2014). Converging genetic and functional brain imaging evidence links neuronal excitability to working memory, psychiatric disease, and brain activity. *Neuron, 81*(5), 1203–1213. doi: 10.1016/j.neuron.2014.01.010

Hertzberg, L., Katsel, P., Roussos, P., Haroutunian, V., & Domany, E. (2015). Integration of gene expression and GWAS results supports involvement of calcium signaling in Schizophrenia. *Schizophrenia Research.* doi: 10.1016/j.schres.2015.02.001

Holzman, P. S., Proctor, L. R., & Hughes, D. W. (1973). Eye-tracking patterns in schizophrenia. *Science, 181*(4095), 179–181.

Hou, L., & Zhao, H. (2013). A review of post-GWAS prioritization approaches. *Frontiers in Genetics, 4,* 280. doi: 10.3389/fgene.2013.00280

Iacono, W. G., Vaidyanathan, U., Vrieze, S. I., & Malone, S. M. (2014). Knowns and unknowns for psychophysiological endophenotypes: integration and response to commentaries. *Psychophysiology, 51*(12), 1339–1347. doi: 10.1111/psyp.12358

Kallmann, F. J., & Rypins, S. J. (1938). *The genetics of schizophrenia; a study of heredity and reproduction in the families of 1,087 scizophrenics.* New York, NY: J.J. Augustin.

Kang, E., Burdick, K. E., Kim, J. Y., Duan, X., Guo, J. U., Sailor, K. A., . . . Ming, G. L. (2011). Interaction between FEZ1 and DISC1 in regulation of neuronal development and risk for schizophrenia. *Neuron,* 72(4), 559–571. doi: 10.1016/j.neuron.2011.09.032

Klein, R. J., Zeiss, C., Chew, E. Y., Tsai, J. Y., Sackler, R. S., Haynes, C., . . . Hoh, J. (2005). Complement factor H polymorphism in age-related macular degeneration. *Science, 308*(5720), 385–389. doi: 10.1126/Science.1109557

Lee, S. H., DeCandia, T. R., Ripke, S., Yang, J., Schizophrenia Psychiatric Genome-Wide Association Study, C., International Schizophrenia, C., . . . Wray, N. R. (2012). Estimating the proportion of variation in susceptibility to schizophrenia captured by common SNPs. *Nature Genetics, 44*(3), 247–250. doi: 10.1038/ng.1108

Lee, S. H., & Wray, N. R. (2013). Novel genetic analysis for case-control genome-wide association studies: quantification of power and genomic prediction accuracy. *Plos One, 8*(8), e71494. doi: 10.1371/journal.pone.0071494

Lencz, T., Knowles, E., Davies, G., Guha, S., Liewald, D. C., Starr, J. M., . . . Malhotra, A. K. (2014). Molecular genetic evidence for overlap between general cognitive ability and risk for schizophrenia: a report from the Cognitive Genomics consorTium (COGENT). *Molecular Psychiatry, 19*(2), 168–174. doi: 10.1038/mp.2013.166

Lichtenstein, P., Yip, B. H., Bjork, C., Pawitan, Y., Cannon, T. D., Sullivan, P. F., & Hultman, C. M. (2009). Common genetic determinants of schizophrenia and bipolar disorder in Swedish families: a population-based study. *Lancet, 373*(9659), 234–239. doi: 10.1016/S0140-6736(09)60072-6

Mah, S., Nelson, M. R., Delisi, L. E., Reneland, R. H., Markward, N., James, M. R., . . . Braun, A. (2006). Identification of the semaphorin receptor PLXNA2 as a candidate for susceptibility to schizophrenia. *Molecular Psychiatry, 11*(5), 471–478. doi: 10.1038/sj.mp.4001785

Mathew, I., Gardin, T. M., Tandon, N., Eack, S., Francis, A. N., Seidman, L. J., . . . Keshavan, M. S. (2014). Medial temporal lobe structures and hippocampal subfields in psychotic disorders: findings from the Bipolar-Schizophrenia Network on Intermediate Phenotypes (B-SNIP) study. *JAMA Psychiatry, 71*(7), 769–777. doi: 10.1001/jamapsychiatry.2014.453

McIntosh, A. M., Gow, A., Luciano, M., Davies, G., Liewald, D. C., Harris, S. E., . . . Deary, I. J. (2013). Polygenic Risk for Schizophrenia Is Associated with Cognitive Change Between Childhood and Old Age. *Biological Psychiatry, 73*(10), 938–943. doi: 10.1016/J.Biopsych.2013.01.011

Meyer-Lindenberg, A., & Weinberger, D. R. (2006). Intermediate phenotypes and genetic mechanisms of psychiatric disorders. *Nature Reviews Neuroscience, 7*(10), 818–827.

Mittal, V. A., Ellman, L. M., & Cannon, T. D. (2008). Gene-environment interaction and covariation in schizophrenia: the role of obstetric complications. *Schizophrenia Bulletin, 34*(6), 1083–1094. doi: 10.1093/schbul/sbn080

Nicodemus, K. K., Law, A. J., Radulescu, E., Luna, A., Kolachana, B., Vakkalanka, R., . . . Weinberger, D. R. (2010). Biological validation of increased schizophrenia risk with NRG1, ERBB4, and AKT1 epistasis via functional neuroimaging in healthy controls. *Archives of General Psychiatry, 67*(10), 991–1001. doi: 10.1001/archgenpsychiatry.2010.117

Ohi, K., Hashimoto, R., Ikeda, M., Yamamori, H., Yasuda, Y., Fujimoto, M., . . . Takeda, M. (2014). Glutamate Networks Implicate Cognitive Impairments in Schizophrenia: Genome-Wide Association Studies of 52 Cognitive Phenotypes. *Schizophrenia Bulletin*. doi: 10.1093/schbul/sbu171

Owens, S. F., Picchioni, M. M., Ettinger, U., McDonald, C., Walshe, M., Schmechtig, A., . . . Toulopoulou, T. (2012). Prefrontal deviations in function but not volume are putative endophenotypes for schizophrenia. *Brain, 135*(Pt 7), 2231–2244. doi: 10.1093/brain/aws138

Plomin, R. (2011). Commentary: Why are children in the same family so different? Non-shared environment three decades later. *International Journal of Epidemiology, 40*(3), 582–592.

Plomin, R., DeFries, J. C., & McClearn, G. E. (2008). *Behavioral genetics*: Worth Pub.

Pogue-Geile, M. F., & Yokley, J. L. (2010). Current Research on the Genetic Contributors to Schizophrenia. *Current Directions in Psychological Science, 19*(4), 214–219. doi: 10.1177/0963721410378490

Purcell, S. M., Moran, J. L., Fromer, M., Ruderfer, D., Solovieff, N., Roussos, P., . . . Sklar, P. (2014). A polygenic burden of rare disruptive mutations in schizophrenia. *Nature, 506*(7487), 185-+. doi:10.1038/Nature12975

Purcell, S. M., Wray, N. R., Stone, J. L., Visscher, P. M., O'Donovan, M. C., Sullivan, P. F., . . . Scolnick, E. M. (2009). Common polygenic variation contributes to risk of schizophrenia and bipolar disorder. *Nature, 460*(7256), 748–752. doi: 10.1038/Nature08185

Reich, D. E., & Lander, E. S. (2001). On the allelic spectrum of human disease. *Trends in Genetics, 17*(9), 502–510.

Ripke, S., O'Dushlaine, C., Chambert, K., Moran, J. L., Kahler, A. K., Akterin, S., . . . Sullivan, P. F. (2013). Genome-wide association analysis identifies 13 new risk loci for schizophrenia. *Nature Genet, 45*(10), 1150–1159. doi: 10.1038/ng.2742

Schizophrenia Working Group of the Psychiatric Genomics, C. (2014). Biological insights from 108 schizophrenia-associated genetic loci. *Nature, 511*(7510), 421–427. doi: 10.1038/nature13595

Schork, A. J., Thompson, W. K., Pham, P., Torkamani, A., Roddey, J. C., Sullivan, P. F., . . . Dale, A. M. (2013). All SNPs are not created equal: genome-wide association studies reveal a consistent pattern of enrichment among functionally annotated SNPs. *PLoS Genet*, *9*(4), e1003449. doi: 10.1371/journal.pgen.1003449

Snitz, B. E., MacDonald, A. W., & Carter, C. S. (2006). Cognitive deficits in unaffected first-degree relatives of schizophrenia patients: a meta-analytic review of putative endophenotypes. *Schizophrenia Bulletin*, *32*(1), 179–194.

Stefansson, H., Meyer-Lindenberg, A., Steinberg, S., Magnusdottir, B., Morgen, K., Arnarsdottir, S., . . . Stefansson, K. (2014). CNVs conferring risk of autism or schizophrenia affect cognition in controls. *Nature*, *505*(7483), 361–366. doi: 10.1038/nature12818

Sullivan, P. F. (2013). Questions about DISC1 as a genetic risk factor for schizophrenia. *Molecular Psychiatry*, *18*(10), 1050–1052. doi: 10.1038/mp.2012.182

Szatkiewicz, J. P., O'Dushlaine, C., Chen, G., Chambert, K., Moran, J. L., Neale, B. M., . . . Sullivan, P. F. (2014). Copy number variation in schizophrenia in Sweden. *Molecular Psychiatry*, *19*(7), 762–773. doi: 10.1038/mp.2014.40

Tan, H. Y., Callicott, J. H., & Weinberger, D. R. (2008). Intermediate phenotypes in schizophrenia genetics redux: is it a no brainer? *Molecular Psychiatry*, *13*(3), 233–238. doi: 10.1038/sj.mp.4002145

Toulopoulou, T., Picchioni, M., Rijsdijk, F., Hua-Hall, M., Ettinger, U., Sham, P., & Murray, R. (2007). Substantial genetic overlap between neurocognition and schizophrenia—Genetic modeling in twin samples. *Archives of General Psychiatry*, *64*(12), 1348–1355. doi: 10.1001/Archpsyc.64.12.1348

Turner, J. A., Calhoun, V. D., Michael, A., van Erp, T. G., Ehrlich, S., Segall, J. M., . . . Wang, L. (2012). Heritability of multivariate gray matter measures in schizophrenia. *Twin Research and Human Genetics*, *15*(3), 324–335. doi: 10.1017/thg.2012.1

van Erp, T. G., Therman, S., Pirkola, T., Tuulio-Henriksson, A., Glahn, D. C., Bachman, P., . . . Cannon, T. D. (2008). Verbal recall and recognition in twins discordant for schizophrenia. *Psychiatry Research*, *159*(3), 271–280. doi: 10.1016/j.psychres.2007.03.003

van Scheltinga, A. F. T., Bakker, S. C., van Haren, N. E. M., Derks, E. M., Buizer-Voskamp, J. E., Boos, H. B. M., . . . Study, P. G.-w. A. (2013). Genetic schizophrenia risk variants jointly modulate total brain and white matter volume. *Biological Psychiatry*, *73*(6), 525–531. doi: 10.1016/J.Biopsych.2012.08.017

van Scheltinga, A. F. T., Bakker, S. C., van Haren, N. E. M., Derks, E. M., Buizer-Voskamp, J. E., Cahn, W., . . . G, P. G.-W. A. S. (2013). Schizophrenia genetic variants are not associated with intelligence. *Psychological Medicine*, *43*(12), 2563–2570. doi: 10.1017/S0033291713000196

Walton, E., Turner, J., Gollub, R. L., Manoach, D. S., Yendiki, A., Ho, B. C., . . . Ehrlich, S. (2013). Cumulative genetic risk and prefrontal activity in patients with schizophrenia. *Schizophrenia Bulletin*, *39*(3), 703–711. doi: 10.1093/schbul/sbr190

Wang, K. S., Liu, X. F., & Aragam, N. (2010). A genome-wide meta-analysis identifies novel loci associated with schizophrenia and bipolar disorder. *Schizophrenia Research*, *124*(1–3), 192–199. doi: 10.1016/j.schres.2010.09.002

Whalley, H. C., Sprooten, E., Hackett, S., Hall, L., Blackwood, D. H., Glahn, D. C., . . . McIntosh, A. M. (2013). Polygenic risk and white matter integrity in individuals at high risk of mood disorder. *Biological Psychiatry*, *74*(4), 280–286. doi: 10.1016/j.biopsych.2013.01.027

Wheeler, A. L., & Voineskos, A. N. (2014). A review of structural neuroimaging in schizophrenia: from connectivity to connectomics. *Frontiers in Human Neuroscience*, *8*, 653. doi: 10.3389/fnhum.2014.00653

Yang, J. A., Benyamin, B., McEvoy, B. P., Gordon, S., Henders, A. K., Nyholt, D. R., . . . Visscher, P. M. (2010). Common SNPs explain a large proportion of the heritability for human height. *Nat Genet*, *42*(7), 565–U131. doi: 10.1038/Ng.608

Zheutlin, A. B., Fortgang, R. G., Sabb, F. W., Bilder, R. M., Freimer, N., London, E., . . . Cannon, T. D. Common variants for schizophrenia ascertained through genome-wide association with a cognitive endophenotype.

/// 9 /// NEUROIMAGING IN SCHIZOPHRENIA

SUZANNE JASBERG and KELVIN O. LIM

INTRODUCTION

Researchers have been profoundly interested in the structure and function of the human brain for centuries. Early scientists relied on post mortem pathology analysis to understand the role of a lesion in human behavior. Very rarely, such as the famous Phineas Gage frontal lobe injury, were scientists able to elucidate how structure related to function in a living brain. Over time, imaging technology began to progress in a way in which scientists could begin to robustly study pathology in living tissue.

Clinically, imaging techniques are used both diagnostically and interventionally in many fields of medicine. In cardiology, imaging guides a clinician to decide if a blockage should be managed with medication or with surgery. Oncologists rely heavily on Positron Emission Technology (PET) to evaluate and track the status of tumors. Neurologists utilize imaging to decide if a stroke is ischemic or hemorrhagic and which treatment modality to pursue.

Comparatively, in psychiatry, imaging is less able to directly manage care. It is used primarily to exclude gross lesions or "organic" and identifiable causes of psychotic illness. As such, imaging is utilized daily in the diagnostic workup of psychosis, which will be explained shortly. The majority of interest lies in the ever-advancing research domains that utilize complex imaging techniques to understand the pathophysiology of psychiatric disease and, specific to this chapter, schizophrenia.

This chapter will first describe the clinical utility of the field's current imaging technology. The remainder of the chapter will focus on numerous imaging modalities, describing the basic science principles and research use of each. By reading this chapter, the student should be able to progress through training with a strong grasp on the utility of clinical imaging and the potentials of imaging research in schizophrenia.

CLINICAL UTILITY

Currently, imaging is utilized in schizophrenia to complete a comprehensive first episode psychosis workup. In a first episode of illness, it is essential to rule out any and all organic forms of psychosis. One must be sure that there is no underlying brain mass or infectious disease that might result in psychotic symptoms.

First-episode psychotic symptoms, as well as prodromal symptoms, warrant a systematic medical workup in order to exclude medical causes of psychosis. The diagnosis of schizophrenia requires there be an absence of a medical condition that could account for the observed and experienced psychopathological signs and symptoms. Massachusetts General Hospital Schizophrenia Program, Harvard Medical School, has compiled a comprehensive clinical laboratory and imaging assessment strategy (Freudenreich, Schulz, & Goff, 2009). The sample screening battery proposed includes neuroimaging to constitute a thorough exam.

Completing such an exam ensures there is no delay in treatment of a medical illness and that schizophrenia is reliably diagnosed. Of note, this examination also includes a thorough medical, family, and social history. A thorough laboratory workup is also essential to rule out any underlying medical condition and to ensure a medical baseline (e.g., metabolic status) is established before beginning treatment.

As stated, this screening battery includes the recommendation to obtain a noncontrast brain magnetic resonance image (MRI). Noncontrast MRI allows the best detection of conditions that might produce psychosis, such as vasculitis or tumor. Computed Tomography (CT) scanning is best utilized to rule out acute stroke, which is unlikely to present without gross neurological signs.

When institutions adopt these screening guidelines, it is inevitable that incidental findings occur. Incidental findings refer to abnormalities discovered on a scan that are not clinically relevant and do not require further follow-up. The purpose of the scan was to investigate whether there was a gross lesion that could be held accountable for said psychotic symptoms. If a lesion is found that is not capable of producing psychotic symptoms, and not in need of further follow-up, the data obtained in the scan is incidental. In an MRI study of 2000 people from the general population who underwent high-resolution structural brain MRI with a 1.5 tesla magnet, 145 people (7.6 percent) had asymptomatic infarcts. Additionally, 1.8 percent had incidental cerebral aneurysms, and 1.6 percent had incidental benign tumors (Vernooji & van der Lugt, 2007). In medicine, it is always important to remember the purpose of the test one orders, and how the outcome of the test helps answer the particular clinical question from which the task was generated. Of note, in a study of patients with schizophrenia versus controls, it was found that 30 percent of the scans had an abnormality, and chronic schizophrenia patients were more likely to have incidental brain abnormalities compared to first-episode psychosis patients or controls (Lubman & McGorry, 2002).

Admittedly, compared to other fields, neuroimaging is not as clinically useful in psychiatry as it is in other specialties. This can be disappointing in a patient visit or while explaining to loving parents exactly why their child has been diagnosed with schizophrenia from a neuroimaging perspective. Psychiatry is akin to cardiology 50 years ago. The developments and discoveries that will take place through a trainee's career are both vast and tremendously impactful. The remainder of the chapter will serve to educate the trainee on the basic science of each imaging technique and how these modalities are used in clinical research.

RESEARCH UTILITY

X-ray

X-ray pneumoencephalograpy, one of the first neuroimaging tools, allowed researchers to inject air into the cerebrospinal fluid to visualize enlarged ventricular sizes in schizophrenia. This technique was powerful, but also quite painful for the patient. Later, X-ray computed tomography (CT) allowed for the study of more complex brain structure, including size, shape, and lesions.

Computed Tomography

CT scanning was the first powerful and easily utilized structural imaging technique. CT was a paramount technological advancement, allowing clinicians to visualize cross-sectional anatomy of the living brain. This major discovery, for which Hounsfield and Cormack won the Nobel Prize in Medicine in 1979, revolutionized care.

The technology is mature and reliable, and remains a very important clinical tool in medicine. We will briefly examine the principles behind CT scanning, because it is historically useful to grasp. Currently, CT scanning is seldom used in psychiatry, outside of determining if there is an acute cortical or subcortical bleed.

CT technology consists of utilizing the degree of x-ray attenuation by various tissues. In X-ray technology, X-rays pass through an object to a background, which obtains only a single projection. CT scanning was able to take multiple projections as the scanner moves about the object, and through mathematical algorithms scientists were able to reconstruct an image with depth rather than just shadows as in x-ray. This allows for the analysis of ventricular size, sulci size, and brain volumes. Additionally, CT scans also allow for the analysis of density. This is an essential function that allows clinicians to identify acute stroke, because the density of blood is drastically different from brain tissue.

CT scanning was used in primary studies to assess ventricular size and total brain size in schizophrenia. In 1976, Johnstone and colleagues reported that lateral ventricles were enlarged in chronic schizophrenia patients. This finding was replicated multiple times and confirmed statistically significant group differences in ventricular sizes between patients and controls (Reveley, 1985).

Magnetic Resonance Imaging

Magnetic Resonance Imaging (MRI) technology was another advancement in the study of living tissue. MRI provides increased soft-tissue contrast, based on nuclear magnetic resonance (NMR) technology. Interestingly, MRI utilizes NMR technology, but the word "nuclear" was dropped to make this imaging modality more appealing to the general population who might not understand the technological application of the word. This imaging technology won Lauterbur and Mansfield the Nobel Prize in 2003. These ideas were based on Block and Purcells 1952 Nobel Prize in physics, awarded for developing the NRM technology on which MRI was based.

NMR is made possible by harnessing "spin," which exists in molecules with an odd number of protons or neutrons. For example C12 exhibits no spin, but C13 isotope, as it is odd, has spin. Hydrogen atoms, with 1 proton, exhibit spin. The high proportion of hydrogen that exists in water allows an image to be obtained quickly.

MRI imaging is completed by applying a magnetic field and matching the magnetic field to the resonance state of hydrogen atoms in any tissue containing water. Atoms affected by a magnetic field can be thought of as spinning tops. Tops, without any external influence would spin randomly. When these tops have been subjected to an external magnetic field, they align vertically to the field. Then, a pulsing frequency is applied to disrupt the tops. This frequency effectively disrupts the spin, and the time it takes to resume normalcy is recorded (McCarley, 2002).

In MRI there are two important measurements, T1 and T2 relaxation times. Again, the spinning tops are aligned by the magnetic force. Then an applied radiofrequency pulse perturbs the vector alignment. The time it takes for the vector alignment to return to 63 percent of its original placement is deemed the T1 relaxation time (McCarley, 2002).

On the other hand, T2 relaxation time depends on the wobble associated with a top being out of alignment. When the spinning tops, or nuclei, are subjected to tilt, the nuclei will wobble about the z axis. At first the tops wobble in chorus, but over time they depart from their harmony and "wobble" at various frequencies. The time it takes for the nuclei to wobble in sequence to eventually wobbling at 37 percent concordance is deemed T2. The time it takes to "de-wobble" (T2) is always less than or equal to the time it takes to return to alignment (T1). MRI began to gain utility when researchers studied the time differences between T1 and T2 in different tissues such as tumor tissue versus normal tissue, which present as different levels of white/black contrast. In schizophrenia, an early notable finding showed that T2 relaxation time was longer in patients with schizophrenia than in controls. This indicated a tissue-specific difference between those with the disease and those without (McCarley, 2002).

Higher strength magnetic fields cause protons to more efficiently absorb the maximum amount of energy. The strength of the magnetic field is rated in Tesla, which ranges from 1 to 3 in clinical applications and up to 9 in research settings. To support such strong magnetic fields, superconducting systems must be set up utilizing helium to cool the system and continue the magnetic field indefinitely.

Individuals with implanted medical devices such as pacemakers or metal objects cannot undergo an MRI. MRI is noninvasive, and does not produce radiation, thus making it a safe technology for repetitive scans. It is also a safe technology for children. The MRI process does require one to lie still in a loud tube type structure for around 30 minutes. Music is often used to calm people during this loud and sometimes claustrophobic process. Additionally, clinicians often premedicate with anxiolytic agents, such as lorazepam, to help comfort the patient during the exam.

Hopefully, the previous section has laid a framework for understanding the basic science of MRI techniques. Next, the science and research application of more sophisticated MRI techniques are discussed. The understanding of the basic principles of MRI will allow one to grasp new advancements in this modality quickly.

Structural MRI

In 1984, Smith and colleagues complete the first structural MRI studies in schizophrenia. We will be able to review only portions of the past 20 years of data and intellectual investment into this technique. Compared to CT studies, MRI allowed researchers to distinguish the importance between grey and white matter as well as between brain parenchyma and CSF.

MRI data was utilized to further characterize brain changes in people with schizophrenia. It was known that ventricular size was increased in individuals with schizophrenia based on CT studies. MRI technology allowed researchers to better understand these brain changes. It was found that there is loss of grey matter in people with schizophrenia. These individuals also show loss of brain volume and compensatory enlargement of the lateral and third ventricles. Temporal lobe volume loss is also prominent in individuals with schizophrenia. Additionally, long duration of untreated psychosis results in increased ventricular volumes and decreased cortical volume (Sadock, 2007).

Functional MRI

Functional MRI (fMRI) technology was first studied in disorders such as stroke or epilepsy. In 1990, Seji Ogawa defined the concept of blood-oxygen-level-dependent contrast, or BOLD. This technology harnessed the difference between oxygenated hemoglobin and deoxygenated hemoglobin in variable blood flow. Increased blood flow in an area results in increased levels of oxygenated hemoglobin and a resultant increased MR signal. Thus, utilizing functional imaging in schizophrenia allows researchers to understand which areas of the brain are metabolizing glucose quickly versus slowly, or utilizing higher or lower amounts of blood flow in specific situations. The ability to visualize resting-state blood flow, as well as blood flow in response to various tasks, has allowed researchers to understand how the brain is functioning differently in patients versus controls. Because of fMRI technology researchers can look beyond structural differences to direct assessment of abnormalities in brain function.

Since BOLD technology simply assesses differences in oxygenated hemoglobin versus deoxygenated hemoglobin, it is completely noninvasive. Other techniques, discussed later, rely on tracer molecules to ascertain functional status of brain areas. The fMRI sequences have no radiation risk and are noninvasive, and thus have the advantage of being safe to repeat time and time again. This allows for sequential measurements in response to external stimuli. Stimuli tested include response to medication, disease progression, task versus rest states and assessments of learning.

For example, in learning, a single patient's brain state can be compared during correct and incorrect trials. This experimental model eliminates confounders that arise based on comparing disease to control (Berman, 2002). Additionally, brain states can be studied before and after learning tasks to assess how cognitive task practice can shape brain function. Similar concepts can be used to track disease progression or response to antipsychotic medications.

Schizophrenia is a complex pathology, and no one pathognomonic abnormality exists. Rather, fMRI studies have helped clarify that schizophrenia is a disease of widespread dysfunction in neural circuitry. Interestingly, when assessing entire brain function as a global measure, patients with schizophrenia looked very similar to controls. Individuals with schizophrenia and controls look similar during many resting-state studies as well. However, when individuals with schizophrenia are scanned during tasks, distinct abnormalities arise compared to controls (Berman, 2002).

Of note, antipsychotic medications have often been questioned as the culprit for brain changes in schizophrenia, and fMRI data has helped to clarify this question. An 18-year follow-up study showed that prefrontal hypofunction was stable in individuals with chronic antipsychotic use (Cantor-Graae, Warkentin, Franzen, Risberg, & Ingvar, 1991; Grace, 1991). Also, the prefrontal hypofunction is not seen in other illnesses where neuroleptics are used, such as the subcortical dementias. A study of monozygotic twins showed that the twin who had less exposure to antipsychotic medication had increased hypofunction of the frontal lobes. And last, frontal lobe hypofunction is seen in first-episode psychosis patients who are neuroleptic naïve (Berman, 2002).

Further studies will continue to assess the effects that neuroleptic medication might have on brain state and structure. The aforementioned studies can be used to facilitate discussion on this point with patients and family. Studies in magnetic resonance spectroscopy, a technique described shortly, also confirmed there were no neuronal composition differences after antipsychotic exposure. In fact, these neuronal-loss markers were present in first-episode patients and appear native to the disease state (Bustillo et al., 2008).

As seen clinically, positive symptoms of schizophrenia such as hallucinations and delusions resolve rapidly with antipsychotic medication. However, patients often continue to suffer profound disability and decreased quality of life, despite resolution of positive symptoms. This loss of functional status is largely contributed to cognitive dysfunction. Data from fMRI has helped examine the root of this cognitive dysfunction, and remains a robust area of research.

Presently, much focus has been given to the prefrontal cortex and frontal lobe circuitry, which has been a long-standing focus of inquiry into the pathology of schizophrenia. Specifically, during working-memory tasks, patients showed abnormal activity in the prefrontal cortex—specifically the dorsolateral prefrontal cortex (DLPFC). Other cognitive tasks, such as verbal recall, showed deficits in the cingulate cortex and frontal-temporal regions (Berman, 2002).

Interestingly, both underactive and hyperactive states have been described in individuals with schizophrenia in response to cognitive tasks. These findings support the dysconnectivity hypothesis. It is hypothesized that some areas of the brain are not responding robustly enough in response to a cognitive task. However, other areas of the brain are over-recruiting in response to a task, rendering the information received jumbled because the circuitry recruited is excessive (Berman, 2002). This highlights the complexity of the illness, as it is not simply a hypofunctional state but rather dysfunctional in its true sense. In general, however, the primary summary in cognitive studies points to hypofunction of the dorsolateral prefrontal cortex. Further studies aim at understanding the cause of the dysfunctional state as it connects to poor cognitive performance.

Another brain structure of interest in fMRI data is the temporal lobe. It is known that diseases that affect the temporal lobe, such as temporal lobe epilepsy can cause psychotic symptoms (Berman, 2002). Data suggests that temporal lobe dysfunction is also found in schizophrenia, although more studies will need to be completed to further sort out reports of hypo- versus hyperfunctionality. Again, as in the frontal lobe, this likely supports the idea that schizophrenia is truly a disease of dysfunction.

Finally, one should note there have been interesting studies pointing to the role of the lateral temporal cortex in the generation of auditory hallucinations (Berman, 2002). This remains an active area of study because this could be a potential specific target for positive symptoms outside of global dopamine dysregulation.

The next step in assessing this data is to synthesize what these areas of abnormal perfusion might mean through correlations with symptomatology. Hypofrontality has been shown in patients with negative symptoms, prominent social withdrawal, and low motivation (Ingvar & Franzen, 1974). Additionally, hypofrontality has been strongly correlated with cognitive deficits. Hallucinations appear to be linked to the sensory area that directs the symptom. For example, auditory hallucinations are associated with brocca's area and left superior temporal cortex (McGuire et al., 1996). Psychomotor retardation has been correlated to decreased activity in the DLPFC. Disorganized thought process has been linked to increased right anterior cingulate activity. Increased medial temporal lobe activity has been connected to reality distortion. Increased temporal lobe activity is associated with thought disorder as well (Berman, 2002).

A final and fascinating area of study in fMRI research is the idea of functional connectivity. As explained, multiple brain regions perform abnormally in response to various tasks or stimuli. This led researchers to ponder how these various abnormalities could be connected: Could these be more than isolated islands of abnormal activity? Could this somehow represent abnormal or aberrant functional connectivity?

The frontal lobe, which has been highlighted in theories of schizophrenia, is highly connected. For example, during a working memory task, patients with schizophrenia showed tight correlation between DLPFC neuronal integrity and cerebral blood flow that was not present in normal controls (Berman, 2002). Additionally, abnormal connectivity between prefrontal and temporal limbic areas has also been studied. Weinberger found that in monozygotic twins discordant for schizophrenia, there was an inverse relationship between hippocampal volume and dorsolateral prefrontal correct activation during cognitive tasks. This finding was important not only because it points out neocortical limbic dysconnectivity, but also because it highlights a neurodevelopmental mechanism of disease (Weinberger, Berman, Suddath, & Torrey, 1992). Working memory tasks showed hypofrontality in conjunction with increased temporal-hippocampal and cerebellar overactivity in patients with schizophrenia (Meyer-Lindenberg et al., 2001). Friston and Frith (1995) also found that prefrontal and temporal coactivation did not occur simultaneously as they should during a verbal fluency test.

In general, MRI technology continues to advance and remains a useful modality. Few psychiatric conditions are linked directly to a brain abnormality at one moment in time. The fMRI technology allows for analysis of dysconnectivity and analysis of change over time.

Diffusion Imaging

Diffusion imaging is an important MRI advancement in schizophrenia research. Diffusion, generically, is the movement of a substance from a higher concentration gradient to a lower gradient. In a substance, such as water, the movement of atoms as they randomly move and collide is called Brownian motion. In a living tissue, water molecules constantly collide with brain structures, such as cell membranes.

Another important topic in this imaging modality is the concept of isotropy and anisotropy. Isotropic diffusion refers to the concept of uniformity in all directions—the molecules would be diffusing equally in all directions. Anisotropic diffusion refers to situations in which molecules are diffusing more in one direction than in others. When an object impedes motion (e.g., walls of an axon), it increases the probability that the solution will be diffusing in an unequal manner.

Diffusion Tensor Imaging, or DTI is measuring water in nerve-fiber tracts. The walls of the nerve tracts collide with water molecules, creating anisotropic diffusion. Water molecules are more likely to flow vertically down the tract, as opposed to other directions. Water molecules in other areas of the brain do not have the strict confines of a nerve track, and have more isotropic diffusion. Various images are compared to visualize in which direction and at what speed the water molecules are moving (de Figueiredo, Borgonovi, & Doring, 2011).

These nerve-fiber tracts and their direction are then reconstructed into beautiful images representing a whole brain nerve-fiber map. Research methods are being developed to more precisely map nerve fibers that cross, because current technology is unable to precisely map diffusion in overlapping fibers. As technology advances, the resolution of the tract paths will improve.

Connectomics

Schizophrenia has been most recently described as both a disorder of both neurotransmitter regulation as well as disordered neural connectivity to describe the lack of integration for major elements in thought disorders. This lack of integration due to abnormalities in brain circuitry has been analyzed through multiple functional and diffusion imaging studies. An additional layer in the assessment of the dysconnectivity hypothesis is currently being investigated through the study of connectomics.

This idea of connectomics harnesses the neuroimaging techniques of MRI and tractography to create a map of interconnected regions. This technique focuses on important regions of interest (nodes) and the nerve tracts that connect them (edges). Connectomics incorporates graph theory methods to elucidate these multiple nodes, which, when connected aberrantly, point toward increased risk of psychotic illness. The idea of looking specifically at this map of nodal networks, the connectome, allows one to further assess brain function, which is difficult to extrapolate from purely structural or blood-flow data. This data assessment technique, developed by Hagmann and Sporns in 2005, most closely simulates the brain to a computer.

Nodes are identified and analyzed for connectedness. Highly connected nodes are deemed hubs. Nodes can cluster and tightly connect with a relatively small number of other nodes. This is called segregation. Nodes can also be distributed in such a way that it is possible to reach multiple nodes in a network by traversing relatively few edges. This concept is called an integrated network, or integration. Often, this integration and segregation is different between control brains and proband brains. This organization can be measured globally or can focus specifically on a certain edge (Griffa & Hagmann, 2013).

Schizophrenia, which has long been described as a disease of dysconnectivity, is a rich area of research in connectomics. Studies in schizophrenia have shown increased path length, altered clustering coefficients, and a loss of frontal hubs (van den Heuvel, Mandl,

Stam, Kahn, & Hulshoff Pol, 2010, Zhang et al., 2012). Additional nodes have also been shown to be less efficient, including areas in the frontal, temporal, paralimbic, limbic, and putamen regions (Wang et al., 2012). Additionally, Wang found an inverse correlation between network efficiency and severity of positive and negative symptoms. This again supports the dysconnectivity hypothesis. The inefficiencies in these important networks also supports the significant processing abnormalities in cognitive impairment found in the disease.

Magnetic Resonance Spectroscopy

Magnetic resonance spectroscopy (MRS) is a chemical assay modality that allows researchers to visualize the concentration of specific molecules in various brain regions. It does not require the injection of radio ligands and does not involve ionizing radiation. Magnetic resonance spectroscopy, similar to MRI, requires a magnetic field. Magnetic resonance spectroscopy technology harnesses the specific spin properties of nuclei with an odd number of protons and neutrons. Similar to MRI, a brief magnetic pulse excites the nuclei to a higher energy state, from which the nuclei then relax. The varying resonance frequencies are detected by a coil, which produces the MR signal. These signals are then localized spatially and mapped. This technology allows for the identification of various organic molecules, including proteins, nucleic acids, and carbohydrates (Weinberger & Laruelle, 2002).

Phosphomonoesters (PME) and phosphodiesters (PDE) were localized and studied in first-episode patients. A highly publicized study reported decreased PME and phosphorous and increased PDE and ATP, which has been interpreted to reflect increased membrane turnover, which is suggestive of increased pruning in brains of early schizophrenia patients. Increased levels of ATP and PDE were also interpreted to reflect decreased frontal lobe functioning, representated by higher unused levels of ATP (Pettegrew, Keshavan, & Minshew, 1993). Scientists are actively working to replicate this study but continue to produce conflicting data. This is a body of literature that, if followed, will continue to yield an exciting story regarding drug effects and neuronal metabolism as the technology progresses.

Nuclear Medicine Imaging

Single photon emission computed tomography (SPECT) and positron emission tomography (PET) both use radioactive compounds, which act as tracers during experiments. The use of tracers allowed for fine-tuning localization. The fMRI data allowed for localization within a few millimeters of brain tissue, but tracer use allowed resolution of receptor occupancy and localization.

The use of these radioactive tracers allows the researcher to study receptors, transporters, and enzymes in brain tissue. The ability to visualize ligand binding allows researchers to answer questions about specific biochemical changes pertaining to symptoms, disease progression and treatment response. In schizophrenia, these techniques are primarily utilized in understanding the dopamine D2 receptor function (Weinberger & Laruelle, 2002).

Single photo emission compound tomography technology requires administration of a radioligand to the blood stream. The bound radioligand then emits radiation based on blood flow, which is captured by a gamma camera. This 2D representation is then constructed into 3D images. In contrast, PET imaging utilizes positron annihilation. In PET scanning a positron emitting radioligand is injected, which binds to an area of interest. As the positron (antiparticle of an electron) decays, it will collide with an electron. This collision results in the release of two gamma photons in opposite directions. The collision of these photons are recorded by a detector, and based on the time of collision and mathematical algorithms, the point of annihilation can be localized.

The first major receptor system studied, not surprisingly, has been the dysregulated dopamine system in schizophrenia. Antipsychotic drugs primarily block D2 receptors and subsequently reduce positive symptoms. Studies showed an increase in D2 receptor concentration in patients with schizophrenia (Weinberger & Laruelle, 2002). Studies also showed that patients with schizophrenia have a larger dopamine release than normal controls following administration of amphetamine. It is also hypothesized that individuals with schizophrenia have an increased affinity for dopamine at D2 receptors compared to controls.

Additionally, studies that induced an acute dopamine depletion state showed that people with schizophrenia have a higher rate of D2 occupancy during an illness exacerbation compared to normal controls. It was then shown that, after dopamine depletion, individuals with schizophrenia demonstrated higher D2 receptor availability. This increased dopamine occupancy finding was interestingly not associated with increase in positive symptoms. Increased occupancy was, however, associated with better treatment response to antipsychotic medication (Weinberger & Laruelle, 2002). These receptor studies support historical theories regarding dopamine's role in the pathophysiology of the disease.

Newer theories of schizophrenia—namely neurodevelopmental and connectivity models—are also studied using PET and SPECT technology. It has been hypothesized that the prefrontal cortex is unable to correctly regulate dopamine neuron firing, resulting in inappropriate subcortical dopamine functioning (Grace, 1991; Weinberger & Laruelle, 2002). Amphetamine challenges have also demonstrated that NMDA receptor hypofunction in patients with schizophrenia may be playing a role in disruption of glutamatergic systems, which should be regulating dopaminergic cell activity. Additionally, PET studies showed that prefrontal cortex D1 receptor densities are decreased in young patients with schizophrenia, and this low-density state was associated with negative symptoms and working memory impairment. These nuclear imaging techniques have allowed researchers to ascertain this detailed information, including receptor occupancy and function, which is a level of detail drastically different than structural techniques.

Additionally, nuclear imaging has been prolifically utilized in understanding receptor occupancy for antipsychotic medications. By studying receptor occupancy, it was found that there is an 80 percent D2 receptor occupancy threshold, at which higher levels of receptor occupancy result in an increased probability of extrapyramidal side effects (Farde et al., 1992). Most studies were performed at clinically established therapeutic doses, which correlated to at least 50 percent receptor occupancy. Interestingly, above this 50 percent threshold, studies showed that there did not seem to be any further correlation between receptor occupancy and symptom reduction. Interestingly, clozapine at therapeutic doses, occupied between 40 percent and 60 percent of the D2 receptor sites. Clozapine's ability to provide clinical response at occupancy levels below the 80 percent threshold explains it's decreased likelihood of producing extrapyramidal symptoms (Pilowsky et al., 1992). The SPECT studies also showed that the atypical antipsychotic clozapine achieved higher cortical D2 occupancy than striatal occupancy. In contrast, typical antipsychotics showed relatively equal occupancy in both sites (Pilowsky et al., 1997).

As the field progresses, a more robust cache of ligands will be developed, which will allow researchers to investigate alternative pathways and second messaging systems. This will remain an important research area, but at present is unlikely to move quickly into the clinical domain. Ligands available are limited, and each imaging sequence is very costly.

Event Related Potentials

Event-related potentials (ERP) is a field of study that provides precise (millisecond) temporal resolution. Other neuroimaging techniques, such as MRI and PET can localize lesions or phenomenon to exact anatomical locations, ERP has the ability to temporally characterize an event. Spatial resolution of ERP is achieved by combining this technology with MRI technologies, to achieve both spatial and temporal localization. Massive amounts of information can be gained by combining ERP technology with specific cognitive tasks. This technology has the ability to detect when information reaches cortex and how the signal can be modified by various stimuli or distractions. This technology has the potential to help differentiate how information is processed differently in controls versus people with schizophrenia. There is tremendous potential for this technique to illuminate further details into the pathophysiology of schizophrenia (Desimone, 2002).

CONCLUSION

Neuroimaging will continue to advance both as a diagnostic tool and as a predictor of disease course. Will the disease have prominent cognitive deficits? Will the disease consist of primarily negative or positive symptoms? Will the individual respond well to antipsychotic medications, or will he or she likely to be a nonresponder and eventually require clozapine?

From a research perspective, scientists will continue to understand the pathophysiological meaning of the differences between control and disease state. Scientists will strive to understand imaging abnormalities as they pertain to tasks, stressors, medication exposure, and neurotransmitter dysregulation. Imaging research will continue to advance as new techniques are developed and modalities are combined to create imaging sequence powerhouses. These research applications are also beginning to translate into clinical use, which will advance the field profoundly.

REFERENCES

Berman, K. (2002). Functional neuroimaging in schizophrenia. In *Neuropsychopharmacology: The 5th Generation of Progress*. Davis, K. L., Charney, D., Coyle, J. T., & Nemeroff, C., Eds. Philadelphia, PA: Lippincott, Williams, & Wilkins. 745–756.

Bustillo, J. R., Rowland, L. M., Jung, R., Brooks, W. M., Qualls, C., Hammond, R., . . . Lauriello, J. (2008). Proton magnetic resonance spectroscopy during initial treatment with antipsychotic medication in schizophrenia. *Neuropsychopharmacology, 33*(10), 2456–2466.

Cantor-Graae, E., Warkentin, S., Franzen, G., Risberg, J., & Ingvar, D. H. (1991). Aspects of stability of regional cerebral blood flow in chronic schizophrenia: an 18-year followup study. *Psychiatry Research,* 40, 253–266.

de Figueiredo, E. H., Borgonovi, A. F., & Doring, T. M. (2011). Basic concepts of MR imaging, diffusion MR imaging, and diffusion tensor imaging. *Magnetic Resonance Imaging Clinic of North America, 19*(1), 1–22. doi: 10.1016/j.mric.2010.10.005

Desimone, R. (2002) Emerging imaging technologies and their application to psychiatric research. In *Neuropsychopharmacology: The 5th Generation of Progress*. Davis, K. L., Charney, D., Coyle, J. T., & Nemeroff, C., Eds. Philadelphia, PA: Lippincott, Williams, & Wilkins. 299–300.

Farde, L., Nordström, A. L., Wiesel, F. A., Pauli, S., Halldin, C., & Sedvall, G. (1992). Positron emission tomography analysis of central D1 and D2 dopamine receptor occupancy in patients treated with classical neuroleptics and clozapine. *Archives of General Psychiatry 49*, 538–544.

Freudenreich, O., Schulz, S. C., & Goff, D. C. (2009). Initial medical work-up of first-episode psychosis: a conceptual review. *Early Interventional Psychiatry*, 3(1), 10–18,

Friston, K. J., & Frith, C. D. (1995). Schizophrenia: A disconnection syndrome? *Clinical Neuroscience, 3*, 89–97.

Griffa, A., & Hagmann, P. (2013). Structural connectomics in brain diseases. *NeuroImage, 80*, 515–526.

Grace, A. A. (1991). Phasic versus tonic dopamine release and the modulation of dopamine system responsivity: A hypothesis for the etiology of schizophrenia. *Neuroscience, 41*, 1–24.

Ingvar, D. H., & Franzen, G. (1974). Abnormalities of cerebral blood flow distribution in patients with chronic schizophrenia. *Acta Psychiatrica Scandanavia, 50*, 425–462.

Lubman, D. I., & McGorry, P. D. (2002). Incidental radiological findings on brain magnetic resonance imaging in first-episode psychosis and chronic schizophrenia *Acta Psychiatrica Scandinavica, 106*, 331–336.

Makris, N., Papadimitriou, G. M., Worth, A. J., Jenkins, B. G., Garrido, L., Sorensen, A. G., . . . Kennedy, D. N. (2002). Diffusion tensor imaging. In: *Neuropsychopharmacology: The 5th Generation of Progress*. Davis, K. L., Charney, D., Coyle, J. T., & Nemeroff, C., Eds. Philadelphia, PA: Lippincott, Williams, & Wilkins. 357–371.

McCarley, R. (2002). Structural magnetic resonance imaging studies in schizophrenia. In *Neuropsychopharmacology: The 5th Generation of Progress*. Davis, K. L., Charney, D., Coyle, J. T., & Nemeroff, C., Eds. Philadelphia, PA: Lippincott, Williams, & Wilkins. 757–774.

Meyer-Lindenberg, A., Poline, J. B., Kohn, P. D., Holt, J. L., Egan, M. F., & Berman, K. F. (2001). Altered cortical functional connectivity during working memory in schizophrenia. *American Journal of Psychiatry, 158(11), 1809-17.*

McGuire, P. K., Silbersweig, D. A., Wright, I., Murray, R. M., Frackowiak, R. S., & Fret, C. D. (1996). The neural correlates of inner speech and auditory verbal imagery in schizophrenia: relationship to auditory verbal hallucinations. *British Journal of Psychiatry, 169*, 148–159.

Pettegrew, J. W., Keshavan, M. S., & Minshew, N. J. (1993). 31P nuclear magnetic resonance spectroscopy: neurodevelopment and schizophrenia. *Schizophrenia Bulletin, 19*, 35–53.

Pilowsky, L. S., Costa, D. C., Ell, P. J., Murray, R. M., Verhoeff, N. P., & Kerwin, R. W. (1992). Clozapine, single photon emission tomography, and the D2 dopamine receptor blockade hypothesis of schizophrenia. *Lancet, 340*, 199–202.

Pilowsky, L. S., Mulligan, R. S., Acton, P. D., Ell, P. J., Costa, D. C., & Kerwin, R. W. (1997). Limbic selectivity of clozapine. *Lancet, 350*, 490–491.

Reveley, M. A. (1985). CT scans in schizophrenia. *British Journal of Psychiatry. 146*, 367–371.

Sadock, B. (2007). Schizophrenia. In Virginia Sadock (Ed.), *Kaplan and Sadock's Synopsis of Psychiatry* (10th ed.) Philadelphia, PA: Lippincott, Williams, & Wilkins. 467–497.

van den Heuvel, M. P., Mandl, R. C., Stam, C. J., Kahn, R. S., & Hulshoff Pol, H. E. (2010). Aberrant frontal and temporal complex network structure in schizophrenia: a graph theoretical analysis. *Journal of Neuroscience, 30*, 15915–15926.

Vernooij, M., & Van Der Lugt, A. (2007). Incidental findings on brain MRI in the general population. *New England Journal of Medicine, 357*(18), 1821–1828.

Wang, Q., Su, T. P., Zhou, Y., Chou, K. H., Chen, I. Y., Jiang, T., . . . Lin, C. P. (2012). Anatomical insights into disrupted small-world networks in schizophrenia. *Neuroimage, 59*(2), 1085–1093.

Weinberger, D. R., Berman, K. F., Suddath, R., & Torrey, E. F. (1992). Evidence of dysfunction of a prefrontal-limbic network in schizophrenia: a magnetic resonance imaging and regional cerebral blood flow study of discordant monozygotic twins. *American Journal of Psychiatry* (1992). *149*, 890–897.

Weinberger, D., & Laruelle, M. (2002). Neurochemical and neuropharmacological imaging in schizophrenia. In *Neuropsychopharmacology: The 5th Generation of Progress*. Davis, K. L., Charney, D., Coyle, J. T., & Nemeroff, C., Eds. Philadelphia, PA: Lippincott, Williams, & Wilkins. 833-855.

Zhang, Y., Lin, L., Lin, C. P., Zhou, Y., Chou, K.-H., Lo, C. Y., . . . Jiang, T. (2012). Abnormal topological organization of structural brain networks in schizophrenia. *Schizophrenia. Research, 141*, 109–118.

/// 10 /// THE ROLE OF NEUROTRANSMITTERS IN SCHIZOPHRENIA

KATHRYN M. GILL and ANTHONY A. GRACE

INTRODUCTION

Schizophrenia is a complex disorder that likely spans dysfunctions across multiple circuits and neurotransmitter systems. As such, there have been reports of numerous biochemical changes in schizophrenia indicative of neurotransmitter dysfunction in multiple systems, among the most prominent being dopamine, glutamate, serotonin, and γ-aminobutyric acid (GABA). The most compelling evidence for each candidate neurotransmitter system associated with schizophrenia will be discussed; including pharmacological mechanisms of psychotomimetic and antipsychotic drug action, postmortem assessment of neurotransmitter-associated proteins and enzymes, in vivo imaging data of neurotransmitter release and receptor binding from patients, correlations with animal models, and genetic vulnerabilities associated with specific neurotransmitter systems. The chapter concludes with a discussion of how a neural network view of the neurochemical aberrations observed in schizophrenia is perhaps more appropriate than focusing on an individual neurotransmitter system.

DOPAMINE

The neurotransmitter system historically most heavily implicated in schizophrenia is the dopamine system. There are four major dopamine pathways in the central nervous system, two of which have been implicated in schizophrenia. The mesolimbic system originates in the midbrain, in the ventral tegmental area (VTA) lying medial and superior to the substantia nigra in rats and in the dorsal aspect of the substantia nigra in humans. Dopamine neurons in the VTA project to the medial brain areas of the limbic system, including the nucleus accumbens/ventral striatum, bed nuclei of the stria terminalis, amygdala, hippocampus, lateral septal nuclei, and the entorhinal cortex. Arvid Carlsson was one of the first to suggest that overactivation of the mesolimbic dopamine system is responsible for the patterns of disordered thought and perception characteristic of schizophrenia. The mesocortical dopamine system also originates in the midbrain and projects to the prefrontal cortex. Mesocortical dopamine projects modulate executive functions, motivation, attention, and social behavior. It is the mesocortical projections to medial and cingulate cortex that are likely involved in generating the negative symptoms of schizophrenia, including loss of motivation and flattened affect. In contrast, the dopamine signaling in the dorsolateral prefrontal cortex (DLPFC) are proposed to be involved in cognitive symptoms of this disorder. Thus, local depletion of dopamine in the DLPFC of monkeys with the toxin 6-hydroxydopamine impairs performance on cognitive tasks. In one model of schizophrenia, Daniel Weinberger and colleagues posited that the mesolimbic and mesocortical dopaminergic projections are disrupted in different ways in schizophrenia (Deutch, 1992; Knable & Weinberger, 1997; D. R. Weinberger, 1987). First, an increase in the mesolimbic pathway (via D2, D3, and D4 receptor activation) is primarily responsible for the generation of positive symptoms. Second, diminished activity in the mesocortical dopamine system would account for the cognitive, and potentially some of the negative, symptoms. According to this model, activity of the mesocortical pathway to prefrontal cortex acts as a brake by inhibiting the mesolimbic pathway. In schizophrenia, this balance is disrupted, and there is uncontrolled disinhibition and overactivity of the mesolimbic dopamine system.

Pharmacological Evidence Implicating the Dopamine System in Schizophrenia

Early pharmacological evidence was pivotal in the development of the dopamine hypothesis of schizophrenia. There are two sources of pharmacologic evidence linking dopamine system activation and psychotic symptoms. Drugs such as amphetamine, L-dihydroxyphenylalanine (L-DOPA), and cocaine are classified as psychotomimetics due to their capacity to generate psychosis-like symptoms in normal individuals and exacerbate psychosis in schizophrenia. For example, amphetamine can cause bizarre, repetitive, stereotyped behaviors in monkeys and enhanced locomotion in rodents. Secondly, the serendipitous discovery of the first generation antipsychotic drugs and their characterization as dopamine antagonists further implicated the dopamine system in modulating or mediating certain symptoms in schizophrenia. Conversely, drugs that deplete dopamine levels, such as reserpine and alpha-methyl-para-tyrosine, can decrease psychotic symptoms (Arnold & Freeman, 1956; Carlsson et al., 1973; Carlsson, 1973; Shepherd & Watt, 1956). This has been further substantiated by PET imaging studies, in which amphetamine-induced dopamine release in the associative striatum was found to correlate with worsening of psychosis (review in (Lieberman, Kane, & Alvir, 1987).

All currently prescribed antipsychotic drugs target the pathological increased activity of the dopamine system. There are five subtypes of the dopamine receptor, with the D2 class (comprising D2, D3, and D4 receptors) being the most associated with the treatment of schizophrenia. The classic or first generation antipsychotic drugs, such as haloperidol, bind primarily to the D2 receptor subtypes. In contrast, the atypical or second-generation antipsychotic drugs, such as clozapine, in addition to also binding D3 and D4 receptors, have been characterized as having a more rapid off-rate from D2 receptors. These drugs also exhibit a more rich pharmacology, also affecting serotonin and adrenergic receptors. This pattern of expression may explain in part the relative greater efficacy of the second-generation antipsychotic drugs without the extrapyramidal side effects associated with the classic agents. Both D2 and D3 receptors are of particular importance because they are expressed on the terminals of dopamine neurons themselves where they exhibit an inhibitory influence on both the firing rate and release of dopamine at the terminals. There is an association between the efficacy of a given antipsychotic drug in ameliorating symptoms and its affinity for dopamine receptors, more specifically a correlation between the drug's affinity for the D2 receptor and the dose required for therapeutic action (Creese, Burt, & Snyder, 1976; Seeman et al., 1976; Seeman & Van Tol, 1995; Seeman, 1995).

Functional Measures of Dopamine Involvement in Schizophrenia

The general efficacy of first generation antipsychotic drugs, which act to block dopamine receptor activation, in ameliorating certain schizophrenia symptoms would suggest that there is an excess dopamine release in the brains of schizophrenia patients. However, there has been little to no evidence of a global increase in dopamine levels in the brains of schizophrenia patients. Despite this lack of evidence for a general increase in dopamine, what would be more interesting is the regional activation of the dopamine system in particular brain areas. Recent advances in brain imaging technology have proven vital in the confirmation of dopamine-system activation changes in schizophrenia patients.

Positron emission tomography (PET) and single-photon emission computerized tomograph (SPECT) studies have proven vital in demonstrating alterations in neurotransmitter release, synthesis, and availability of postsynaptic receptors. As opposed to providing direct measurements of dopamine levels, instead, changes in dopamine release are inferred from alterations in the binding of radiolabeled receptor selective compounds during PET scans. Since the radioligands compete with endogenous dopamine (DA), it is assumed that displacement of the radiotracer binding potential is correlated with the synaptic dopamine level. These measurements can provide either basal or dynamic measures of dopamine system activation. Under dynamic conditions, dopamine release is evoked by the administration of a DA-releasing drug. In these experiments, it is the reduction of the radiotracer binding potential that signifies an increase in dopamine system activity.

The synthesis of dopamine can be assessed by administering radiolabeled f fluorodopa and measuring its uptake into dopamine terminals in the cortex and striatum, measured via PET scans conducted after the administration of L-3,4dihydroxyphenylalanine (L-DOPA), is increased in neuroleptic-free schizophrenia patients (Dao-Castellana et al., 1997), consistent with increased dopamine neuron activity (Howes et al., 2013).

Studies by Anissa Abi-Dhargham and Marc Laruelle have been the most influential in exploring the complex alterations of dopamine transmission in schizophrenia and their relationship to clinical symptoms, cognition, and response to treatment. PET and SPECT studies have both been used to show increases in striatal dopamine release in response to amphetamine administration in neuroleptic-free, first-episode psychotic patients. Previously, in vivo brain imaging of the binding of D2-selective ligands as a means of assessing the density of dopamine D2 receptors in neuroleptic-free patients with schizophrenia had yielded inconsistent results (Farde et al., 1990; Nordstrom et al., 1995; Wong et al., 1997). Thus, studies using the high-affinity drug [11C]methylspiperone have shown elevated D2 receptors in schizophrenia (Nordstrom et al., 1995; Wong et al., 1997). In contrast, studies utilizing the low-affinity compound [11C]raclopride fail to display such an elevation (Farde et al., 1990). This discrepancy appears to be due in part to the quantitatively different effects of endogenous dopamine on [11C]methylspiperone and [11C]raclopride binding (Seeman & Tallerico, 1999). In a meta-analysis, (D. Weinberger & Laruelle, 2001) compared 17 studies utilizing radiotracers selective for D2 receptors in schizophrenia patients who were both antipsychotic drug free and antipsychotic drug naive and their matched healthy controls. They concluded that there is a small but significant increase in striatal D2 receptor density. To bypass the potential limitation of competition between the radioligand and endogenous DA, novel studies have conducted D2 imaging while subjects are in a state of acute dopamine depletion, accomplished by the administration of the tyrosine hydroxylase inhibitor AMPT beforehand. By measuring the D2 levels in the depleted state, it is now possible to unmask D2 receptors that were bound by endogenous dopamine at baseline. Using this approach with SPECT and the D2 radiotracer [123I]IBZM, Abi-Dargham and colleagues were able to show an increase in striatal D2 receptor availability in patients with schizophrenia after acute dopamine depletion (Abi-Dargham et al., 1998; Abi-Dargham et al., 2000). It was concluded that there was an increased occupancy of striatal D2 receptors by dopamine at baseline in schizophrenia patients. Interestingly, there was an amelioration of positive symptoms following AMPT administration in patients (Abi-Dargham et al., 2009).

A more recent study by Abi-Dhargham (Slifstein et al., 2015) utilizes the PET D2/3 radiotracer carbon 11-labeled FLB457 in combination with the amphetamine-induced displacement of the tracer as a means of extrapolating changes in dopamine release in the prefrontal cortex, associative striatum, and extrastriatal regions of patients with schizophrenia. In contrast to the striatal increases in dopamine release, there is a reduction in dopamine release in the DLPFC and extrastriatal regions in schizophrenia patients. This would suggest a heterogeneous condition in schizophrenia in which alterations in dopamine release are region specific. Supporting this possibility, the blunted prefrontal cortical activation in schizophrenia patients during working memory performance can be normalized following the administration of a dopamine agonist, contrary to a generalized hyperactivity of the dopamine system observed subcortically in schizophrenia patients.

Postmortem Evidence of Dopamine System Involvement in Schizophrenia

Postmortem examination of the brains of schizophrenia patients has been vital in establishing the structural and biochemical alterations occurring with this disorder. This has been particularly evident in studies examining receptor subunit expression. This includes an increase in presynaptic dopamine D2 autoreceptors, along with a decrease in postsynaptic variants, in the dorsolateral prefrontal cortex of schizophrenia brains measured postmortem (Kaalund et al., 2014). Dopamine D2 receptors exist in monomer, dimer, and oligomeric forms. It has been proposed that D2 receptor dimerization is altered in schizophrenia such that not only is the density of D2 receptors increased, but they are also preferentially expressed in the monomer form (Seeman & Kapur, 2000; Zawarynski et al., 1998).

Although numerous postmortem studies have consistently revealed D2 receptors to be elevated in the striatum of patients with schizophrenia, a major caveat to these data involves the prior treatment with antipsychotic drugs in a majority of patients donating postmortem tissues, raising the probability that the drugs themselves contributed to the elevation of D2 receptors.

There is also evidence for decreases in postmortem tyrosine hydroxylase immunolabeling, the rate-limiting enzyme for the synthesis of dopamine, in the prefrontal cortex of schizophrenia patients. A more recent postmortem study staining for tyrosine-hydroxylase has shown that dopamine is increased in the substantia nigra of schizophrenia patients (Howes et al., 2013). This would suggest that in addition to changes in postsynaptic dopamine receptor density, there are also subregional alterations in dopamine synthesis in schizophrenia patients.

Genetic Models

Genetic polymorphisms related to the dopamine system have been shown to contribute to a vulnerability to the development of schizophrenia. There is evidence for an association between the dopamine D2 receptor gene and schizophrenia. A single amino-acid substitution (Cys311) in the dopamine D2 receptor gene is associated both with a schizophrenia diagnosis as well as a favorable treatment response (Itokawa, Arinami, & Toru, 2010). Catechol-O-methyltransferase (COMT) is a catabolic enzyme involved in the degradation of a number of molecules, including but not limited to dopamine. The *COMT* gene is located in a fragment on chromosome 22q11, the deletion of which yields a myriad of psychiatric conditions, including schizophrenia (reviewed in (Williams, Owen, & O'Donovan, 2007)). In the brain, *COMT* encodes the membrane-bound isoform MB-COMT. In the prefrontal cortex, unlike the nucleus accumbens, dopamine released into the synapse is primarily metabolized by COMT or cleared by reuptake into noradrenergic terminals. Consequently, COMT can have a greater regionally specific impact on PFC function. The coding sequence of *COMT* contains a common G>A polymorphism (rs4680) that results in the valine-to-methionine (VAL/MET) polymorphism. The amino acid change to the VAL phenotype results in a higher activity of COMT. It has been postulated that the high-activity MET variant would have greater association with schizophrenia due to greater dopamine metabolism in the cortex and consequent disruption of cognitive ability. Microdeletions occurring on chromosome 22q11.2 encompassing the *COMT* gene can yield a psychiatric condition referred to as velocardiofacial syndrome (VCFS). Subjects with VCFS have a prevalence rate as high as 25 percent for developing psychosis. However, a recent meta-analysis of the case-control literature has failed to find a significant effect at the Val/Met locus and subsequent schizophrenia (Munafo et al., 2005), making a single locus effect of the Val/Met polymorphism on schizophrenia unlikely. There has been recent work done illustrating that the COMT genetic variation alone may not have a substantial impact on the development of schizophrenia. However, when the COMT mutation is combined with cannabis use there is a significant increased risk of schizophrenia (Ermis et al., 2015).

Critical Interpretation of the Dopamine Hypothesis of Schizophrenia

Overall, it would appear that alterations in normal dopamine-system function are associated primarily with the positive symptoms, delusions grandiosity, and so forth in schizophrenia. However, PET imaging studies have supported a link between prefrontal cortical activity, functional dopamine release, and working memory performance in schizophrenia patients. Schizophrenia patients also demonstrate increased sensitivity to dopaminergic agonist/releasing drugs, indicative of an increased basal activation of the dopamine system. Validated animal models of the sensorimotor gating deficits characteristic of schizophrenia include neurochemical changes in dopamine, glutamate, and GABA substrates (Bast & Feldon, 2003; Bolton et al., 2012; Brown et al., 2015; Carboni et al., 2004; Francois et al., 2009; Hauser et al., 2005; Heldt, Green, & Ressler, 2004; Nguyen et al., 2014; Swerdlow et al., 2001a; Swerdlow et al., 2001b; Swerdlow et al., 2005; Young, Randall, & Wilcox, 1995). The methylazoxymethanol acetate (MAM) neurodevelopmental model of schizophrenia (further details provided later) have demonstrated increases in dopaminergic activity along with enhanced behavioral responses to amphetamine as well as altered sensorimotor gating, similar to what has been observed in schizophrenia patients (Gill et al., 2011; Lodge, Behrens, & Grace, 2009).

Despite the dominance of the dopamine hypothesis in schizophrenia research, there are some discrepancies that would suggest the involvement of other neurotransmitter systems. It was indicated earlier that despite the increase in responsivity of the dopamine system to amphetamine, there is no direct evidence of a global increase in dopamine release in schizophrenia patients at baseline. Indeed, amphetamine-induced psychosis elevates dopamine nearly 30-fold over baseline; much higher than has been reported in disease states. Even the compelling imaging data of alterations in dopamine release or receptor binding have a major caveat of being a corollary extrapolated from a measure of bound receptors of a radioligand.

In addition, the primary treatments for schizophrenia that center on altering dopamine system activation are only effective in treating certain symptom classes, mainly the positive symptoms. The negative and cognitive symptoms associated with schizophrenia are only marginally improved by medications that primarily target the dopamine system. Cognitive impairments that are largely neglected by first-generation antipsychotic drugs include attention, learning, memory, and executive functions. Furthermore, nearly a third of schizophrenia patients fail to respond to the first generation antipsychotic drug treatments despite high levels of D2 receptor occupancy. This raises the possibility of a subtype of schizophrenia that is "nondopaminergic."

Caution should be used when attributing the action of a therapeutic agent to the causal mechanisms of the disease. Compensatory changes initiated by the pharmacologic agent may compensate for deficiencies related to the disease without directly treating the cause for the altered mechanism itself. Although antipsychotic drugs occupy D2 receptors very rapidly, the maximal therapeutic effects are often delayed, bolstering the likelihood for compensatory mechanisms underlying the therapeutic benefit. One delayed consequence of long-term dopamine blockade is a phenomenon known as dopamine supersensitivity, or an increase in dopamine receptors per cell and thus an increased sensitivity to dopamine release. In addition, chronic antipsychotic drug treatment can lead to a persistent alteration in the activity of the dopamine system referred to as depolarization block. Electrophysiological recordings from dopamine neurons in rats have shown that chronic antipsychotic drug treatment results in the time-dependent reduction in neuron firing resulting from an *overexcitation*, or depolarization block. Additionally, antipsychotic drugs with the greatest therapeutic efficacy selectively diminish dopamine neuron firing via depolarization block in the mesolimbic dopamine neurons in the ventral tegmental area (Gill et al., 2014; Grace & Bunney, 1986; Grace et al., 1997; Hollerman et al., 1992). In contrast, drugs that precipitate unwanted extra-pyramidal side effects cause depolarization block of mesostriatal dopamine neurons in the substantia nigra (Grace, 1992). Interestingly, in the MAM model of schizophrenia, in which a hyperdopaminergic state is already present, antipsychotic drugs rapidly induce depolarization block; this is consistent with clinical experience showing that patients with the highest (dopamine-dependent) positive symptoms respond rapidly to antipsychotic drug treatment (Valenti et al., 2011).

Long-term treatment can also impact other neurotransmitter systems, such as a decrease in the serotonin 5-HT2 receptor. In rodents, repeated haloperidol treatment increases 5HT-2A receptor expression in the striatum while decreasing 5-HT-2A expression in the cingulate cortex.

A substantial proportion of patients (20 percent) does not respond to the first-generation antipsychotic drugs but do show improvements following second-generation agents, like clozapine, that bind only weakly to D2 receptors. Clozapine is known to block serotonin 5-HT2A receptors, as well as alpha1 epinephrine and H1 histamine receptors. Even so, these drugs are given at higher doses to achieve similar levels of D2 occupancy. Consequently, the mechanisms of antipsychotic drugs may not be attributed to a single molecular target.

GLUTAMATE

Glutamate is the primary excitatory neurotransmitter in the brain and is the sole neurotransmitter released from cortical projections. Glutamate arrived on the scene as a potential alterative to the dopamine model of schizophrenia in 1980. A reduction in cerebral spinal fluid levels of glutamate was observed in patients with schizophrenia (Kim et al., 1980). Although the reproducibility of this result has been contested, it prompted further exploration of the role glutamate may play in psychosis. In addition, the psychotomimetic properties of glutamatergic-drugs like phencyclidine (PCP) bolstered this claim.

There are two broad glutamate receptor classes: ionotropic (α-amino-3-hydroxy-5-methyl-4-isoxazolepropionate (AMPA))/kainate (non-NMDA) and and the G-protein-coupled metabotropic (N-methyl-D-aspartate (NMDA)) (mGluR 1-8 subtypes) receptors. Ionotropic receptors are permeable to sodium and/or calcium and facilitate rapid depolarization. In contrast, metabotropic glutamate receptors mediate a slower form of synaptic transmission by virtue of their G-protein coupled mechanisms. NMDA receptors are permeable to calcium and have a unique mechanism requiring the coincident binding of glutamate with a depolarizing shift to become activated. The evidence for glutamate participation in the molecular, cellular, and behavioral abnormalities of schizophrenia is presented later. More specifically, the role of NMDA receptors as likely candidates for mediating glutamate's effects in schizophrenia is discussed. In addition, the therapeutic potential for mGluR2/3 receptor selective antipsychotic drugs is explored. The glutamate hypothesis of schizophrenia has focused chiefly on the compromised function of the NMDA receptor, particularly in the frontal cortex.

Pharmacological Evidence of Glutamate System Involvement in Schizophrenia

Both ketamine and PCP exhibit the potential to induce dose-dependent schizophrenia-like effects encompassing positive (delusions and hallucinations), negative (avolition and apathy), and cognitive (memory and attention deficiencies) symptom dimensions. Normal subjects given PCP report a depersonalization, as well as a disconnection from their environment. Both drugs share a mechanism with NMDA-receptor antagonism. PCP and ketamine also greatly exacerbate preexisting symptoms in schizophrenia patients (Javitt & Zukin, 1991; Krystal et al., 1994; Lahti et al., 1995a; Lahti et al., 1995b). This would seem to suggest a baseline deficit in glutamate signaling in patients with schizophrenia.

The mechanism by which NMDA antagonism leads to downstream increases in glutamate and cumulative neurotoxicity has not been fully defined, but there is some evidence supporting the involvement of GABAergic interneurons. NMDA antagonists can reduce GABA interneuron function, which could subsequently enhance pyramidal cell firing due to disinhibition in both the prefrontal cortex and hippocampus.

A recent directive for novel antipsychotic drugs that has produced mixed results has been treatment with mGluR2/3 receptor agonists. There has been a long association of mGluR2/3 receptors and schizophrenia. It has been hypothesized that for the long-term regulation of an abnormal glutamate system, targeting mGlu receptors is a more tenable solution than targeting NMDA receptors directly (Moghaddam, 2004). It has been postulated that presynaptic mGluR 2/3 receptors modulate the release of glutamate via inhibition of inhibition of the adenylate cyclase-cAMP-PKA pathway (reviewed in M. L. Li et al., 2015). In rats, activation of mGluR 2/3 receptors with the mGluR 2/3 receptor agonist LY354740 can reverse the electrophysiological alterations in prefrontal cortical neurons that were induced by the NMDA receptor antagonist MK-801 (Homayoun, Jackson, & Moghaddam, 2005). In rodent models of schizophrenia, mGluR 2/3 agonist treatment can reverse the cognitive impairments, sensory gating disturbances, stereotopy, enhanced locomotion, as well as cortical glutamate efflux (Cartmell, Monn, & Schoepp, 1999; Cartmell & Schoepp, 2000; Chartoff, Heusner, & Palmiter, 2005; Hikichi et al., 2013; Moghaddam & Adams, 1998; Woolley et al., 2008; Xi et al., 2011). Despite this promising preclinical data, Phase III clinical trials with the mGluR2/3 agonist LY2140023 (pomaglumetad methionil) have failed to meet primary endpoints based on the positive and negative syndrome scale (PNASS) (Downing et al., 2014; Stauffer et al., 2013). However, this may be a consequence of a system that has been altered by prior D2 antagonist antipsychotic drug treatment (Gill et al., 2014).

Postmortem Evidence of Glutamate System Involvement in Schizophrenia

There has been inconsistent postmortem data supporting decreases in glutamate signaling in schizophrenia. Studies utilizing quantitative autoradiography have shown both increases and decreases of AMPA-receptor expression in the caudate nucleus (Noga et al., 1997; Noga & Wang, 2002). There are simultaneous decreases reported in NR1 subunit expression in the hippocampus and cortex. Subregion-specific reductions in kainite as well as AMPA, but not NMDA, receptors have been observed in the hippocampus (Meador-Woodruff & Healy, 2000).

Genetic Evidence of Glutamate System Involvement in Schizophrenia

Polymorphisms in the genes that encode neuregulin-1 and its receptor ErbB4 have been associated with increased risk for the development of schizophrenia (review in (Mei & Xiong, 2008). Briefly, detailed breakdown of the 8p locus and haplotype-association analysis of families with increased susceptibility for schizophrenia narrowed the region to 8p12–8p21, and NRG1, which lies in this region, was identified as a candidate gene for schizophrenia (Stefansson et al., 2002; Stefansson et al., 2003). Neuregulin-1 can influence the expression of NMDA receptors via activation of ErbB4 receptors. Neuregulin-1 stimulation has been shown to suppress NMDA receptor activation in both human and rodent prefrontal cortex (Hahn et al., 2006; Pitcher et al., 2011). Neuregulin-1-induced suppression of NMDA receptor activation is more pronounced in schizophrenia subjects than in controls, consistent with enhanced neuregulin-1 binding at the ErbB4 receptor in patients. (B. Li et al., 2007) Neuregulin-1, likely via ErbB4 receptors, modulates synaptic plasticity but not baseline synaptic transmission in hippocampal slices (B. Li et al., 2007; Pitcher et al., 2008). In addition, neuregulin-1 participates in neural development, specifically axon guidance of thalamocortical projections, as well as glial cell proliferation and migration. Expression of the risk allele SNP8NRG243177 of NRG1 in particular is associated with decreased frontal cortex and temporal-lobe activation, increased likelihood of psychotic symptoms, and diminished IQ (Hall et al., 2006). There is also evidence for single-nucleotide polymorphisms in the type-2 and 3 metobotropic glutamate receptor gene that is associated with both cognitive performance and prefrontal cortical activity in schizophrenia patients (Bishop et al., 2015; Chen et al., 2005; Egan et al., 2004; Joo, 2008).

Functional Measures of Glutamate Involvement in Schizophrenia

NMDA receptors mediate slow excitatory postsynaptic potentials (EPSPs) considered critical for the expression of complex behaviors. In imaging studies comparing healthy volunteers with schizophrenia patients, ketamine administration yields similar patterns of hypofrontality (Breier et al., 1997; Lahti et al., 1995b). Compared to studies involving DA, there are scant imaging studies exploring glutamate or NMDA receptor binding in schizophrenia. However, a SPECT study demonstrated reduced hippocampal NMDA receptor binding in antipsychotic drug-free schizophrenia patients.

Proton magnetic resonance spectroscopy has been used as a means of measuring glutamate and glutamine levels in individuals at high risk of psychosis, as well as acutely psychotic or chronic schizophrenia. There are cortical and striatal increases in glutamine and glutamate, predominately in individuals with a high familial risk of developing schizophrenia or in the early stages of the illness (Modinos et al., 2015; Stone et al., 2009).

SEROTONIN

Pharmacological Evidence Implicating Serotonin System in Schizophrenia

Similar to the pharmacological evidence supporting dopamine involvement in schizophrenia, the mechanisms of the second-generation antipsychotic drugs, such as clozapine and risperidone, have implicated serotonin. The efficacy of second-generation antipsychotic drugs, such as clozapine, is not attributed solely to dopamine receptor activity. Indeed, clozapine binds relatively weakly to the dopamine D2 receptor. Instead, clozapine binds mainly to the D3 and D4 receptors, which happen to be weakly expressed in the basal ganglia. Consequently, clozapine is associated with fewer extrapyramidal side effects that plague the first generation antipsychotic drugs. In addition to its modulation of the dopamine system, clozapine also impacts serotonergic activity as a partial antagonist at the 5-HT2 subunit. Indeed, second-generation antipsychotic drugs like clozapine have a relatively higher affinity for 5-HT2A receptors than D2 receptors in vitro and in vivo. Both acute and chronic clozapine treatment reduces 5-HT2 receptor subunit expression in the rat frontal cortex (Buckland et al., 1997; Burnet et al., 1996).

Additional pharmacological support for the role of serotonin in mediating particular symptoms in schizophrenia stems from the hallucinatory capacity of psychedelic drugs. Although there is little evidence supporting direct effects on the firing of serotonergic neurons in the dorsal raphe, the psychotomimetic capacity of the indoleamine and phenethylamine hallucinogens correlates with their shared affinity for the 5-HT2 receptor subtype. This would suggest the potential for excessive serotonin activity in schizophrenia patients. However, there is no evidence for endogenous indoleamines or phenethylamines being involved in the pathophysiology of schizophrenia. The hallucinogenic compound psilocybin is rapidly converted to psilocin after ingestion. Psilocin binds to and activates serotonin receptors, particularly but not exclusively 5-HT2A receptors. PET imaging with fluordeoxyglucose after psiloin administration in humans has shown metabolic reduction in anterior cingulate and other cortical areas consistent with "hypofrontality" (Vollenweider et al., 1997).

Postmortem Evidence of Serotonin System Involvement in Schizophrenia

There have been mixed reports regarding changes in 5-HT2 receptor binding observed postmortem in schizophrenia patients. Increased (Whitaker, Crow, & Ferrier, 1981), decreased (Arora & Meltzer, 1991; Bennett et al., 1979; Mita et al., 1986) or normal (Mackay et al., 1978; Owen et al., 1981; Reynolds, Rossor, & Iversen, 1983) 5-HT2 binding has been reported in the frontal cortex of neuroleptic-treated schizophrenic patients. These alterations were unlikely to be the result of neuroleptic treatment since two studies failed to find any differences between the 5-HT2 binding in the frontal cortex of neuroleptic-treated and unmedicated schizophrenic patients (Laruelle et al., 1993; Mita et al., 1986). Perhaps unsurprisingly, a PET study from young, neuroleptic-free schizophrenia patients found no significant difference in 5-HT2A receptor density (Trichard et al., 1998).

Genetic Associations with Serotonin and Schizophrenia

The most compelling polymorphisms associated with serotonin conferring increased risk of schizophrenia involve the 5HT-2A receptor gene. The clinical response in schizophrenia patients to clozapine treatment is associated with polymorphisms in the promoter and coding regions of the 5-HT2A receptor (Arranz et al., 1998). There have also been reports of an association between schizophrenia diagnosis and the T102C and the -1438A/G polymorphisms of the 5-HT2A receptor gene (Gu et al., 2013). However, as was observed with the Val/Met polymorphism, a recent meta-analysis failed to find a significant association between the T102C polymorphism on the 5-HT2A gene and schizophrenia (Tan et al., 2014).

Functional Measures of Serotonin Involvement in Schizophrenia

Autoradiographic studies have shown the distribution of 5-HT2A receptors throughout the cerebral cortex (particularly medial prefrontal cortex), the olfactory bulb, the claustrum, the nucleus accumbens, the olfactory tubercle, and the n. tractus solitaries (reviewed in Aghajanian & Marek, 2000). Of particular interest, immunocytochemcial studies have shown 5-HT2A receptors are densely expressed at the apical dendrites of cortical pyramidal neurons. The effect of hallucinogens on complex processes like cognition, perception, and mood indicate the likely involvement of cerebral cortex. Indeed, the application of 5-HT in cortical areas produces an increase in postsynaptic potentials that are 5-HT2A mediated. Although 5-HT can increase the amplitude of spontaneous EPSCs via a postsynaptic mechanism, there is evidence for presynaptic enhancement of the release of glutamate that involves 5-HT2A receptors and a subsequent indirect retrograde messenger. However, a recent PET study in young antipsychotic-free and antipsychotic drug-naïve schizophrenia patients failed to bring about any significant alteration in 5-HT2A receptor density. PET imaging has demonstrated selective binding of the antipsychotic drug clozapine to both dopamine D1 and serotonin 5-HT2 receptors localized in the frontal cortex (Lundberg et al., 1996).

GABA

γ-Aminobutyric acid (GABA) is the primary inhibitory neurotransmitter in the brain and is a more recent target of schizophrenia research. The activity of inhibitory interneurons is especially important for modulating working memory. For example, fast-spiking GABA interneurons in the monkey DLPFC are active during the delay period during working memory performance, and are required for task-related neuronal firing of pyramidal neurons during working memory (Rao, Williams, & Goldman-Rakic, 2000). In addition, local infusions of GABA antagonists in the PFC can impair working memory performance. Cortical GABA interneurons are a heterogeneous population that can be separated based on morphological, physiological, or biochemical attributes. The PFC interneurons most implicated in schizophrenia are the parvalbumin-(PV) expressing chandelier (axo-axonic) and wide arbor basket cells (axo-cell body or axo-dendritic). It is unclear how GABA neurotransmission is impacted at the synapse in schizophrenia, so alternatively the focus is shifted to the postsynaptic effect of GABA. $GABA_A$ receptors are the primary postsynaptic target of GABA released from chandelier neurons in the cortex. In addition, $GABA_A$ receptors are also present on pyramidal cells in the hippocampus.

The $GABA_A$ receptor is a pentameric anion-selective ion channel that is composed of different classes of subunits (α1-6, β1-3, γ1-3, δ, θ, ρ, and ε) (McKernan & Whiting, 1996). The α2 $GABA_A$ receptor subunit is present at >95 percent of inhibitory synapses onto pyramidal neuron initial segments in the PFC (Nusser et al., 1996). The α5 containing $GABA_A$ receptors represent a small proportion of all $GABA_A$ receptors—less than 5 percent. In contrast to the dominate role of the α2 $GABA_A$ receptor subunit in PFC, the α5 $GABA_A$ receptor subunit is unique in its relatively confined distribution in the HPC, and to a lesser extent in the cortex and thalamus (Heldt et al., 2004; Ramos et al., 2004; Serwanski et al., 2006).

Postmortem Evidence of GABA System Involvement in Schizophrenia

Perhaps the most robust, consistent, and extensively reported biochemical alteration measured postmortem in the brains of schizophrenia patients have been reductions in GABA-related molecules. Initially, deficits in some specific morphological subtypes of interneurons in the frontal cortex in schizophrenia were reported (Benes, Vincent, & Todtenkopf, 2001). First, mRNA levels for the 67-kilodalton isoform of glutamic acid decarboxylase (GAD67), an enzyme principally responsible for GABA synthesis, and the GABA membrane transporter GAT1, which regulates the reuptake of synaptically released GABA, were shown to be decreased in a subset of GABA neurons (Curley et al., 2013; Hoftman et al., 2013). Second, affected GABA neurons include those that express the calcium-binding protein parvalbumin (PV), because PV mRNA levels are decreased in the prefrontal cortex of subjects with schizophrenia and GAD67 mRNA is undetectable in almost half of PV-containing neurons (Gonzalez-Burgos & Lewis, 2012). These changes are accompanied by decreased GAT1 expression in the presynaptic terminals of PV-containing neurons and by the previously mentioned increased postsynaptic α2 GABAA receptor subunit expression at the axon initial segments of pyramidal neurons (Beneyto et al., 2010; Lewis, 2000). Further research elucidated that this reduction was specific to a subgroup of GABAergic interneurons containing parvalbumin (PV), which is found in the fast-firing cells providing inhibitory control of the cortico-fugal pyramidal cells (Zhang, Sun, & Reynolds, 2002). The developmental expression of PV relatively late identifies a potentially vulnerable interneuron subpopulation in the progression of schizophrenia (Fish et al., 2013).

In the DLPFC of individuals with schizophrenia, the density of α2 $GABA_A$ immunoreactivty is increased (Volk et al., 2002). Since there is a decrease in PV mRNA-expression (in both chandelier and basket neurons) in the middle cortical layers of schizophrenia patients, this could potentially represent a compensatory overexpression of $GABA_A$ receptors at the soma and axon initial segment locally. Antagonism or genetic deletion of α5 $GABA_A$ R has behavioral consequences that resemble some of the behavioral abnormalities seen in schizophrenia, including reduced prepulse inhibition to startle (Hauser et al., 2005) and impaired latent inhibition (Gerdjikov et al., 2008). Alterations in α5 $GABA_A$ receptor binding in the hippocampus of schizophrenia patients have also been reported. PET scans of [11C]Ro15-4513, a GABAA/benzodiazepine compound with high affinity for the binding α5 $GABA_A$ receptor, in schizophrenia patients revealed a negative correlation between negative symptom severity and α5 $GABA_A$ binding in PFC and HPC (Asai et al., 2008).

Functional Measures of GABA System Involvement in Schizophrenia

Interneurons are proposed to underlie functional rhythmic events in the brain. Computational models of synchronous oscillatory activity that occurs across disparate brain regions has assigned a unique role for PV-expressing, fast-spiking interneurons. Oscillatory activity between cortical and subcortical regions such as the hippocampus and the amygdala has been implicated in normal cognitive processes and relies on intact GABAergic activity, via $GABA_A$ receptors, of interneurons (Mann, Radcliffe, & Paulsen, 2005; Mann & Paulsen, 2007; Whittington, Traub, & Jeffreys, 1995). Gamma oscillations (30–80 Hz) correlate with cognitive processes including perceptual binding, attention, arousal, and object recognition. Oscillations in the theta range (4-10Hz) serve complementary cognitive functions with gamma oscillations, in particular episodic memory formation. Both gamma and theta oscillations are observed independently in cortex and HPC (Buhl, Tamas, & Fisahn, 1998; Penttonen et al., 1998; Wang & Buzsaki, 1996). However, gamma oscillations in both regions are modulated by, and embedded within, theta oscillations (Bragin et al., 1995; Chrobak & Buzsaki, 1998; Lisman & Idiart, 1995). Oscillatory activity in general, and gamma oscillations in particular, are believed to represent the functional state and coordinated activity within neuronal systems (Fisahn et al., 1998). Gamma oscillations are reported to correspond most closely to functional imaging studies of metabolic activation in brain regions, and as such are likely a better index of function than is neuronal firing. Gamma oscillations are induced and sustained in the DLPFC during the delay period of working memory tasks. In addition, as working memory load increases, there are corresponding increases in the power, or strength, of gamma band oscillations in DLPFC PV-expressing neurons in the middle cortical layers mediate oscillatory activity in the gamma band range. A different cell subpopulation located in the superficial layers, and expressing both PV and calbindin, is involved in theta frequency oscillations (4–7 Hz) (reviewed in Lewis, Hashimoto, & Volk, 2005).

PV is a calcium-binding protein whose expression in interneurons releasing GABA uniquely depends on the level of neuronal activity—a quality not shared by nonfast spiking interneurons (Jiang & Swann, 2005; Patz et al., 2004; Sun, 2009). The loss of PV corresponds with a pathological alteration in oscillatory activity with broad consequences on network dynamics between brain regions. In schizophrenia patients, phase locking of gamma activity to task-relevant stimuli is impaired. There are also reductions in the power of gamma-band oscillations during the delay period of a working memory task in schizophrenia patients. Gamma oscillations in the HPC also require $GABA_A$ receptor activity (Whittington et al., 1995), and there is a loss of evoked gamma oscillatory activity both in in the MAM rodent model of schizophrenia and in humans in regions showing

PV neuron decreases (Gonzalez-Burgos, Hashimoto, & Lewis, 2010; Lodge et al., 2009; Minzenberg et al., 2010). In addition, more specifically α5 $GABA_A$ receptors are also important for regulating gamma oscillatory activity in HPC slice preparations (Glykys & Mody, 2006; Glykys, Mann, & Mody, 2008; Towers et al., 2004). Genetic reduction of α5 $GABA_A$ receptor expression can increase the occurrence of spontaneous gamma in the CA3 pyramidal layer (Glykys et al., 2008), as well as the power of kainite-induced frequency oscillations (Glykys & Mody, 2006). Thus, it appears that α5 $GABA_A$ receptor acts to limit increases in gamma power.

Genetic Evidence of GABA System Involvement in Schizophrenia

Based on the strong postmortem evidence, GABA receptor subunit genes are plausible candidate genes for schizophrenia. However, researchers have found weak evidence of linkage between this gene and schizophrenia (Papadimitriou et al., 2001). Other markers of GABA neurotransmission have been explored for potential genetic risk of schizophrenia. It has been shown that the mRNA expression for the GABA membrane transporter GAT-1 is relatively unaltered in most prefrontal cortex GABA neurons in patients with schizophrenia but is reduced below a detectable level in a subset of GABA neurons (Volk et al., 2001).

Therapeutic Potential of Targeting GABAergic System in Schizophrenia

There has been some exciting work done recently, demonstrating that pharmacologically targeting the GABA system or preventing the decrease in PV-expressing neurons can prevent either dopamine system pathology or aberrant behaviors in animal models of schizophrenia. In the MAM rodent model, treatment with a novel benzodiazepine-positive allosteric modulator (PAM), selective for the α5 subunit of the $GABA_A$ receptor, SH-053-2'F-R-CH3, can target abnormal HPC output likely arising from reductions in the number of PV-expressing neurons, which in turn normalizes downstream dopaminergic neuronal activity as well as amphetamine-induced locomotor activity (Gill et al., 2011; Gill et al., 2014). In a separate study, peripubertal administration of the antianxiety agent diazepam, a less selective positive allosteric modulator of $GABA_A$ receptors, was found to prevent the increase in dopamine neuron activity and blunt the behavioral hyperresponsivity to amphetamine adult MAM animals (Du & Grace, 2013).

It has been suggested that a dysregulation of the oxidative, neuroimmune, and glutamatergic systems due to genetic and early-life environmental risk factors contribute to the reductions of PV interneurons in schizophrenia, ultimately impacting cognition, social competence, and affective behavior (Steullet et al., 2010).

CONVERGING ALTERATIONS AMONG MULTIPLE NEUROTRANSMITTER SYSTEMS

Evidence has been presented for dysfunctions within multiple neurotransmitter systems; however, it is clear that these systems function in a highly integrated manner. Glutamate neurons regulate the function of other neurons, including GABAergic and dopaminergic neurons that have also been implicated in schizophrenia. NMDA receptors modulate the activity of GABAergic interneurons in the cortex, a cell population known to exhibit altered morphology in schizophrenia patients. Selectively ablating NMDA receptors on PV-positive interneurons in the hippocampus in a genetic mouse model has demonstrated both hippocampal-network disturbances as well as behavioral deficits, including impaired spatial working memory and spatial recognition memory (Korotkova et al., 2010). These data substantiate a role for PV-expressing interneurons, via an NMDA-receptor mediated mechanism, in regulating hippocampal oscillatory activity and subsequent behaviors pertaining to disorders such as schizophrenia. Further complicating the action of glutamate in schizophrenia is the observation that dopamine D2 receptors are also localized on presynaptic glutamate terminals and can inhibit the release of glutamate.

Another example of crosstalk between neurotransmitter systems is the enhancement by hallucinogens (via 5-HT2A receptors) of glutamate release. The increase in the frequency of EPSPs induced by hallucinogens is blocked mGluR II/III agonists acting presynaptically as well as by AMPA antagonists acting postsynaptically at non-NMDA glutamate receptors. NMDA antagonists elevate extracellular brain levels of 5-HT as well as its metabolite 5-HIAA in prefrontal cortex. 5-HT2 antagonists can block some of the behavioral effects produced by NMDA antagonism (e.g,. head twitch and hyperlocomotion). In rodents the increase in prefrontal cortical activation produced by ketamine is blocked by clozapine, but not haloperidol, perhaps owing to the 5-HT2A antagonist properties of clozapine that haloperidol lacks (Duncan et al., 1998).

Network Disturbance

Given the nature and complexity of the symptoms associated with schizophrenia, it is clear that disturbance in a single transmitter system cannot explain all the varied pathophysiology of this disorder. A more suitable model would incorporate disturbances within nodes of a distributed neural network encompassing multiple brain areas and, therefore, would not be limited to an individual neurochemical. Consequently, the primary deficiency in schizophrenia may be a general loss of connectivity as opposed to a direct lesion of a given neurotransmitter system.

For example, aberrant hippocampal activity as a central contributor to dopamine pathology in schizophrenia is supported by evidence from both human schizophrenia patients and animal models (Figure 10.1). Despite the indication of hippocampal hypermetabolism and volume reduction in patients with schizophrenia, without these measures having been assessed in the same patient population, it was previously unresolved whether hippocampal functional alterations preceded the morphological changes and subsequent symptom onset (Schobel et al., 2009; Schobel et al., 2013). Recent work with subjects categorized as "clinical high risk" for developing schizophrenia has shown progressive alterations in hippocampal function when subjects were longitudinally assessed with both cerebral blood volume-fMRI and structural MRI measures (Modinos et al., 2015). By following the same individuals, a subset of which went on to develop schizophrenia, it was concluded that the hippocampal hyperactivation preceded symptom onset. When morphological changes were mapped onto the activation images, it was also determined that the regions of greatest activation, CA1 and subicular subregions, demonstrated the greatest morphological changes and volumetric reduction. In order to address the potential of a glutamatergic mechanism underlying the hippocampal pathology, the authors employed a repeated ketamine animal model of psychosis. As was observed in the schizophrenia patients, ketamine-treated animals demonstrated subregion specific increases in hippocampal activation that preceded atrophy. These data are consistent with both animal models of schizophrenia attributing dopamine system hyperactivation to aberrant hippocampal output (Lodge & Grace, 2007) as well as previous reports from ultrahigh-risk patients showing a negative correlation between hippocampal glutamate levels and striatal dopamine activity (Stone et al., 2010).

The nucleus accumbens is a central region of the limbic system that integrates inputs from other limbic areas, including the hippocampus, the amygdala entorhinal cortex, and the anterior cingulate. Importantly, these are all regions implicated in schizophrenia. Aberrant changes in output from the accumbens, perhaps resulting from increased hippocampal activity, can have a deleterious impact on downstream mesolimbic dopamine activity. A further complication is the impact of dopamine on the integration of inputs on the nucleus accumbens itself (Figure 10.2) and the modulation of output to other limbic regions such as the ventral pallidum, septum, hypothalamus, anterior cingulate, and frontal cortex.

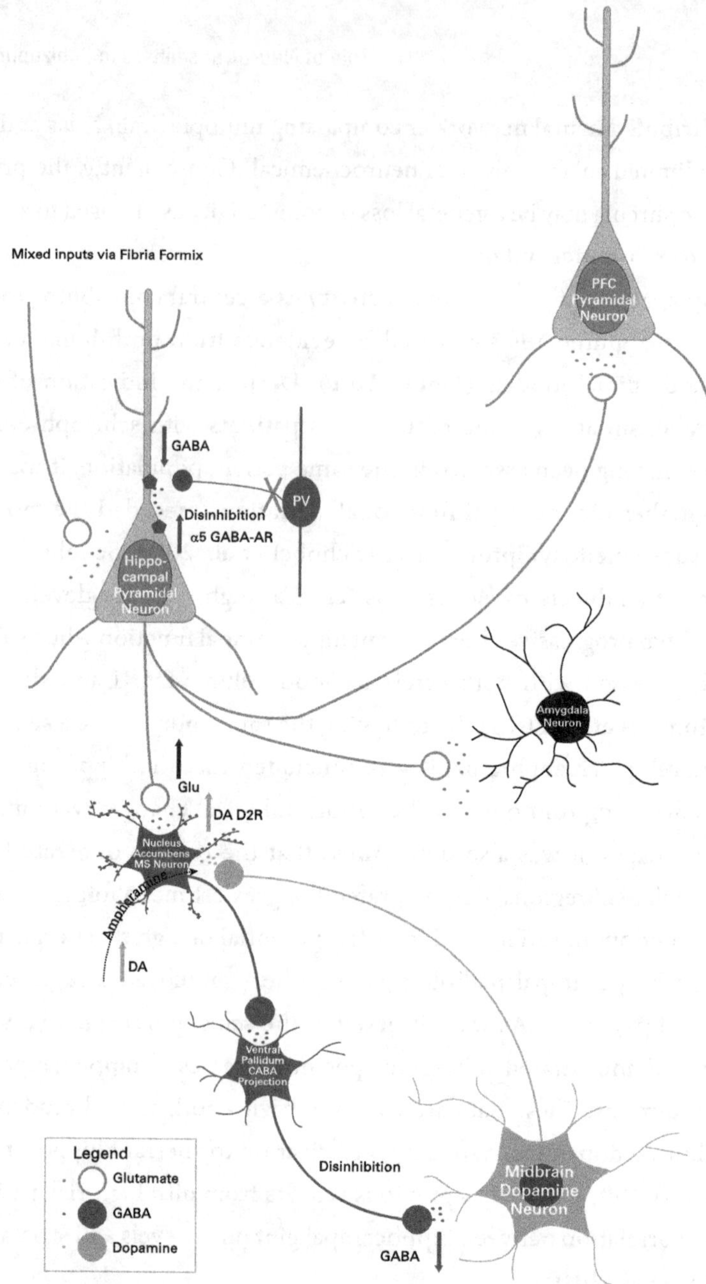

FIGURE 10.1 Widespread impact of hippocampal hyperactivity in schizophrenia. Aberrant increases in hippocampal output, likely resulting from a disinhibition arising from reduced PV interneurons, can impact activity across multiple circuits. First, there are likely increases in glutamate release at hippocampal projections to amygdala and prefrontal cortex, which could impact negative and cognitive symptom domains. Secondly, increased dopamine release from the midbrain is a consequence of enhanced glutamate release from hippocampal projections to the nucleus accumbens. As a result, there is an increase in inhibitory projections from the nucleus accumbens to the ventral pallidum, which will ultimately disinhibit dopamine neural activity downstream, leading to the dopamine-dependent positive psychotic symptoms. As a psychotomimetic, amphetamine could act in a similar fashion by increasing dopamine release onto medium spiny neurons in the nucleus accumbens and increasing their output.

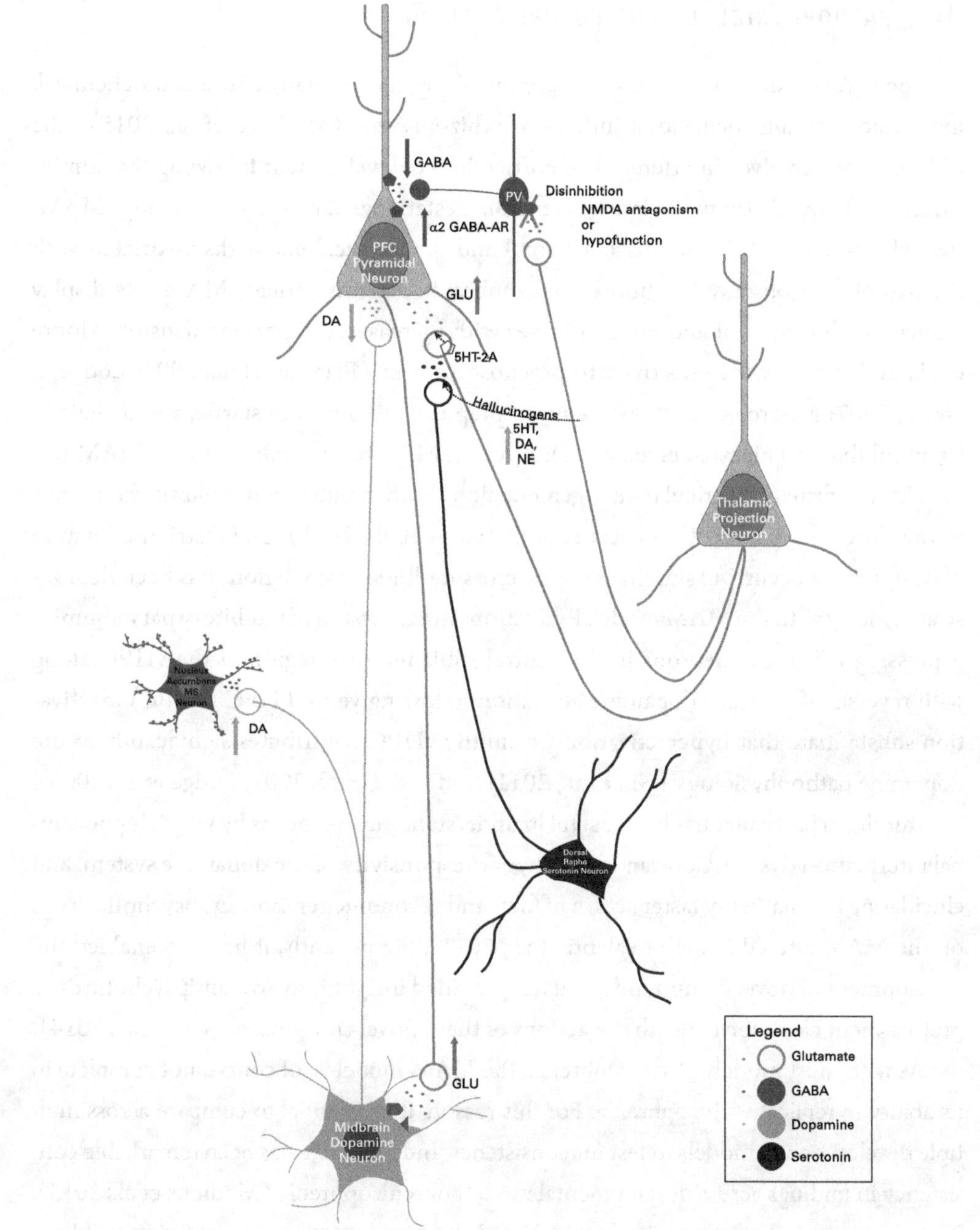

FIGURE 10.2 Alterations in prefrontal cortical activity in schizophrenia. Similar to the hippocampus, abnormal changes in prefrontal cortical activation is a consequence of destabilized interneuron networks resulting from reductions in PV. This would change the response of cortical neurons to glutamatergic input arising from the thalamus. NMDA antagonism selectively acting at GABAergic interneurons in the PFC, or hypofunction occurring at these neurons presynaptically, could lead to an imbalance of thalamic input such that cortical output neurons are inappropriately selectively engaged. Serotonergic hallucinogens likely act via 5HT-2A receptors to increase the release of glutamate presynaptically and subsequently enhance cortical postsynaptic responses. Increased PFC output can increase mesolimbic dopamine release (e.g. nucleus accumbens), but decrease mesocortical dopamine release.

The MAM rodent model of schizophrenia recapitulates many of the neurochemical, morphological, and behavioral indices of schizophrenia (Modinos et al., 2015). The MAM model involves interference of corticolimbic development following the administration of the DNA methylating agent on gestational day 17. Importantly, MAM-treated offspring exhibit similar behavioral and biochemical hallmarks associated with the pathologies observed in human schizophrenia patients. Briefly, MAM rats display reduced limbic cortical and HPC volumes with increased cell-packing density (Moore et al., 2006), increased sensitivity to psychostimulants (Flagstad et al., 2004; Lodge & Grace, 2007; Moore et al., 2006), reduced prepulse inhibition to startle, and deficits in latent inhibition (Flagstad et al., 2004). A recent MRI study conducted with MAM rats has also confirmed ventricular enlargement along with simultaneous volume reductions in the HPC and paraHPC cortical regions (Chin et al., 2011). The distributed nature of dysfunction occurring simultaneously across multiple brain regions has been demonstrated nicely with the MAM model. Reductions in expression of inhibitory parvalbumin-expressing (PV) interneurons in the ventral subiculum subregion of the vHPC along with reversal of aberrant dopamine activation following ventral HPC (vHPC) inactivation substantiate that hyperactivation within the vHPC contributes significantly to the dopamine pathophysiology (Gill et al., 2011; Lodge & Grace, 2007; Lodge et al., 2009). This model in particular has been useful in understanding the means by which hippocampal interneuron dysfunction can lead to hyper-responsivity of the dopamine system, and elucidating the markedly faster action of first- and second-generation antipsychotic drugs on the MAM-altered system (Valenti et al., 2011). Significantly, it has also enabled the development of novel compounds, and has provided insight into how antipsychotic drug pretreatment can interfere with the actions of these novel compounds (Gill et al., 2014).

As with most models of schizophrenia, the MAM model is, of course, not complete in its ability to replicate schizophrenia. For this reason, it is essential to compare across multiple developmental models to test for consistency. Indeed, there has been remarkable consistency in findings across developmental models of schizophrenia (Modinos et al., 2015). This convergence between animal models and the human patient has been invaluable in advancing our understanding of the circuitry of schizophrenia and in identifying novel sites of intervention for the treatment and ultimately prevention of schizophrenia in humans.

ACKNOWLEDGMENTS

This work was supported by United States Public Health Service Grant MH57440 (A.A.G.)

REFERENCES

Abi-Dargham, A., Gil, R., Krystal, J., Baldwin, R. M., Seibyl, J. P., Bowers, M., . . . Laruelle, M. (1998). Increased striatal dopamine transmission in schizophrenia: confirmation in a second cohort. *Am J Psychiatry, 155*(6), 761–767. doi: 10.1176/ajp.155.6.761

Abi-Dargham, A., Rodenhiser, J., Printz, D., Zea-Ponce, Y., Gil, R., Kegeles, L. S., . . . Laruelle, M. (2000). Increased baseline occupancy of D2 receptors by dopamine in schizophrenia. *Proc Natl Acad Sci U S A, 97*(14), 8104–8109.

Abi-Dargham, A., van de Giessen, E., Slifstein, M., Kegeles, L. S., & Laruelle, M. (2009). Baseline and amphetamine-stimulated dopamine activity are related in drug-naive schizophrenic subjects. *Biol Psychiatry, 65*(12), 1091–1093. doi: 10.1016/j.biopsych.2008.12.007

Aghajanian, G. K., & Marek, G. J. (2000). Serotonin model of schizophrenia: emerging role of glutamate mechanisms. *Brain Res Brain Res Rev, 31*(2–3), 302–312.

Arnold, A. L., & Freeman, H. (1956). Reserpine in hospitalized psychotics; a controlled study on chronically disturbed women. *AMA Arch Neurol Psychiatry, 76*(3), 281–285.

Arora, R. C., & Meltzer, H. Y. (1991). Serotonin2 (5-HT2) receptor binding in the frontal cortex of schizophrenic patients. *J Neural Transm Gen Sect, 85*(1), 19–29.

Arranz, M. J., Munro, J., Sham, P., Kirov, G., Murray, R. M., Collier, D.A. . . . Kerwin, R. W. (1998). Meta-analysis of studies on genetic variation in 5-HT2A receptors and clozapine response. *Schizophr Res, 32*(2), 93–99.

Asai, Y., Takano, A., Ito, H., Okubo, Y., Matsuura, M., Otsuka, A., . . . Suhara, T. (2008). GABAA/Benzodiazepine receptor binding in patients with schizophrenia using [11C]Ro15-4513, a radioligand with relatively high affinity for alpha5 subunit. *Schizophr Res, 99*(1–3), 333–340. doi: 10.1016/j.schres.2007.10.014

Bast, T., & Feldon, J. (2003). Hippocampal modulation of sensorimotor processes. *Prog Neurobiol, 70*(4), 319–345.

Benes, F. M., Vincent, S. L., & Todtenkopf, M. (2001). The density of pyramidal and nonpyramidal neurons in anterior cingulate cortex of schizophrenic and bipolar subjects. *Biol Psychiatry, 50*(6), 395–406.

Beneyto, M., Abbott, A., Hashimoto, T., & Lewis, D. A. (2011). Lamina-specific alterations in cortical GABA(A) receptor subunit expression in schizophrenia. *Cereb Cortex, 21*(5), 999–1011. doi: 10.1093/cercor/bhq169

Bennett, J. P., Jr., Enna, S. J., Bylund, D. B., Gillin, J. C., Wyatt, R. J., & Snyder, S. H. (1979). Neurotransmitter receptors in frontal cortex of schizophrenics. *Arch Gen Psychiatry, 36*(9), 927–934.

Bishop, J. R., Reilly, J. L., Harris, M. S., Patel, S. R., Kittles, R., Badner, J. A., . . . Sweeney, J. A. (2015). Pharmacogenetic associations of the type-3 metabotropic glutamate receptor (GRM3) gene with working memory and clinical symptom response to antipsychotics in first-episode schizophrenia. *Psychopharmacology (Berl), 232*(1), 145–154. doi: 10.1007/s00213-014-3649-4

Bolton, M. M., Heaney, C. F., Sabbagh, J. J., Murtishaw, A. S., Magcalas, C. M., & Kinney, J. W. (2012). Deficits in emotional learning and memory in an animal model of schizophrenia. *Behav Brain Res, 233*(1), 35–44. doi: 10.1016/j.bbr.2012.04.049

Bragin, A., Jando, G., Nadasdy, Z., Hetke, J., Wise, K., & Buzsaki, G. (1995). Gamma (40-100 Hz) oscillation in the hippocampus of the behaving rat. *J Neurosci, 15*(1 Pt 1), 47–60.

Breier, A., Malhotra, A. K., Pinals, D. A., Weisenfeld, N. I., & Pickar, D. (1997). Association of ketamine-induced psychosis with focal activation of the prefrontal cortex in healthy volunteers. *Am J Psychiatry, 154*(6), 805–811. doi: 10.1176/ajp.154.6.805

Brown, J. A., Ramikie, T. S., Schmidt, M. J., Baldi, R., Garbett, K., Everheart, M. G., . . . Mirnics, K. (2015). Inhibition of parvalbumin-expressing interneurons results in complex behavioral changes. *Mol Psychiatry, 20*(12), 1499–1507. doi: 10.1038/mp.2014.192

Buckland, P. R., D'Souza, U., Maher, N. A., & McGuffin, P. (1997). The effects of antipsychotic drugs on the mRNA levels of serotonin 5HT2A and 5HT2C receptors. *Brain Res Mol Brain Res, 48*(1), 45–52.

Buhl, E. H., Tamas, G., & Fisahn, A. (1998). Cholinergic activation and tonic excitation induce persistent gamma oscillations in mouse somatosensory cortex in vitro. *J Physiol, 513(Pt 1)*, 117–126.

Burnet, P. W., Chen, C. P., McGowan, S., Franklin, M., & Harrison, P. J. (1996). The effects of clozapine and haloperidol on serotonin-1A, -2A and -2C receptor gene expression and serotonin metabolism in the rat forebrain. *Neuroscience, 73*(2), 531–540.

Carboni, G., Tueting, P., Tremolizzo, L., Sugaya, I., Davis, J., Costa, E., . . . Guidotti, A. (2004). Enhanced dizocilpine efficacy in heterozygous reeler mice relates to GABA turnover downregulation. *Neuropharmacology, 46*(8), 1070–1081. doi: 10.1016/j.neuropharm.2004.02.001

Carlsson, A. (1973). [Mode of action of tricyclic antidepressants]. *Tidsskr Nor Laegeforen, 93*(17), 1300–1302.

Carlsson, A., Roos, B. E., Walinder, J., & Skott, A. (1973). Further studies on the mechanism of antipsychotic action: potentiation by alpha-methyltyrosine of thioridazine effects in chronic schizophrenics. *J Neural Transm, 34*(2), 125–132.

Cartmell, J., Monn, J. A., & Schoepp, D. D. (1999). The metabotropic glutamate 2/3 receptor agonists LY354740 and LY379268 selectively attenuate phencyclidine versus d-amphetamine motor behaviors in rats. *J Pharmacol Exp Ther, 291*(1), 161–170.

Cartmell, J., & Schoepp, D. D. (2000). Regulation of neurotransmitter release by metabotropic glutamate receptors. *J Neurochem, 75*(3), 889–907.

Chartoff, E. H., Heusner, C. L., & Palmiter, R. D. (2005). Dopamine is not required for the hyperlocomotor response to NMDA receptor antagonists. *Neuropsychopharmacology, 30*(7), 1324–1333. doi: 10.1038/sj.npp.1300678

Chen, Q., He, G., Chen, Q., Wu, S., Xu, Y., Feng, G., . . . He, L. (2005). A case-control study of the relationship between the metabotropic glutamate receptor 3 gene and schizophrenia in the Chinese population. *Schizophr Res, 73*(1), 21–26. doi: 10.1016/j.schres.2004.07.002

Chin, C. L., Curzon, P., Schwartz, A. J., O'Connor, E. M., Rueter, L. E., Fox, G. B., . . . Basso, A. M. (2011). Structural abnormalities revealed by magnetic resonance imaging in rats prenatally exposed to methylazoxymethanol acetate parallel cerebral pathology in schizophrenia. *Synapse, 65*(5), 393–403. doi: 10.1002/syn.20857

Chrobak, J. J., & Buzsaki, G. (1998). Gamma oscillations in the entorhinal cortex of the freely behaving rat. *J Neurosci, 18*(1), 388–398.

Creese, I., Burt, D. R., & Snyder, S. H. (1976). Dopamine receptor binding predicts clinical and pharmacological potencies of antischizophrenic drugs. *Science, 192*(4238), 481–483.

Curley, A. A., Eggan, S. M., Lazarus, M. S., Huang, Z. J., Volk, D. W., & Lewis, D. A. (2013). Role of glutamic acid decarboxylase 67 in regulating cortical parvalbumin and GABA membrane transporter 1 expression: implications for schizophrenia. *Neurobiol Dis, 50*, 179–186. doi: 10.1016/j.nbd.2012.10.018

Dao-Castellana, M. H., Paillere-Martinot, M. L., Hantraye, P., Attar-Levy, D., Remy, P., Crouzel, C., . . . Martinot, J. L. (1997). Presynaptic dopaminergic function in the striatum of schizophrenic patients. *Schizophr Res, 23*(2), 167–174. doi: 10.1016/S0920-9964(96)00102-8

Downing, A. M., Kinon, B. J., Millen, B. A., Zhang, L., Liu, L., Morozova, M. A., . . . Gomez, J. C. (2014). A double-blind, placebo-controlled comparator study of LY2140023 monohydrate in patients with schizophrenia. *BMC Psychiatry, 14*, 351. doi: 10.1186/s12888-014-0351-3

Du, Y., & Grace, A. A. (2013). Peripubertal diazepam administration prevents the emergence of dopamine system hyperresponsivity in the MAM developmental disruption model of schizophrenia. *Neuropsychopharmacology, 38*(10), 1881–1888. doi: 10.1038/npp.2013.101

Duncan, G. E., Leipzig, J. N., Mailman, R. B., & Lieberman, J. A. (1998). Differential effects of clozapine and haloperidol on ketamine-induced brain metabolic activation. *Brain Res, 812*(1–2), 65–75.

Egan, M. F., Straub, R. E., Goldberg, T. E., Yakub, I., Callicott, J. H., Hariri, A. R., . . . Weinberger, D. R. (2004). Variation in GRM3 affects cognition, prefrontal glutamate, and risk for schizophrenia. *Proc Natl Acad Sci U S A, 101*(34), 12604–12609. doi: 10.1073/pnas.0405077101

Ermis, A., Erkiran, M., Dasdemir, S., Turkcan, A. S., Ceylan, M. E., Bireller, E. S., . . . Cakmakoglu, B. (2015). The relationship between catechol-O-methyltransferase gene Val158Met (COMT) polymorphism and premorbid cannabis use in Turkish male patients with schizophrenia. *In Vivo, 29*(1), 129–132.

Farde, L., Wiesel, F. A., Stone-Elander, S., Halldin, C., Nordstrom, A. L., Hall, H., . . . Sedvall, G. (1990). D2 dopamine receptors in neuroleptic-naive schizophrenic patients. A positron emission tomography study with [11C]raclopride. *Arch Gen Psychiatry, 47*(3), 213–219.

Fisahn, A., Pike, F. G., Buhl, E. H., & Paulsen, O. (1998). Cholinergic induction of network oscillations at 40 Hz in the hippocampus in vitro. *Nature, 394*(6689), 186–189. doi: 10.1038/28179

Fish, K. N., Hoftman, G. D., Sheikh, W., Kitchens, M., & Lewis, D. A. (2013). Parvalbumin-containing chandelier and basket cell boutons have distinctive modes of maturation in monkey prefrontal cortex. *J Neurosci, 33*(19), 8352–8358. doi: 10.1523/JNEUROSCI.0306-13.2013

Flagstad, P., Mork, A., Glenthoj, B. Y., van Beek, J., Michael-Titus, A. T., & Didriksen, M. (2004). Disruption of neurogenesis on gestational day 17 in the rat causes behavioral changes relevant to positive and negative schizophrenia symptoms and alters amphetamine-induced dopamine release in nucleus accumbens. *Neuropsychopharmacology, 29*(11), 2052–2064. doi: 10.1038/sj.npp.1300516

Francois, J., Ferrandon, A., Koning, E., Angst, M. J., Sandner, G., & Nehlig, A. (2009). Selective reorganization of GABAergic transmission in neonatal ventral hippocampal-lesioned rats. *Int J Neuropsychopharmacol, 12*(8), 1097–1110. doi: 10.1017/S1461145709009985

Gerdjikov, T. V., Rudolph, U., Keist, R., Mohler, H., Feldon, J., & Yee, B. K. (2008). Hippocampal alpha 5 subunit-containing GABA A receptors are involved in the development of the latent inhibition effect. *Neurobiol Learn Mem, 89*(2), 87–94. doi: 10.1016/j.nlm.2007.06.003

Gill, K. M., & Grace, A. A. (2014). The role of alpha5 GABAA receptor agonists in the treatment of cognitive deficits in schizophrenia. *Curr Pharm Des, 20*(31), 5069–5076.

Gill, K. M., Lodge, D. J., Cook, J. M., Aras, S., & Grace, A. A. (2011). A novel alpha5GABA(A)R-positive allosteric modulator reverses hyperactivation of the dopamine system in the MAM model of schizophrenia. *Neuropsychopharmacology, 36*(9), 1903–1911. doi: 10.1038/npp.2011.76

Glykys, J., Mann, E. O., & Mody, I. (2008). Which GABA(A) receptor subunits are necessary for tonic inhibition in the hippocampus? *J Neurosci, 28*(6), 1421–1426. doi: 10.1523/JNEUROSCI.4751-07.2008

Glykys, J., & Mody, I. (2006). Hippocampal network hyperactivity after selective reduction of tonic inhibition in GABA A receptor alpha5 subunit-deficient mice. *J Neurophysiol, 95*(5), 2796–2807. doi: 10.1152/jn.01122.2005

Gonzalez-Burgos, G., Hashimoto, T., & Lewis, D. A. (2010). Alterations of cortical GABA neurons and network oscillations in schizophrenia. *Curr Psychiatry Rep, 12*(4), 335–344. doi: 10.1007/s11920-010-0124-8

Gonzalez-Burgos, G., & Lewis, D. A. (2012). NMDA receptor hypofunction, parvalbumin-positive neurons, and cortical gamma oscillations in schizophrenia. *Schizophr Bull, 38*(5), 950–957. doi: 10.1093/schbul/sbs010

Grace, A. A. (1992). The depolarization block hypothesis of neuroleptic action: implications for the etiology and treatment of schizophrenia. *J Neural Transm Suppl, 36*, 91–131.

Grace, A. A., & Bunney, B. S. (1986). Induction of depolarization block in midbrain dopamine neurons by repeated administration of haloperidol: analysis using in vivo intracellular recording. *J Pharmacol Exp Ther, 238*(3), 1092–1100.

Grace, A. A., Bunney, B. S., Moore, H., & Todd, C. L. (1997). Dopamine-cell depolarization block as a model for the therapeutic actions of antipsychotic drugs. *Trends Neurosci, 20*(1), 31–37. doi: 10.1016/S0166-2236(96)10064-3

Gu, L., Long, J., Yan, Y., Chen, Q., Pan, R., Xie, X., . . . Su, L. (2013). HTR2A-1438A/G polymorphism influences the risk of schizophrenia but not bipolar disorder or major depressive disorder: a meta-analysis. *J Neurosci Res, 91*(5), 623–633. doi: 10.1002/jnr.23180

Hahn, C. G., Wang, H. Y., Cho, D. S., Talbot, K., Gur, R. E., Berrettini, W. H., . . . Arnold, S. E. (2006). Altered neuregulin 1-erbB4 signaling contributes to NMDA receptor hypofunction in schizophrenia. *Nat Med, 12*(7), 824–828. doi: 10.1038/nm1418

Hall, J., Whalley, H. C., Job, D. E., Baig, B. J., McIntosh, A. M., Evans, K. L., . . . Lawrie, S. M. (2006). A neuregulin 1 variant associated with abnormal cortical function and psychotic symptoms. *Nat Neurosci, 9*(12), 1477–1478. doi: 10.1038/nn1795

Hauser, J., Rudolph, U., Keist, R., Mohler, H., Feldon, J., & Yee, B. K. (2005). Hippocampal alpha5 subunit-containing GABAA receptors modulate the expression of prepulse inhibition. *Mol Psychiatry, 10*(2), 201–207. doi: 10.1038/sj.mp.4001554

Heldt, S. A., Green, A., & Ressler, K. J. (2004). Prepulse inhibition deficits in GAD65 knockout mice and the effect of antipsychotic treatment. *Neuropsychopharmacology, 29*(9), 1610–1619. doi: 10.1038/sj.npp.1300468

Hikichi, H., Kaku, A., Karasawa, J., & Chaki, S. (2013). Stimulation of metabotropic glutamate (mGlu) 2 receptor and blockade of mGlu1 receptor improve social memory impairment elicited by MK-801 in rats. *J Pharmacol Sci, 122*(1), 10–16.

Hoftman, G. D., Volk, D. W., Bazmi, H. H., Li, S., Sampson, A. R., & Lewis, D. A. (2015). Altered cortical expression of GABA-related genes in schizophrenia: illness progression vs developmental disturbance. *Schizophr Bull, 41*(1), 180–191. doi: 10.1093/schbul/sbt178

Hollerman, J. R., Abercrombie, E. D., & Grace, A. A. (1992). Electrophysiological, biochemical, and behavioral studies of acute haloperidol-induced depolarization block of nigral dopamine neurons. *Neuroscience, 47*(3), 589–601.

Homayoun, H., Jackson, M. E., & Moghaddam, B. (2005). Activation of metabotropic glutamate 2/3 receptors reverses the effects of NMDA receptor hypofunction on prefrontal cortex unit activity in awake rats. *J Neurophysiol, 93*(4), 1989–2001. doi: 10.1152/jn.00875.2004

Howes, O. D., Williams, M., Ibrahim, K., Leung, G., Egerton, A., McGuire, P. K., . . . Turkheimer, F. (2013). Midbrain dopamine function in schizophrenia and depression: a post-mortem and positron emission tomographic imaging study. *Brain, 136*(Pt 11), 3242–3251. doi: 10.1093/brain/awt264

Itokawa, M., Arinami, T., & Toru, M. (2010). Advanced research on dopamine signaling to develop drugs for the treatment of mental disorders: Ser311Cys polymorphisms of the dopamine D2-receptor gene and schizophrenia. *J Pharmacol Sci, 114*(1), 1–5.

Javitt, D. C., & Zukin, S. R. (1991). Recent advances in the phencyclidine model of schizophrenia. *Am J Psychiatry, 148*(10), 1301–1308. doi: 10.1176/ajp.148.10.1301

Jiang, M., & Swann, J. W. (2005). A role for L-type calcium channels in the maturation of parvalbumin-containing hippocampal interneurons. *Neuroscience, 135*(3), 839–850. doi: 10.1016/j.neuroscience.2005.06.073

Joo, Y. H. (2008). Neurophyisological and neurocognitive endophenotypes for schizophrenia genetics research. *Psychiatry Investig, 5*(4), 199–202. doi: 10.4306/pi.2008.5.4.199

Kaalund, S. S., Newburn, E. N., Ye, T., Tao, R., Li, C., Deep-Soboslay, A., . . . Kleinman, J. E. (2014). Contrasting changes in DRD1 and DRD2 splice variant expression in schizophrenia and affective disorders, and associations with SNPs in postmortem brain. *Mol Psychiatry, 19*(12), 1258–1266. doi: 10.1038/mp.2013.165

Kim, J. S., Kornhuber, H. H., Schmid-Burgk, W., & Holzmuller, B. (1980). Low cerebrospinal fluid glutamate in schizophrenic patients and a new hypothesis on schizophrenia. *Neurosci Lett, 20*(3), 379–382.

Knable, M. B., & Weinberger, D. R. (1997). Dopamine, the prefrontal cortex and schizophrenia. *J Psychopharmacol, 11*(2), 123–131.

Korotkova, T., Fuchs, E. C., Ponomarenko, A., von Engelhardt, J., & Monyer, H. (2010). NMDA receptor ablation on parvalbumin-positive interneurons impairs hippocampal synchrony, spatial representations, and working memory. *Neuron, 68*(3), 557–569. doi: 10.1016/j.neuron.2010.09.017

Krystal, J. H., Karper, L. P., Seibyl, J. P., Freeman, G. K., Delaney, R., Bremner, J. D., . . . Charney, D. S. (1994). Subanesthetic effects of the noncompetitive NMDA antagonist, ketamine, in humans. Psychotomimetic, perceptual, cognitive, and neuroendocrine responses. *Arch Gen Psychiatry, 51*(3), 199–214.

Lahti, A. C., Holcomb, H. H., Medoff, D. R., & Tamminga, C. A. (1995). Ketamine activates psychosis and alters limbic blood flow in schizophrenia. *Neuroreport, 6*(6), 869–872.

Lahti, A. C., Koffel, B., LaPorte, D., & Tamminga, C. A. (1995). Subanesthetic doses of ketamine stimulate psychosis in schizophrenia. *Neuropsychopharmacology, 13*(1), 9–19. doi: 10.1016/0893-133X(94)00131-I

Laruelle, M., Abi-Dargham, A., Casanova, M. F., Toti, R., Weinberger, D. R., & Kleinman, J. E. (1993). Selective abnormalities of prefrontal serotonergic receptors in schizophrenia. A postmortem study. *Arch Gen Psychiatry, 50*(10), 810–818.

Lewis, D. A. (2000). GABAergic local circuit neurons and prefrontal cortical dysfunction in schizophrenia. *Brain Res Brain Res Rev, 31*(2–3), 270–276.

Lewis, D. A., Hashimoto, T., & Volk, D. W. (2005). Cortical inhibitory neurons and schizophrenia. *Nat Rev Neurosci, 6*(4), 312–324. doi: 10.1038/nrn1648

Li, B., Woo, R. S., Mei, L., & Malinow, R. (2007). The neuregulin-1 receptor erbB4 controls glutamatergic synapse maturation and plasticity. *Neuron, 54*(4), 583–597. doi: 10.1016/j.neuron.2007.03.028

Li, M. L., Hu, X. Q., Li, F., & Gao, W. J. (2015). Perspectives on the mGluR2/3 agonists as a therapeutic target for schizophrenia: Still promising or a dead end? *Prog Neuropsychopharmacol Biol Psychiatry, 60*, 66–76. doi: 10.1016/j.pnpbp.2015.02.012

Lieberman, J. A., Kane, J. M., & Alvir, J. (1987). Provocative tests with psychostimulant drugs in schizophrenia. *Psychopharmacology (Berl), 91*(4), 415–433.

Lisman, J. E., & Idiart, M. A. (1995). Storage of 7 +/- 2 short-term memories in oscillatory subcycles. *Science, 267*(5203), 1512–1515.

Lodge, D. J., Behrens, M. M., & Grace, A. A. (2009). A loss of parvalbumin-containing interneurons is associated with diminished oscillatory activity in an animal model of schizophrenia. *J Neurosci, 29*(8), 2344–2354. doi: 10.1523/JNEUROSCI.5419-08.2009

Lodge, D. J., & Grace, A. A. (2007). Aberrant hippocampal activity underlies the dopamine dysregulation in an animal model of schizophrenia. *J Neurosci, 27*(42), 11424–11430. doi: 10.1523/JNEUROSCI.2847-07.2007

Lundberg, T., Lindstrom, L., Hartvig, P., Reibring, L., Agren, H., Lundqvist, H., . . . Langstrom, B. (1996). Serotonin-2 and dopamine-1 binding components of clozapine in frontal cortex and striatum in the human brain visualized by positron emission tomography. *Psychiatry Res, 67*(1), 1–10.

Mackay, A. V., Yates, C. M., Wright, A., Hamilton, P., & Davies, P. (1978). Regional distribution of monoamines and their metabolites in the human brain. *J Neurochem, 30*(4), 841–848.

Mann, E. O., & Paulsen, O. (2007). Role of GABAergic inhibition in hippocampal network oscillations. *Trends Neurosci, 30*(7), 343–349. doi: 10.1016/j.tins.2007.05.003

Mann, E. O., Radcliffe, C. A., & Paulsen, O. (2005). Hippocampal gamma-frequency oscillations: from interneurones to pyramidal cells, and back. *J Physiol, 562*(Pt 1), 55–63. doi: 10.1113/jphysiol.2004.078758

McKernan, R. M., & Whiting, P. J. (1996). Which GABAA-receptor subtypes really occur in the brain? *Trends Neurosci, 19*(4), 139–143.

Meador-Woodruff, J. H., & Healy, D. J. (2000). Glutamate receptor expression in schizophrenic brain. *Brain Res Brain Res Rev, 31*(2–3), 288–294.

Mei, L., & Xiong, W. C. (2008). Neuregulin 1 in neural development, synaptic plasticity and schizophrenia. *Nat Rev Neurosci, 9*(6), 437–452. doi: 10.1038/nrn2392

Minzenberg, M. J., Firl, A. J., Yoon, J. H., Gomes, G. C., Reinking, C., & Carter, C. S. (2010). Gamma oscillatory power is impaired during cognitive control independent of medication status in first-episode schizophrenia. *Neuropsychopharmacology, 35*(13), 2590–2599. doi: 10.1038/npp.2010.150

Mita, T., Hanada, S., Nishino, N., Kuno, T., Nakai, H., Yamadori, T., . . . Tanaka, C. (1986). Decreased serotonin S2 and increased dopamine D2 receptors in chronic schizophrenics. *Biol Psychiatry, 21*(14), 1407–1414.

Modinos, G., Allen, P., Grace, A. A., & McGuire, P. (2015). Translating the MAM model of psychosis to humans. *Trends Neurosci, 38*(3), 129–138. doi: 10.1016/j.tins.2014.12.005

Moghaddam, B. (2004). Targeting metabotropic glutamate receptors for treatment of the cognitive symptoms of schizophrenia. *Psychopharmacology (Berl), 174*(1), 39–44. doi: 10.1007/s00213-004-1792-z

Moghaddam, B., & Adams, B. W. (1998). Reversal of phencyclidine effects by a group II metabotropic glutamate receptor agonist in rats. *Science, 281*(5381), 1349–1352.

Moore, H., Jentsch, J. D., Ghajarnia, M., Geyer, M. A., & Grace, A. A. (2006). A neurobehavioral systems analysis of adult rats exposed to methylazoxymethanol acetate on E17: implications for the neuropathology of schizophrenia. *Biol Psychiatry, 60*(3), 253–264. doi: 10.1016/j.biopsych.2006.01.003

Munafo, M. R., Bowes, L., Clark, T. G., & Flint, J. (2005). Lack of association of the COMT (Val158/108 Met) gene and schizophrenia: a meta-analysis of case-control studies. *Molecular Psychiatry*, 10(8), 765–770.

Nguyen, R., Morrissey, M. D., Mahadevan, V., Cajanding, J. D., Woodin, M. A., Yeomans, J. S., . . . Kim, J. C. (2014). Parvalbumin and GAD65 interneuron inhibition in the ventral hippocampus induces distinct behavioral deficits relevant to schizophrenia. *J Neurosci*, *34*(45), 14948–14960. doi: 10.1523/JNEUROSCI.2204-14.2014

Noga, J. T., Hyde, T. M., Herman, M. M., Spurney, C. F., Bigelow, L. B., Weinberger, D. R., . . . Kleinman, J. E. (1997). Glutamate receptors in the postmortem striatum of schizophrenic, suicide, and control brains. *Synapse*, 27(3), 168–176. doi: 10.1002/(SICI)1098-2396(199711)27:3<168::AID-SYN2>3.0.CO;2-B

Noga, J. T., & Wang, H. (2002). Further postmortem autoradiographic studies of AMPA receptor binding in schizophrenia. *Synapse*, *45*(4), 250–258. doi: 10.1002/syn.10106

Nordstrom, A. L., Farde, L., Eriksson, L., & Halldin, C. (1995). No elevated D2 dopamine receptors in neuroleptic-naive schizophrenic patients revealed by positron emission tomography and [11C]N-methylspiperone. *Psychiatry Res*, *61*(2), 67–83.

Nusser, Z., Sieghart, W., Benke, D., Fritschy, J. M., & Somogyi, P. (1996). Differential synaptic localization of two major gamma-aminobutyric acid type A receptor alpha subunits on hippocampal pyramidal cells. *Proc Natl Acad Sci U S A*, *93*(21), 11939–11944.

Owen, F., Cross, A. J., Crow, T. J., Lofthouse, R., & Poulter, M. (1981). Neurotransmitter receptors in brain in schizophrenia. *Acta Psychiatr Scand Suppl*, *291*, 20–28.

Papadimitriou, G., Dikeos, D., Daskalopoulou, E., Karadima, G., Avramopoulos, D., Contis, C., . . . Stefanis, C. (2001). Association between GABA-A receptor alpha 5 subunit gene locus and schizophrenia of a later age of onset. *Neuropsychobiology*, *43*(3), 141–144. doi: 54882

Patz, S., Grabert, J., Gorba, T., Wirth, M. J., & Wahle, P. (2004). Parvalbumin expression in visual cortical interneurons depends on neuronal activity and TrkB ligands during an Early period of postnatal development. *Cereb Cortex*, *14*(3), 342–351.

Penttonen, M., Kamondi, A., Acsady, L., & Buzsaki, G. (1998). Gamma frequency oscillation in the hippocampus of the rat: intracellular analysis in vivo. *Eur J Neurosci*, *10*(2), 718–728.

Pitcher, G. M., Beggs, S., Woo, R. S., Mei, L., & Salter, M. W. (2008). ErbB4 is a suppressor of long-term potentiation in the adult hippocampus. *Neuroreport*, *19*(2), 139–143. doi: 10.1097/WNR.0b013e3282f3da10

Pitcher, G. M., Kalia, L. V., Ng, D., Goodfellow, N. M., Yee, K. T., Lambe, E. K., . . . Salter, M. W. (2011). Schizophrenia susceptibility pathway neuregulin 1-ErbB4 suppresses Src upregulation of NMDA receptors. *Nat Med*, *17*(4), 470–478. doi: 10.1038/nm.2315

Ramos, B., Lopez-Tellez, J. F., Vela, J., Baglietto-Vargas, D., del Rio, J. C., Ruano, D., . . . Vitorica, J. (2004). Expression of alpha 5 GABAA receptor subunit in developing rat hippocampus. *Brain Res Dev Brain Res*, *151*(1–2), 87–98. doi: 10.1016/j.devbrainres.2004.04.003

Rao, S. G., Williams, G. V., & Goldman-Rakic, P. S. (2000). Destruction and creation of spatial tuning by disinhibition: GABA(A) blockade of prefrontal cortical neurons engaged by working memory. *J Neurosci*, *20*(1), 485–494.

Reynolds, G. P., Rossor, M. N., & Iversen, L. L. (1983). Preliminary studies of human cortical 5-HT2 receptors and their involvement in schizophrenia and neuroleptic drug action. *J Neural Transm Suppl*, *18*, 273–277.

Schobel, S. A., Chaudhury, N. H., Khan, U. A., Paniagua, B., Styner, M. A., Asllani, I., . . . Small, S. A. (2013). Imaging patients with psychosis and a mouse model establishes a spreading pattern of hippocampal dysfunction and implicates glutamate as a driver. *Neuron*, *78*(1), 81–93. doi: 10.1016/j.neuron.2013.02.011

Schobel, S. A., Kelly, M. A., Corcoran, C. M., Van Heertum, K., Seckinger, R., Goetz, R., . . . Malaspina, D. (2009). Anterior hippocampal and orbitofrontal cortical structural brain abnormalities in association with cognitive deficits in schizophrenia. *Schizophr Res*, *114*(1–3), 110–118. doi: 10.1016/j.schres.2009.07.016

Seeman, P. (1995). Therapeutic receptor-blocking concentrations of neuroleptics. *Int Clin Psychopharmacol*, *10 Suppl* 3, 5–13.

Seeman, P., & Kapur, S. (2000). Schizophrenia: more dopamine, more D2 receptors. *Proc Natl Acad Sci U S A, 97*(14), 7673–7675.

Seeman, P., Lee, T., Chau-Wong, M., & Wong, K. (1976). Antipsychotic drug doses and neuroleptic/dopamine receptors. *Nature, 261*(5562), 717–719.

Seeman, P., & Tallerico, T. (1999). Rapid release of antipsychotic drugs from dopamine D2 receptors: an explanation for low receptor occupancy and early clinical relapse upon withdrawal of clozapine or quetiapine. *Am J Psychiatry, 156*(6), 876–884. doi: 10.1176/ajp.156.6.876

Seeman, P., & Van Tol, H. H. (1995). Deriving the therapeutic concentrations for clozapine and haloperidol: the apparent dissociation constant of a neuroleptic at the dopamine D2 or D4 receptor varies with the affinity of the competing radioligand. *Eur J Pharmacol, 291*(2), 59–66.

Serwanski, D. R., Miralles, C. P., Christie, S. B., Mehta, A. K., Li, X., & De Blas, A. L. (2006). Synaptic and nonsynaptic localization of GABAA receptors containing the alpha5 subunit in the rat brain. *Journal of Comparative Neurology, 499*(3), 458–470. doi: 10.1002/cne.21115

Shepherd, M., & Watt, D. C. (1956). A controlled clinical study of chlorpromazine and reserpine in chronic schizophrenia. *Journal of Neurology, Neurosurgery, and Psychiatry, 19*(3), 232–235.

Slifstein, M., van de Giessen, E., Van Snellenberg, J., Thompson, J. L., Narendran, R., Gil, R., . . . Abi-Dargham, A. (2015). Deficits in prefrontal cortical and extrastriatal dopamine release in schizophrenia: a positron emission tomographic functional magnetic resonance imaging study. *JAMA Psychiatry, 72*(4), 316–324. doi: 10.1001/jamapsychiatry.2014.2414

Stauffer, V. L., Millen, B. A., Andersen, S., Kinon, B. J., Lagrandeur, L., Lindenmayer, J. P., . . . Gomez, J. C. (2013). Pomaglumetad methionil: no significant difference as an adjunctive treatment for patients with prominent negative symptoms of schizophrenia compared to placebo. *Schizophrenia Research, 150*(2–3), 434–441. doi: 10.1016/j.schres.2013.08.020

Stefansson, H., Sarginson, J., Kong, A., Yates, P., Steinthorsdottir, V., Gudfinnsson, E., . . . St Clair, D. (2003). Association of neuregulin 1 with schizophrenia confirmed in a Scottish population. *American Journal of Human Genetics, 72*(1), 83–87.

Stefansson, H., Sigurdsson, E., Steinthorsdottir, V., Bjornsdottir, S., Sigmundsson, T., Ghosh, S., . . . Stefansson, K. (2002). Neuregulin 1 and susceptibility to schizophrenia. *American Journal of Human Genetics, 71*(4), 877–892. doi: 10.1086/342734

Steullet, P., Cabungcal, J. H., Kulak, A., Kraftsik, R., Chen, Y., Dalton, T. P., . . . Do, K. Q. (2010). Redox dysregulation affects the ventral but not dorsal hippocampus: impairment of parvalbumin neurons, gamma oscillations, and related behaviors. *Journal of Neuroscience, 30*(7), 2547–2558. doi: 10.1523/JNEUROSCI.3857-09.2010

Stone, J. M., Day, F., Tsagaraki, H., Valli, I., McLean, M. A., Lythgoe, D. J., . . . Oasis. (2009). Glutamate dysfunction in people with prodromal symptoms of psychosis: relationship to gray matter volume. *Biological Psychiatry, 66*(6), 533–539. doi: 10.1016/j.biopsych.2009.05.006

Stone, J. M., Howes, O. D., Egerton, A., Kambeitz, J., Allen, P., Lythgoe, D. J., . . . McGuire, P. (2010). Altered relationship between hippocampal glutamate levels and striatal dopamine function in subjects at ultra high risk of psychosis. *Biological Psychiatry, 68*(7), 599–602. doi: 10.1016/j.biopsych.2010.05.034

Sun, Q. Q. (2009). Experience-dependent intrinsic plasticity in interneurons of barrel cortex layer IV. Journal of Neurophysiology, *102*(5), 2955–2973. doi: 10.1152/jn.00562.2009

Swerdlow, N. R., Hanlon, F. M., Henning, L., Kim, Y. K., Gaudet, I., & Halim, N. D. (2001). Regulation of sensorimotor gating in rats by hippocampal NMDA: anatomical localization. *Brain Research, 898*(2), 195–203.

Swerdlow, N. R., Platten, A., Kim, Y. K., Gaudet, I., Shoemaker, J., Pitcher, L., . . . Auerbach, P. (2001). Sensitivity to the dopaminergic regulation of prepulse inhibition in rats: evidence for genetic, but not environmental determinants. *Pharmacology Biochemistry and Behavior, 70*(2–3), 219–226.

Swerdlow, N. R., Shoemaker, J. M., Bongiovanni, M. J., Neary, A. C., Tochen, L. S., & Saint Marie, R. L. (2005). Reduced startle gating after D1 blockade: effects of concurrent D2 blockade. *Pharmacology Biochemistry and Behavior, 82*(2), 293–299. doi: 10.1016/j.pbb.2005.08.018

Tan, J., Chen, S., Su, L., Long, J., Xie, J., Shen, T., . . . Gu, L. (2014). Association of the T102C polymorphism in the HTR2A gene with major depressive disorder, bipolar disorder, and schizophrenia. *American Journal of Medical Genetics Part B: Neuropsychiatric Genetics, 165B*(5), 438–455. doi: 10.1002/ajmg.b.32248

Towers, S. K., Gloveli, T., Traub, R. D., Driver, J. E., Engel, D., Fradley, R., . . . Whittington, M. A. (2004). Alpha 5 subunit-containing GABAA receptors affect the dynamic range of mouse hippocampal kainate-induced gamma frequency oscillations in vitro. *Journal of Physiology, 559*(Pt 3), 721–728. doi: 10.1113/jphysiol.2004.071191

Trichard, C., Paillere-Martinot, M. L., Attar-Levy, D., Blin, J., Feline, A., & Martinot, J. L. (1998). No serotonin 5-HT2A receptor density abnormality in the cortex of schizophrenic patients studied with PET. *Schizophrenia Research, 31*(1), 13–17.

Valenti, O., Cifelli, P., Gill, K. M., & Grace, A. A. (2011). Antipsychotic drugs rapidly induce dopamine neuron depolarization block in a developmental rat model of schizophrenia. *Journal of Neuroscience, 31*(34), 12330–12338. doi: 10.1523/JNEUROSCI.2808-11.2011

Volk, D., Austin, M., Pierri, J., Sampson, A., & Lewis, D. (2001). GABA transporter-1 mRNA in the prefrontal cortex in schizophrenia: decreased expression in a subset of neurons. *American Journal of Psychiatry, 158*(2), 256–265. doi: 10.1176/appi.ajp.158.2.256

Volk, D. W., Pierri, J. N., Fritschy, J. M., Auh, S., Sampson, A. R., & Lewis, D. A. (2002). Reciprocal alterations in pre- and postsynaptic inhibitory markers at chandelier cell inputs to pyramidal neurons in schizophrenia. *Cerebal Cortex, 12*(10), 1063–1070.

Vollenweider, F. X., Leenders, K. L., Scharfetter, C., Maguire, P., Stadelmann, O., & Angst, J. (1997). Positron emission tomography and fluorodeoxyglucose studies of metabolic hyperfrontality and psychopathology in the psilocybin model of psychosis. *Neuropsychopharmacology, 16*(5), 357–372. doi: 10.1016/S0893-133X(96)00246-1

Wang, X. J., & Buzsaki, G. (1996). Gamma oscillation by synaptic inhibition in a hippocampal interneuronal network model. *J Neuroscience, 16*(20), 6402–6413.

Weinberger, D., & Laruelle, M. (2001). Neurochemical and neuropharmacological imaging in schizophrenia. In K. L. Davis (Ed.), *Neuropsychopharmacology: The Fifth Generation of Progress* (pp. 833–856). New York, NY: Lippincott, Williams, & Wilkins.

Weinberger, D. R. (1987). Implications of normal brain development for the pathogenesis of schizophrenia. *Archives of General Psychiatry, 44*(7), 660–669.

Whitaker, P. M., Crow, T. J., & Ferrier, I. N. (1981). Tritiated LSD binding in frontal cortex in schizophrenia. *Archives of General Psychiatry, 38*(3), 278–280.

Whittington, M. A., Traub, R. D., & Jefferys, J. G. (1995). Synchronized oscillations in interneuron networks driven by metabotropic glutamate receptor activation. *Nature, 373*(6515), 612–615. doi: 10.1038/373612a0

Williams, H. J., Owen, M. J., & O'Donovan, M. C. (2007). Is COMT a susceptibility gene for schizophrenia? *Schizophrenia Bulletin, 33*(3), 635–641. doi: 10.1093/schbul/sbm019

Wong, D. F., Pearlson, G. D., Tune, L. E., Young, L. T., Meltzer, C. C., Dannals, R. F., . . . Gjedde, A. (1997). Quantification of neuroreceptors in the living human brain: IV. Effect of aging and elevations of D2-like receptors in schizophrenia and bipolar illness. *Journal of Cerebral Blood Flow & Metabolism, 17*(3), 331–342. doi: 10.1097/00004647-199703000-00010

Woolley, M. L., Pemberton, D. J., Bate, S., Corti, C., & Jones, D. N. (2008). The mGlu2 but not the mGlu3 receptor mediates the actions of the mGluR2/3 agonist, LY379268, in mouse models predictive of antipsychotic activity. *Psychopharmacology (Berlin), 196*(3), 431–440. doi: 10.1007/s00213-007-0974-x

Xi, D., Li, Y. C., Snyder, M. A., Gao, R. Y., Adelman, A. E., Zhang, W., . . . Gao, W. J. (2011). Group II metabotropic glutamate receptor agonist ameliorates MK801-induced dysfunction of NMDA receptors via the Akt/GSK-3beta pathway in adult rat prefrontal cortex. *Neuropsychopharmacology, 36*(6), 1260–1274. doi: 10.1038/npp.2011.12

Young, K. A., Randall, P. K., & Wilcox, R. E. (1995). Startle and sensorimotor correlates of ventral thalamic dopamine and GABA in rodents. *Neuroreport, 6*(18), 2495–2499.

Zawarynski, P., Tallerico, T., Seeman, P., Lee, S. P., O'Dowd, B. F., & George, S. R. (1998). Dopamine D2 receptor dimers in human and rat brain. *FEBS Letters, 441*(3), 383–386.

Zhang, Z., Sun, J., & Reynolds, G. P. (2002). A selective reduction in the relative density of parvalbumin-immunoreactive neurons in the hippocampus in schizophrenia patients. *Chinese Medical Journal (English Edition), 115*(6), 819–823.

/// 11 /// THE ROLE OF NEUROPEPTIDES IN SCHIZOPHRENIA

WANLOP ATSARIYASING
and MORRIS GOLDMAN

> *For schizophrenia our knowledge base in 2010 is mostly based on clinical observation... we still do not have a basic understanding of the pathophysiology of the disorder and therefore lack the tools for curative treatment.*
>
> Thomas Insel, MD; Director NIMH; Nature (2010) 468, 187

> *In order for research on mental disorders to more fully harness the scientific power of brain-behavior science, sound efforts must be made to redefine mental disorders into dimensions or components of observable behaviors that are more closely aligned with the biology of the brain.*
>
> NIMH Strategic Plan, Objective 1

INTRODUCTION

Neuropeptides contain 5–50 amino acids arranged linearly (i.e., polypeptides). They are synthesized as ribosomal preprohormones, cleaved and then typically post-translationally modified. Most neuropeptides are coreleased with classic neurotransmitters, albeit under more restricted conditions and at much lower concentrations. Neuropeptides function as neurohormones, neurotransmitters, growth factors, and inflammatory mediators in the central nervous system (CNS), some having additional roles in the periphery (Hoyer & Bartfai, 2012). Acute release typically occurs in response to challenges (e.g., physical or psychological stress, physical injury, substance injection), and receptors are more localized than those of classic neurotransmitters. Neuropeptide receptors are generally G-protein coupled seven-transmembrane proteins (GPCRs), and typically have several subtypes and splice variants. Technological advances in the past decade have enhanced the ability to systematically "deorphanaize" neuropeptides and their receptors, which has accelerated the discovery and localization of new neuropeptides (Griebel & Holsboer, 2012). Together these observations indicate neuropeptides and their receptors can potentially localize neuropathology and provide targeted treatment of neuropsychiatric disorders (Hoyer & Bartfai, 2012).

OBSERVATIONS PROMPTING THEN TEMPERING ENTHUSIASM FOR STUDIES OF PATHOPHYSIOLOGY

This potential utility of neuropeptides seems particularly relevant to schizophrenia. Many neuropeptides are found in dopamine neurons located in structures implicated in schizophrenia (i.e., the nucleus accumbens, the amygdala, the prefrontal cortex, the ventral tegmental area) and alterations in neuropeptide activity have been reported to covary with neural functions thought relevant to the pathophysiology of the illness (Caceda, Kinkead, & Nemeroff, 2007; McGonigle, 2012). Concentrations of neuropeptides and their precursors in the cerebrospinal fluid (CSF) or brain tissue are often reported to differ in persons with and without schizophrenia. Box 11.1 lists some of these findings for different neuropeptide families; recent reviews provide more detail about individual neuropeptide systems (Caceda et al., 2007; Hoyer & Bartfai, 2012).

The findings in Box 1 are not necessarily consistent across studies (Caceda et al., 2007), but in any event have led to few insights into the pathophysiology or treatment options for schizophrenia. A 2007 comprehensive review concluded that "Overall, the clinical data implicating a preeminent role for one or another neuropeptide in schizophrenia is not strong," and "a clear role . . . in the etiology, pathophysiology and treatment . . . has not been consistently demonstrated" (Caceda et al., 2007). No major advances relevant to schizophrenia, per se, have been noted since that time. Why, given the likely involvement of neuropeptide activity in limbic functions relevant to schizophrenia and the more than 1200 scientific articles on the subject, has progress been so limited? Barriers specific to neuropeptide research (Box 11.2), as well as problems

BOX 11.1

OBSERVATIONS IMPLICATING NEUROPEPTIDES IN SCHIZOPHRENIA

- Localized in limbic structures implicated in schizophrenia.[a,b,d,e,f,g, h, j]
- Differences from controls in cerebral spinal fluid levels of neuropeptides.[a,b,c,d,f]
  - Some of these differences parallel psychopathology (e.g., negative symptoms).[c, d]
- Postmortem differences in concentration of neuropeptides, associated mRNAs or their receptor binding in brain structures associated with schizophrenia.[a,b,d,e,f,g, i]
- Functional interactions with dopamine activity in mammals.[a,c,d,g, j]
- Polymorphisms in the promoter region or introns of neuropeptides or their receptors genetically linked to schizophrenia.[a,c,i]
- Neuropeptide activation/reduction reproduce features of the mental disorder in humans or animal models.[c,d,j]
  - Some of these are reversed by antipsychotics/peptide activation.[j]

---

[a] *Cholecystokinin (CCK)*
[b] *corticotropin-releasing factor (CRF)*
[c] *interleukins(IL)*
[d] *neurotensin (NT)*
[e] *Neuropeptide Y (NPY)*
[f] *opiod peptides*
[g] *neurokinins (NK)*
[h] *hypocretin/orexin*
[i] *neuroregulan (NRG1)*
[j] *oxytocin*

associated with the prevailing research paradigm in biological psychiatry are thought to be responsible (Kapur, Phillips, & Insel, 2012; Keshavan, Nasrallah, & Tandon, 2011). Examples of the former include the absence of reproducible marked differences in neuropeptide density in the brains of schizophrenia patients (e.g., analogous to the diminished hypocretin density found in narcolepsy[i]) and the absence of PET ligands for many neuropeptide receptors. As a consequence, investigators have been unable to identify specific neuropeptides or localize neuropathology to discrete neurons. In living humans, neuropeptide levels are typically measured in CSF. Our limited understanding of neuropeptide function and inability to localize abnormal activity is a major barrier to interpreting this data.

BOX 11.2

ISSUES TEMPERING ENTHUSIASM FOR ROLE OF NEUROPEPTIDES IN SCHIZOPHRENIA

- Absence of clear differences in neuropeptide distribution in patients versus controls.
  - Especially in mesolimbic dopamine pathways.
- Inadequate methods of measuring activity in humans (particularly antemortem).
  - Problems interpreting cerebrospinal fluid levels and post-mortem concentrations.
- Relatively weak genetic linkage of neuropeptides to schizophrenia.
  - Possible exception being neuroregulin1 (NRG1).

OBSERVATIONS PROMPTING THEN TEMPERING ENTHUSIASM FOR DEVELOPING PEPTIDE ANALOGUES

Many pharmaceutical trials for schizophrenia over the past 40 years focused on the dopamine D2 receptor, despite accumulating evidence that this target was unlikely to yield new agents with greater efficacy (Pratt, Winchester, Dawson, & Morris, 2012; Sarter & Tricklebank, 2012). The limited response of the illness and adverse effects of available antipsychotics has left a tremendous burden on society (Hyman, 2012; T. R. Insel, 2010) and fueled efforts to identify novel therapies. Unfortunately, subsequent efforts to modulate other neurotransmitters have not provided new therapies, as exemplified by results from two highly publicized trials of glutamatergic agents in schizophrenia (Griebel & Holsboer, 2012; Sarter & Tricklebank, 2012).

Several properties of neuropeptides, in addition to the findings summarized in Box 11.1, have encouraged development of neuropeptide analogues as potential therapies for schizophrenia (Box 11.3). The results of these efforts have also been disappointing. Thus, subsequent to the discovery in the late 1980s that cholecystokinin (CCK) induces panic attacks in many normal subjects (as well as nearly everyone with panic disorder) (Bowers, Choi, & Ressler, 2012), CCK antagonists were found to be ineffective for both anxiety disorders and schizophrenia (Caceda et al., 2007; Griebel & Holsboer, 2012). At about the same time, preliminary evidence that some opioid peptides appeared to be effective treatments in schizophrenia could not be reproduced (Caceda et al., 2007). Negative results of these studies were attributed to heterogeneity of the disorders, inadequate dosing, poor absorption, pharmacokinetic parameters and specificity of the compounds.

BOX 11.3

FACTORS PROMPTING DEVELOPMENT OF NEUROPEPTIDE THERAPIES FOR SCHIZOPHRENIA

- Some neuropeptide effects resemble effects of antipsychotics.
- More localized to CNS structures implicated in severe mental illness than classical neurotransmitters.
- Activity more restricted to psychologically relevant stimuli than classic neurotransmitters.
- Highly preserved across mammalian species.
- Rapid advances in understanding structure and regulation of neuropeptide genes, their transcription and translation.
- Receptor class (i.e., G protein coupled: GPCR) is particularly amenable to pharmacologic manipulation.
- Existence of highly selective neuropeptide receptor sub-type agonists and antagonists.
- Low synaptic concentration (relative to classic neurotransmitters) means less of a challenge to deliver drug.
- Redundancy of function of other peptides diminishes likelihood of adverse effects.

In 1998, the antidepressant effects of a neurokinin (NK) 1 (aka Substance P) antagonist were demonstrated in a placebo-controlled trial in depressed patients (Griebel & Holsboer, 2012). By this time, medicinal chemists were able to synthesize nonpeptidergic analogues, which addressed some of the earlier problems [i.e. improved absorption, distribution, metabolism, excretion (ADME)], thus encouraging further study. A host of trials in schizophrenia patients of NKs and other neuropeptides (i.e. tachykinins, vasopressin (AVP), corticotrophin-releasing factor (CRF), neurotensin) were initiated. Early results typically showed promise, but not the later and larger studies. In particular, NK3 receptor antagonists, which are known to modulate dopaminergic function, were found to be ineffective in three separate trials (Griebel & Holsboer, 2012). Neurotensin analogues, which exhibit antipsychotic properties in animal models, also provided inconclusive results (Meltzer, Arvanitis, Bauer, Rein, & Meta-Trial Study, 2004). As of 2014, only seven of the current ~100 phase II/III trials for neuropsychiatric disorders target neuropeptide receptors [AVP (3), NK (2), CRF (1) nociopeptin (1)], and only one is for persons with schizophrenia (NK1/3 antagonist; Griebel & Holsboer, 2012). Again, it appears specific barriers to developing effective neuropeptide analogues (Box 11.4) as well as limitations of the prevailing research paradigm (see the following section) are likely responsible (McGonigle, 2012; Smith et al., 2014).

BOX 11.4

CHALLENGES TO DEVELOPMENT OF NEUROPEPTIDE THERAPIES FOR SCHIZOPHRENIA

- Screening until now largely based on modifying indices of dopamine activity, which likely reflect a small part of the disease's responsiveness to treatment and have no face validity.
- Synthesis of compounds absorbed from the GI tract, resistant to gut and circulatory peptidases, and capable of crossing into the brain is a daunting task.
    - Particularly for larger structurally complex neuropeptides.
- Receptor properties in rodents and primates frequently differ.
- Some targets are likely heterodimers complicating identification of potentially active agents in animal models.
- Internalization of receptors can lead to rapid desensitization.
- Activity of multiple neuropeptides at same receptor can dilute efficacy.

RECENT TECHNOLOGICAL ADVANCES AND A REVISED RESEARCH PARADIGM RENEW ENTHUSIASM

Although initial enthusiasm for neuropeptide research in schizophrenia is diminished, the future holds promise (Griebel & Holsboer, 2012; Hoyer & Bartfai, 2012). Some of the barriers noted in Boxes 11.2 and 11.4 reflect problems with synthesis and screening of selective and efficacious novel agents. Recent advances summarized in Box 11.5 should help overcome these issues. For instance, advances in X-ray crystallography now provide the structure of agonist-GPCR and antagonist-GPCR complexes, other discoveries enhance drug delivery into the blood stream and brain, and others prolong drug half-life (McGonigle, 2012; Sarter & Tricklebank, 2012).

Perhaps the major barrier to progress, however, has been the conceptual framework underlying the prevailing research paradigm for schizophrenia (Hyman, 2012; Sarter & Tricklebank, 2012). Thus, research subjects are typically grouped by *DSM* disease criteria, despite acknowledgment of heterogeneity across diagnoses and growing awareness that genetic contributions (and thus the pathophysiology) rarely adhere to *DSM* catagories (Keshavan et al., 2011; Rapoport, Giedd, & Gogtay, 2012). According to the prevailing paradigm, unexplained differences between healthy controls and patients are typically interpreted as abnormalities, despite awareness of the complexity and plasticity of the human brain. Given these properties, the vast majority of findings are more likely to instead reflect the following: adaptations, compensations, epiphenomena or

BOX 11.5

RECENT TECHNOLOGIC ADVANCES FURTHERING NEUROPEPTIDE RESEARCH

- Structure-based drug design facilitated by agonist-receptor and antagonist-receptor GPCR x-ray crystallography of G-protein (GP).
- Structural modification of peptides with D-amino acids, N-terminal acetylation, C-amidation, beta or gamma amines, attachment of fatty acid or PEG, cyclization prolong drug half-life.
- Advances in delivery technology (e.g. injectable microspheres, intranasal insufflation, transdermal, liposomal encapsulation) of peptides.
- Enhanced brain delivery by linking compounds to ligands/antibodies that undergo receptor-mediated transport across the blood-brain barrier.
- New animal models not based on dopaminergic neurotransmitter bioassays.
- Recognition of the diversity of GPCR functions and how they can be modified.
- New technologies of high throughput screening for peptides/nonpeptides.
- Recombinant DNA technology enhancing production of large quantities of peptides.
- Transgenic animals permit testing of localized changes in neuropeptide activity.
  - Particularly important since synthesis of bioavailable, brain-penetrating agents is complicated.

downstream consequences of the abnormalities (Karatsoreos & McEwen, 2011). The approach to each of these categories should be very different but is rarely acknowledged.

The directors of the NIMH have been particularly vocal about these issues (Hyman, 2012; Kapur et al., 2012), as well as serving as major contributors to the revised conceptual framework (Insel & Gogtay, 2014). These revisions are particularly apparent in the new research domain criteria (RDoC) (T. Insel et al., 2010) as well as the expectations for trials with potentially novel therapeutic agents (T. R. Insel & Gogtay, 2014). Differences between the prevailing and revised paradigms are particularly striking when considering strategies for identifying new treatments for schizophrenia (Box 11.6). The prevailing model sees schizophrenia as a consequence of disrupted higher cortical functions unique to humans. To effectively treat schizophrenia, one focuses on psychosis, which cannot be reproduced in animal models. Altered neurotransmitter activity (e.g., elevated dopamine activity, diminished GABA activity, diminished NMDA activity) in limbic neurons is posited to produce psychosis (Sarter & Tricklebank, 2012). Markers of this neurotransmitter activity are identified to evaluate therapeutic efficacy in animals, but the mechanisms that account for the biomarkers is of little interest. The biomarkers themselves are not thought to reflect relevant features of the mental illness, and indeed

BOX 11.6

PREVAILING AND REVISED RESEARCH PARADIGMS

- Prevailing: Schizophrenia is a product of altered neurotransmitter function.
  - Revised: Schizophrenia is product of disrupted functional neural circuits.
- Prevailing: Schizophrenia is caused by disruption of higher order cortical functions.
  - Revised: Schizophrenia is a heterogeneous disorder that in some cases may be caused by dysfunction in circuits common to all mammals.
- Prevailing: Animal models cannot reproduce the pathophysiology of schizophrenia
  - Revised: Animal models can reproduce features of the illness.
- Prevailing: Psychosis is a direct reflection of the pathologic process.
  - Psychosis may be a downstream consequence of the pathologic process.
- Prevailing: Symptom clusters, particularly psychosis, should be the focus of pathophysiologic studies.
  - Schizophrenia must be broken down into different features associated with characterized functional circuitry and associated biomarkers.
- Prevailing: Mechanisms of animal behaviors are of limited interest because other mammals can exhibit psychosis.
  - Revised: Clarifying mechanisms of features of the illness in other mammals is critical to understanding and treating schizophrenia.
- Prevailing: If demographic and treatment variables are accounted for, otherwise unexplained differences between patients and controls reflect abnormal function.
  - Revised: Most findings are compensations, epiphenomenon or downstream consequences of the core pathology.

the prevailing paradigm stresses that animal models are incapable of demonstrating key features of the illness.

In contrast, the revised paradigm seeks to identify particular features of the psychiatric illness (e.g., impaired neuropeptide function, impaired affect recognition, enhanced social withdrawal, increased aggression, increased fear, diminished stress tolerance, working memory), which can be modeled in other mammals (Sarter & Tricklebank, 2012; Tandon & Goldman, 2014). This requires "deconstructing the concept of schizophrenia, and then reconstructing the defined elements" (Tandon, Nasrallah, & Keshavan, 2009). Such an effort it is hoped will result in a research-based description of the key elements of mental disorders, providing even greater traction on the potential mechanisms that can cause mental suffering and targets for more effective preemption and treatment. A major goal is the identification of biomarkers for this neurocircuit activity and dysfunction (Hyman, 2012; Sarter & Tricklebank, 2012). Treatments will then be directed to dysfunctional circuits and their biomarkers (Insel & Gogtay, 2014). These elements are unlikely to adhere to *DSM* categories and, thus, schizophrenia is likely the "final common pathway" for different neuropathologic processes. As a consequence, the core pathology in at least some instance may be located in neurosystems common to all mammals, whereas psychosis results from the impact this pathology has on higher cortical functions unique to humans

APPLICATION OF THE REVISED PARADIGM TO NEUROPEPTIDE RESEARCH

It is readily apparent the revised paradigm relies on mechanisms and animal models. The neuropeptide research literature is beginning to reflect this shift. For example, a recent review addresses how neuropeptides associated with schizophrenia (i.e., urocortins, nocicptin, substance P, neuropeptide S, Neuorpeptide Y, and dynorphin) act at different nodes of the neurocircuitry modulating responses to psychological stress (Schank, Ryabinin, Giardino, Ciccocioppo, & Heilig, 2012). Similarly, another recent review addresses how neuropeptide findings (CCK, Neuropeptide Y, nociptin, and other compounds active at opioid receptors) may reflect neurocircuit effects on fear expression and extinction (Bowers et al., 2012). A recent study applies optogenetics to characterize how hypocretins modulate arousal circuitry and interact with other key modulators of arousal (e.g., norepinephrine) (de Lecea, Carter, & Adamantidis, 2012).

CAPITALIZING ON FEATURES OF OXYTOCIN AND VASOPRESSIN REGULATION AND ACTION

The remaining parts of this chapter summarize a series of studies involving the neurohypophyseal neuropeptides, oxytocin and vasopressin (see review by Goldman 2009, 2014 for additional details). The studies relied on the conceptual framework of the revised paradigm, and thus may offer some insights into its advantages and limitations. Some of the features of the revised paradigm include the focus on a distinct subset of schizophrenia patients with a clearly abnormal finding; research designs based on our understanding of neurocircuit functions common to mammals; utilization of animal models to assess mechanisms; and the inclusion of other schizophrenia patients, rather than healthy normals as controls. Properties of the neurohypophyseal systems provide ideal conditions for peripheral peptide levels to function as biomarkers of central circuit activity and functions. Furthermore, recognized modulators of peptide activity can often be identified. Therefore, specific abnormalities can be identified and those findings reflecting compensatory responses can be eliminated.

PROPERTIES OF CENTRAL/PERIPHERAL VASOPRESSIN AND OXYTOCIN

Oxytocin and vasopressin are nearly identical, phylogenetically preserved nonapeptides that are synthesized in adjacent hypothalamic magnocellular neurons in the paraventricular (PVN) and supraoptic nuclei (SON). Their axons terminate in blood vessels in the posterior pituitary (neurohypophysis), thereby gaining direct access to the peripheral blood stream (Figure 11.1). Thus, unlike other neuropeptides, peripheral vasopressin levels are a direct reflection of CNS function. Vasopressin is tightly regulated because it determines salt concentration in plasma (as well as in other extracellular fluids), which is normally maintained within a very narrow band (± 2 percent). Vasopressin secretion from the brain is primarily regulated by plasma sodium levels detected in the third ventricle, but secretion is modulated by other neural circuits involved in physical and psychological stress responsiveness. Many of these influences are well characterized and their influence on vasopressin secretion can be measured or controlled (Robertson, 2006). Hence, peripheral vasopressin provides a biomarker, which can potentially assess the integrity of a number of CNS circuits that modulate its secretion.

In addition to the peripheral blood stream, the dendrites of the same magnocellular neurons also release vasopressin directly into the brain. Within the brain, vasopressin modulates memory, anxiety, and aspects of male social behaviors (Insel, 2010). Some of these functions are disrupted in schizophrenia and thus vasopressin actions in the brain could be relevant to the psychiatric disorder. However, peripheral vasopressin cannot serve as a biomarker for central vasopressin effects because most central vasopressin is not derived from magnocellular dendrites, central and peripheral release of vasopressin seem independent of each other, and central vasopressin functions have not been characterized in humans (Meyer-Lindenberg, Domes, Kirsch, & Heinrichs, 2011).

Peripheral oxytocin, in contrast to vasopressin, although not as tightly regulated (its only constitutive function is to facilitate milk letdown) can serve as a biomarker for central oxytocin effects. Like vasopressin, oxytocin is released into the brain from the dendrites of magnocellular neurons (Figure 11.1). Although their peripheral actions are unrelated, central oxytocin and vasopressin both alter social behavior. Oxytocin's central effects are generally opposite to those seen with vasopressin, leading to the notation that they are "yin and yang" CNS hormones (Legros, 2001). Oxytocin enhances social awareness and behavior as well as diminishes the responses to most psychological stressors (Insel, 2010). Unlike vasopressin, some of these oxytocin effects in humans have been characterized. Again, unlike vasopressin, magnocellular release of oxytocin appears to account for most of the oxytocin in the brain, (Landgraf & Neumann, 2004) and furthermore, central release appears to be correlated with peripheral oxytocin activity

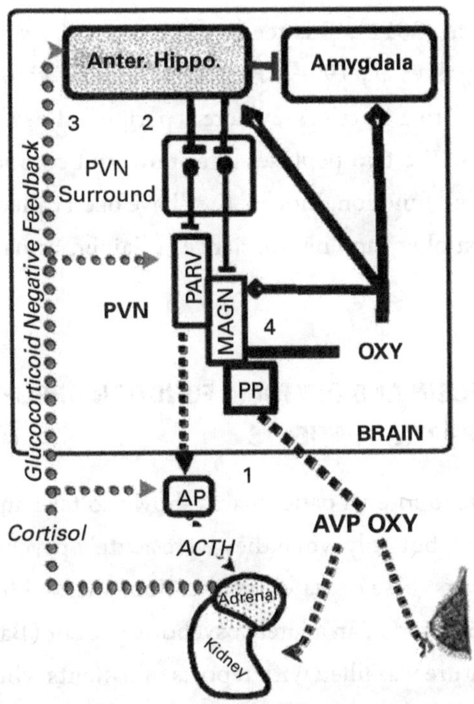

FIGURE 11.1 Model of neurocircuitry underlying central and peripheral neuropeptide dysfunction in schizophrenia patients with water imbalance. (1) Neuroendocrine secretion from hypothalamic magnocellular neurons in the paraventricular (and supraoptic—not shown) nuclei release vasopressin and oxytocin directly into the peripheral circulation. These closely related neuropeptides regulate water excretion and lactation, respectively. Peripheral vasopressin levels are tightly regulated by salt concentration in plasma as well as several other factors (e.g. blood pressure, blood volume), which can be measured or controlled. Stress-hormone secretagogues are released from adjacent PVN neurons into the hypophyseal circulation where they modulate cortisol secretion by inducing adrenocorticotropin release from the anterior pituitary. (2) Projections from the lateral anterior hippocampus (AH) relay in the "PVN surround" and terminate in the paraventricular nucleus where they restrain vasopressin and stress-hormone activity during psychological stress. This pathway may also modulate oxytocin release. Because peripheral vasopressin secretion is directly regulated by the brain, it provides a means of assessing the integrity of this central pathway. (3) The hippocampal influence on the PVN is partly regulated by glucocorticoid negative feedback, which can also be indexed by altering peripheral stress hormone activity. (4) The dendrites on magnocellular neurons also release vasopressin and oxytocin directly into the brain where these peptides modulate responses to psychological stress and other social stimuli. Dendritic release accounts for most of the oxytocin in the brain, and this release parallels peripheral oxytocin secretion, especially during psychological stress. Oxytocin acts at the hippocampus and amygdala to enhance social behaviors, which are disrupted in schizophrenia, particularly in those with water imbalance. Oxytocin's effects on specific social related activity predictive of functional disability in schizophrenia, can be quantified in patients. For these reasons, peripheral oxytocin provides a marker of oxytocin's influence on social function. The involvement of oxytocin can be further assessed by intranasal administration. Abbreviations: PVN–paraventricular nucleus of the hypothalamus; PVN–surround: area around the PVN, which relays subcortical afferents to the PVN; OXY– oxytocin; AVP– vasopressin; AP– anterior pituitary; ACTH– adrenocorticotropin; PARV–parvocellular neurons; MAGN–magnocellular neurons.

(Meyer-Lindenberg et al., 2011). This seems to be particularly apparent following psychological stress (Wotjak et al., 1998). Hence, peripheral vasopressin is a biomarker for neurocircuits modulating its release, whereas peripheral oxytocin is a biomarker for central oxytocin effects. The two peptides offer powerful complementary measures of limbic circuit activity and function. Indeed, they have been called the "veritable Rosetta stone for neuroendocrinology and neuroscience" (Gainer, Yamashita, Fields, House, & Rusnak, 2002).

STUDIES OF VASOPRESSIN AND OXYTOCIN FUNCTION APPLIED TO A SUBSET OF SCHIZOPHRENIA PATIENTS

In 1923, a subset of schizophrenia patients was shown to take an abnormally long time to excrete ingested water, but only when they were acutely psychotic (Targowla, 1923). Fifteen years later, the first case of water intoxication (marked hyponatremia, seizures, coma, or death) was observed in an acutely psychotic patient (Barahal, 1938). Over the next 40 years, the literature was filled with reports of patients whose salt concentrations were abnormally low (i.e. hyponatremic) during exacerbations of their psychotic illness (de Leon, Verghese, Tracy, Josiassen, & Simpson, 1994).

Shortly after the radioimmunoassay for vasopressin was developed in 1975, patients with hyponatremia were observed to have inappropriately elevated plasma vasopressin levels (Raskind, Orenstein, & Christopher, 1975). Subsequently, in 1988, the vasopressin finding was confirmed to be a subtle and unexplained shift in the relationship between plasma sodium and plasma vasopressin (i.e., syndrome of inappropriate antidiuretic hormone secretion (SIADH), type C; Goldman, Luchins, & Robertson, 1988). About 10 years later, another study showed that this shift could be induced in these (but not other schizophrenia patients) by acute psychosis (M. B. Goldman, Robertson, Luchins, Hedeker, & Pandey, 1997). These studies linked an abnormality in vasopressin regulation to altered neurocircuit influences exacerbated by psychosis.

A concurrent brain-imaging study in 1997 suggested that anterior hippocampal volume was diminished in these patients relative to others with schizophrenia (Luchins, Nettles, & Goldman, 1997). Converging evidence had begun to link this part of the hippocampus to schizophrenia and to stress hormone regulation (Herman, Dolgas, & Carlson, 1998). Previous studies had identified enhanced stress hormone activity in patients with, relative to those without, water imbalance, thereby raising the possibility that neuroendocrine dysfunction was not limited to vasopressin (M. B. Goldman, 2009). Research had shown that the hippocampal influence on stress hormone activity involved a projection to the hypothalamus, which restrained stress hormone activity only during psychological stressors. The neurons responsible for stress hormone activity are in the PVN, adjacent to the neurons that secrete vasopressin and oxytocin (Risold & Swanson, 1996). Hence, it seemed plausible that this projection also influenced these neuropeptides. Animal studies confirmed this prediction (Figure 11.1) (Nettles, Pesold, & Goldman, 2000), and indeed these findings were reproduced in an animal model of schizophrenia, which disrupts neurodevelopment of this hippocampal segment. Together these observations raised the possibility that anterior hippocampal pathology might underlie the neurocircuit dysfunction responsible for the vasopressin abnormality.

ASSESSING HIPPOCAMPAL MODULATION OF STRESS HORMONE AND VASOPRESSIN ACTIVITY

Three studies were designed to test this hypothesis. The first demonstrated, as predicted, that vasopressin and stress hormone responses to psychological (but not physical) stress were enhanced in hyponatremic patients. The effect on vasopressin secretion resembled that seen following acute psychosis, suggesting that the psychological stress of acute psychosis may have produced the reset osmostat (M. B. Goldman, 2009). In contrast to patients with hyponatremia, other patients with schizophrenia demonstrated blunted vasopressin and stress-hormone responses, which appeared to be a physiologic adaptation to chronic stress (M. B. Goldman, 2014). The second study characterized hippocampal-mediated glucocorticoid negative feedback, which provides a means of assessing hippocampal restraint of stress hormone activity (Figure 11.1). As predicted, this function was markedly impaired in hyponatremic patients. A third study analyzed the shape of the hippocampus. The study identified deformations in hyponatremic patients with and without polydipsia on the hippocampal surface (anterior lateral) that modulates neuroendocrine responses to stress. Patients without water imbalance exhibited deformations on other hippocampal surfaces (M. B. Goldman, Wang, et al., 2011). The severity of the deformations in the patients with water imbalance was proportional to the extent of their enhanced vasopressin secretion. Together these studies provided strong support that hippocampal pathology is responsible for the abnormal vasopressin regulation in patients with water imbalance.

PERIPHERAL OXYTOCIN INDEXES CENTRAL OXYTOCIN FUNCTIONS THAT ARE LINKED TO SCHIZOPHRENIA

The relationship of the neuroendocrine dysfunction to the underlying mental illness was, however, unclear. Thus, even if the hippocampal deformations were linked to the underlying mental illness, the neuropeptide findings could just as easily be a nonspecific byproduct (i.e., "collateral damage") as they could be biomarkers of central neuropeptide dysfunction integral to the mental illness. Studies with peripheral vasopressin were unlikely to clarify this issue, since peripheral vasopressin cannot provide a measure of central vasopressin activity.

Peripheral oxytocin, however, is such a biomarker. Peripheral oxytocin appears to be modulated by the same hippocampal pathway that influences peripheral vasopressin and stress hormone activity (though this has not been confirmed) (Figure 11.1). Peripheral oxytocin levels predict cognitive and social function measures that are impaired in schizophrenia. These impairments are particularly prominent in those with water imbalance (M. B. Goldman, Wang, et al., 2011). Among these measures is the ability to distinguish facial emotions (Marsh, Yu, Pine, & Blair, 2010), which is consistently linked to core features of the mental illness (Addington, Girard, Christensen, & Addington, 2010).

Plasma oxytocin levels were obtained and found to be lower in patients with, but not without, water imbalance. Furthermore, lower levels of oxytocin were found in those with more impaired facial affect recognition (M. Goldman, Marlow-O'Connor, Torres, & Carter, 2008). In addition, the lower oxytocin levels in the patients with water imbalance were proportional to the size of the deformations on the anterior lateral hippocampus (M. B. Goldman, Wang, et al., 2011). To further test the possibility that diminished central oxytocin activity linked to the hippocampal pathology contributes to impaired facial affect recognition in patients with water imbalance, patients received intranasal oxytocin prior to assessing facial affect recognition. Intranasal oxytocin increases central oxytocin levels (Dal Monte, Noble, Turchi, Cummins, & Averbeck, 2014) and has been found to enhance social cognition, emotion recognition, and social interaction while it diminishes stress responses (Bartz, Zaki, Bolger, & Ochsner, 2011). This pilot study revealed that facial affect recognition was better in patients without water imbalance during the placebo condition. Intranasal oxytocin improved affect recognition in those with water imbalance, but it tended to get worse in those without water imbalance. Most prominent was that recognition of fearful faces was nearly normalized in those with water imbalance (M. B. Goldman, Gomes, Carter, & Lee, 2011). Together these findings linked the vasopressin abnormality to the mental illness, thus raising the possibility that the pathogenesis of their psychiatric disorder differs from that of others with schizophrenia.

LINKING NEUROPEPTIDE FINDINGS TO NEURAL CIRCUIT DYSFUNCTION

The strategic plan for the NIMH states, "Mental illnesses are now studied as brain disorders, specifically as disorders of brain circuits (National Institute of Mental Health, 2008)." The restoration of fear perception by oxytocin suggested that the amygdala may be part of a dysfunctional circuit that includes the anterior lateral hippocampus and hypothalamus. Oxytocin's salutary effects on social behaviors and especially fear responses involve this structure (Lischke et al., 2012), and the previously summarized shape analyses also revealed deformations on the dorsal medial surface of the right amygdala as well as outward deformations on the third ventricle adjacent to the SON and PVN in the anterior hypothalamus (M. B. Goldman, Wang, et al., 2011). Again, patients without water imbalance demonstrated distinct nonoverlapping deformations on other amygdala surfaces. The deformations on the left anterior hippocampus were proportional to their amygdala and third ventricle deformations. The three substructures (i.e., anterior lateral hippocampus, dorsal medial amygdala; anterior hypothalamus) are highly interconnected and modulate both activation and restraint of neuroendocrine responses to psychological stress (Goldman, 2014). Finally, the amygdala deformation was proportional to the enhanced vasopressin response and diminished basal oxytocin levels, whereas the third ventricle deformation was proportional to the enhanced-stress-hormone response. These observations identify a disordered neurocircuit, which may contribute to the distinct psychiatric illness in psychotic persons with water imbalance.

As an initial test of this possibility, resting-state functional magnetic resonance imaging (rs-fMRI) was obtained to examine the functional connectivity of the hippocampus with other brain structures implicated in schizophrenia. The correlation between neural activity (as indexed by the BOLD response) in different structures at rest provides a measure of coordinated functional activity (Unschuld et al., 2014). Our primary interest was the six functional connections between the bilateral hippocampus to the hypothalamus and bilateral amygdala. We predicted the strength of these connections would differ in patients with and without water imbalance

The results demonstrated that the relative functional connection strengths among the hippocampus and the amygdale and hypothalamus were significantly greater in the subset with water imbalance, than those without, ($P < .0007$; M. B. Goldman et al., 2014). These results provided additional evidence of altered neurocircuit activity relevant to the psychiatric disorder in patients with water imbalance

Subsequent research in this subset may further examine the broader efficacy of oxytocin treatment, and explore the possibility of a distinct stress diathesis in those with water imbalance since this may have clear implications for development psychosocial interventions. Other interventions of potential interest include deep brain stimulation, as well as efforts to target specific GABAergic receptors (M. B. Goldman, 2014).

SUMMARY

Although the validity and ultimate utility of this particular body of research remains to be established, the series of studies in patients with schizophrenia with water imbalance demonstrate how the revised research paradigm may offer greater insights into the mechanism and potential treatment of severe mental illness. Given the unique advantages of the neurohypophyseal peptides, one might question if this strategy can be applied to other neuropeptide systems. At least some systems may have the required elements. For instance, altered immune activity is apparent in a subset of schizophrenia patients. This in turn could be a reflection of central immune activity arising from central cytokine dysfunction (Bergink, Gibney, & Drexhage, 2014). Altered central immune activity has been shown to underlie autoimmune-encephalitis, which typically presents symptoms indistinguishable from schizophrenia (Pollak, McCormack, Peakman, Nicholson, & David, 2014). In fact, these antibodies are found in about 10 percent of patients, and very rarely in healthy normals (Pearlman & Najjar, 2014). Central immune activity is regulated by microglia, which resemble monocytes in the periphery. Both cell types produce cytokines, and accumulating evidence suggests peripheral cytokine levels provide an index of central cytokine activity (Bergink et al., 2014; Girgis, Kumar, & Brown, 2014). Evidence indicates that peripheral interleukin-6 (IL-6) and tumor necrosis factor (TNF) levels parallel psychiatric symptomatology, and peripheral IL levels have been reported to predict white-matter density (Najjar & Pearlman, 2015). Finally, preliminary studies indicate that the salutary effect of cytokine modulators on peripheral indices of immune function predict their ability to diminish psychiatric symptoms (Girgis et al., 2014). Hence, further studies into the mechanism of the peripheral changes in immune function could provide insights into targeted therapies for another distinct subset of the severely mentally ill.

CONCLUSIONS

Neuropeptides would appear to be especially useful in characterizing the pathophysiology as well as providing novel treatments for severe mental illness. Although research to date has not led to fundamental changes in our understanding of the illnesses, ongoing technological advances and a reconceptualization of the research paradigm may enable more definitive experiments on the mechanisms and therapy of psychosis.

REFERENCES

Addington, J., Girard, T. A., Christensen, B. K., & Addington, D. (2010). Social cognition mediates illness-related and cognitive influences on social function in patients with schizophrenia-spectrum disorders. *Journal of Psychiatry & Neuroscience, 35*(1), 49–54.

Barahal, H. S. (1938). Water intoxication in a mental case. *Psychiatry Quarterly, 12*(4), 767–771.

Bartz, J. A., Zaki, J., Bolger, N., & Ochsner, K. N. (2011). Social effects of oxytocin in humans: context and person matter. *Trends in Cognitive Sciences, 15*(7), 301–309.

Bergink, V., Gibney, S. M., & Drexhage, H. A. (2014). Autoimmunity, inflammation, and psychosis: a search for peripheral markers. *Biological Psychiatry, 75*(4), 324–331.

Bowers, M. E., Choi, D. C., & Ressler, K. J. (2012). Neuropeptide regulation of fear and anxiety: Implications of cholecystokinin, endogenous opioids, and neuropeptide Y. *Physiology of Behavior, 107*(5), 699–710.

Caceda, R., Kinkead, B., & Nemeroff, C. B. (2007). Involvement of neuropeptide systems in schizophrenia: human studies. *International Review of Neurobiology, 78*, 327–376.

Dal Monte, O., Noble, P. L., Turchi, J., Cummins, A., & Averbeck, B. B. (2014). CSF and blood oxytocin concentration changes following intranasal delivery in macaque. *PLoS One, 9*(8), e103677.

de Lecea, L., Carter, M. E., & Adamantidis, A. (2012). Shining light on wakefulness and arousal. *Biological Psychiatry, 71*(12), 1046–1052.

de Leon, J., Verghese, C., Tracy, J. I., Josiassen, R. C., & Simpson, G. M. (1994). Polydipsia and water intoxication in psychiatric patients: a review of the epidemiological literature. *Biological Psychiatry, 35*(6), 408–419.

Gainer, H., Yamashita, M., Fields, R. L., House, S. B., & Rusnak, M. (2002). The magnocellular neuronal phenotype: cell-specific gene expression in the hypothalamo-neurohypophysial system. *Progress in Brain Research, 139*, 1–14.

Girgis, R. R., Kumar, S. S., & Brown, A. S. (2014). The cytokine model of schizophrenia: emerging therapeutic strategies. *Biological Psychiatry, 75*(4), 292–299.

Goldman, M., Marlow-O'Connor, M., Torres, I., & Carter, C. S. (2008). Diminished plasma oxytocin in schizophrenic patients with neuroendocrine dysfunction and emotional deficits. *Schizophrenia Research, 98*(1–3), 247–255.

Goldman, M. B. (2009). The mechanism of life-threatening water imbalance in schizophrenia and its relationship to the underlying psychiatric illness. *Brain Reseaarch Review, 61*(2), 210–220.

Goldman, M. B. (2014). Brain circuit dysfunction in a distinct subset of chronic psychotic patients. *Schizophrenia Research, 157*(1–3), 204–213.

Goldman, M. B., Gomes, A. M., Carter, C. S., & Lee, R. (2011). Divergent effects of two different doses of intranasal oxytocin on facial affect discrimination in schizophrenic patients with and without polydipsia. *Psychopharmacology (Berlin), 216*(1), 101–110.

Goldman, M. B., Heidinger, L., Schroeder, M. P., Wang, L., Parish, T., & Smith, M. (2014). *Does the brain circuit which modulates neuroendocrine responses to psychological stress differ in polydipsic and nonpolydipsic achizophrenia patients? Does this reflect a generalized stress diathesis?* Paper presented at the Annual Meeting of the American College of Neuropharmacology, Phoenix, Arizona.

Goldman, M. B., Luchins, D. J., & Robertson, G. L. (1988). Mechanisms of altered water metabolism in psychotic patients with polydipsia and hyponatremia. *New England Journal of Medicine, 318*(7), 397–403.

Goldman, M. B., Robertson, G. L., Luchins, D. J., Hedeker, D., & Pandey, G. N. (1997). Psychotic exacerbations and enhanced vasopressin secretion in schizophrenic patients with hyponatremia and polydipsia. *Archives of General Psychiatry, 54*(5), 443–449.

Goldman, M. B., Wang, L., Wachi, C., Daudi, S., Csernansky, J., Marlow-O'Connor, M., ...Torres, I. (2011). Structural pathology underlying neuroendocrine dysfunction in schizophrenia. *Behavior and Brain Research, 218*(1), 106–113.

Grace, A. A. (2012). Dopamine system dysregulation by the hippocampus: implications for the pathophysiology and treatment of schizophrenia. *Neuropharmacology, 62*(3), 1342–1348.

Griebel, G., & Holsboer, F. (2012). Neuropeptide receptor ligands as drugs for psychiatric diseases: the end of the beginning? *Nature Reviews Drug Discovery, 11*(6), 462–478.

Herman, J. P., Dolgas, C. M., & Carlson, S. L. (1998). Ventral subiculum regulates hypothalamo-pituitary-adrenocortical and behavioural responses to cognitive stressors. *Neuroscience, 86*(2), 449–459.

Hoyer, D., & Bartfai, T. (2012). Neuropeptides and neuropeptide receptors: drug targets, and peptide and non-peptide ligands: a tribute to Prof. Dieter Seebach. *Chem Biodiversity, 9*(11), 2367–2387.

Hyman, S. E. (2012). Revolution stalled. *Science Transllational Medicine, 4*(155), 155cm111.

Insel, T., Cuthbert, B., Garvey, M., Heinssen, R., Pine, D. S., Quinn, K., . . . Wang, P. (2010). Research domain criteria (RDoC): toward a new classification framework for research on mental disorders. *American Journal of Psychiatry, 167*(7), 748–751.

Insel, T. R. (2010). The challenge of translation in social neuroscience: a review of oxytocin, vasopressin, and affiliative behavior. *Neuron, 65*(6), 768–779.

Insel, T. R., & Gogtay, N. (2014). National Institute of Mental Health clinical trials: new opportunities, new expectations. *JAMA Psychiatry, 71*(7), 745–746.

Kapur, S., Phillips, A. G., & Insel, T. R. (2012). Why has it taken so long for biological psychiatry to develop clinical tests and what to do about it? *Molecular Psychiatry, 17*(12), 1174–1179.

Karatsoreos, I. N., & McEwen, B. S. (2011). Psychobiological allostasis: resistance, resilience and vulnerability. *Trends in Cognitive Science, 15*(12), 576–584.

Keshavan, M. S., Nasrallah, H. A., & Tandon, R. (2011). Schizophrenia, "Just the Facts" 6. Moving ahead with the schizophrenia concept: from the elephant to the mouse. *Schizophrenia Research, 127*(1–3), 3–13.

Landgraf, R., & Neumann, I. D. (2004). Vasopressin and oxytocin release within the brain: a dynamic concept of multiple and variable modes of neuropeptide communication. *Frontiers in Neuroendocrinology, 25*(3–4), 150–176.

Legros, J. J. (2001). Inhibitory effect of oxytocin on corticotrope function in humans: are vasopressin and oxytocin ying-yang neurohormones? *Psychoneuroendocrinology, 26*(7), 649–655.

Lischke, A., Gamer, M., Berger, C., Grossmann, A., Hauenstein, K., Heinrichs, M., ...Domes, G. (2012). Oxytocin increases amygdala reactivity to threatening scenes in females. *Psychoneuroendocrinology, 37*(9), 1431–1438.

Luchins, D. J., Nettles, K. W., & Goldman, M. B. (1997). Anterior medial temporal lobe volumes in polydipsic schizophrenic patients with and without hypo-osmolemia: a pilot study. *Biological Psychiatry, 42*(9), 767–770.

Marsh, A. A., Yu, H. H., Pine, D. S., & Blair, R. J. (2010). Oxytocin improves specific recognition of positive facial expressions. *Psychopharmacology (Berlin), 209*(3), 225–232.

McGonigle, P. (2012). Peptide therapeutics for CNS indications. *Biochemical Pharmacology, 83*(5), 559–566.

Meltzer, H. Y., Arvanitis, L., Bauer, D., Rein, W., & Meta-Trial Study, G. (2004). Placebo-controlled evaluation of four novel compounds for the treatment of schizophrenia and schizoaffective disorder. *American Journal of Psychiatry, 161*(6), 975–984.

Meyer-Lindenberg, A., Domes, G., Kirsch, P., & Heinrichs, M. (2011). Oxytocin and vasopressin in the human brain: social neuropeptides for translational medicine. *Natinal Review of Neuroscience, 12*(9), 524–538.

Najjar, S., & Pearlman, D. M. (2015). Neuroinflammation and white matter pathology in schizophrenia: systematic review. *Schizophrenia Research, 161*(1), 102–112.

National Institute of Mental Health. (2008). NIMH Strategic Plan, 2008. from http://www.nimh.nih.gov/about/strategic-planning-reports/index.shtml

Nettles, K. W., Pesold, C., & Goldman, M. B. (2000). Influence of the ventral hippocampal formation on plasma vasopressin, hypothalamic-pituitary-adrenal axis, and behavioral responses to novel acoustic stress. *Brain Research, 858*(1), 181–190.

Pearlman, D. M., & Najjar, S. (2014). Meta-analysis of the association between N-methyl-d-aspartate receptor antibodies and schizophrenia, schizoaffective disorder, bipolar disorder, and major depressive disorder. *Schizophrenia Research, 157*(1–3), 249–258.

Pollak, T. A., McCormack, R., Peakman, M., Nicholson, T. R., & David, A. S. (2014). Prevalence of anti-N-methyl-D-aspartate (NMDA) receptor [corrected] antibodies in patients with schizophrenia and related psychoses: a systematic review and meta-analysis. *Psychology Medicine, 44*(12), 2475–2487.

Pratt, J., Winchester, C., Dawson, N., & Morris, B. (2012). Advancing schizophrenia drug discovery: optimizing rodent models to bridge the translational gap. *Nat Rev Drug Discovery, 11*(7), 560–579.

Rapoport, J. L., Giedd, J. N., & Gogtay, N. (2012). Neurodevelopmental model of schizophrenia: update 2012. *Molecular Psychiatry, 17*(12), 1228–1238.

Raskind, M. A., Orenstein, H., & Christopher, T. G. (1975). Acute psychosis, increased water ingestion, and inappropriate antidiuretic hormone secretion. *American Journal of Psychiatry, 132*(9), 907–910.

Risold, P. Y., & Swanson, L. W. (1996). Structural evidence for functional domains in the rat hippocampus. *Science, 272*(5267), 1484–1486.

Robertson, G. L. (2006). Regulation of arginine vasopressin in the syndrome of inappropriate antidiuresis. *American Journal of Medicine, 119*(7 Suppl 1), S36–S42.

Salvador, R., Sarro, S., Gomar, J. J., Ortiz-Gil, J., Vila, F., Capdevila, A., ,,,Pomarol-Clotet, E. (2010). Overall brain connectivity maps show cortico-subcortical abnormalities in schizophrenia. *Human Brain Mapping, 31*(12), 2003–2014.

Sarter, M., & Tricklebank, M. (2012). Revitalizing psychiatric drug discovery. *Nature Reviews Drug Discoveries, 11*(6), 423–424.

Schank, J. R., Ryabinin, A. E., Giardino, W. J., Ciccocioppo, R., & Heilig, M. (2012). Stress-related neuropeptides and addictive behaviors: beyond the usual suspects. *Neuron, 76*(1), 192–208.

Smith, C. M., Walker, A. W., Hosken, I. T., Chua, B. E., Zhang, C., Haidar, M., ...Gundlach, A.L. (2014). Relaxin-3/RXFP3 networks: an emerging target for the treatment of depression and other neuropsychiatric diseases? *Frontiers in Pharmacology, 5*, 46.

Tandon, R., & Goldman, M. B. (2014). Overview of Neurobiology. In P. Janical, M. Goldman, R. Tandon & S. Marder (Eds.), *Schizophrenia: Recent advances in diagnosis and treatment*. New York, NY: Springer.

Tandon, R., Nasrallah, H. A., & Keshavan, M. S. (2009). Schizophrenia, "just the facts" 4. Clinical features and conceptualization. *Schizophrenia Research, 110*(1–3), 1–23.

Targowla, R. (1923). Des troubles fonctionnel du rein dans les maladies mentals. L'excretion del'eau (Kidney malfufunction in mental illness: water excretion). *Bulletins et Mémoires de la Societé Médical des Hôpitaux de Paris, 47*(9), 1711–1715.

Unschuld, P. G., Buchholz, A. S., Varvaris, M., van Zijl, P. C., Ross, C. A., Pekar, J. J., ...Schretlen, D.J. (2014). Prefrontal brain network connectivity indicates degree of both schizophrenia risk and cognitive dysfunction. *Schizophrenia Bulletin, 40*(3), 653–664.

Williamson, P. C., & Allman, J. M. (2012). A framework for interpreting functional networks in schizophrenia. *Frontiers in Human Neuroscience, 6*, 184.

Wotjak, C. T., Ganster, J., Kohl, G., Holsboer, F., Landgraf, R., & Engelmann, M. (1998). Dissociated central and peripheral release of vasopressin, but not oxytocin, in response to repeated swim stress: new insights into the secretory capacities of peptidergic neurons. *Neuroscience, 85*(4), 1209–1222.

/// 12 ///

BRAIN STRUCTURAL ABNORMALITIES AND ANIMAL MODELS OF SCHIZOPHRENIA

A Neurodevelopmental Perspective

S. HOSSEIN FATEMI, TIMOTHY D. FOLSOM, and AFSHAN ANJUM

INTRODUCTION

Schizophrenia is a heterogenous neurodevelopmental disease of the brain that affects 1 percent of the adult population in the world (Fatemi & Folsom, 2009, 2016). The incidence is about 0.2/1000 per year. Risk factors other than family history of schizophrenia include parental age, ethnicity, cannabis use, obstetric complications, prenatal infections, urbanicity, and modernization.

The concept of schizophrenia as a neurodevelopmental brain disorder dates back to original descriptions provided by Kraepelin and Bleuler who mentioned presence of premorbid signs and deficits in social interaction in children who later developed schizophrenia. However, neuropathologic changes in the brains of subjects with schizophrenia were subtle and not as prominent as postmortem findings from disorders such as Huntington's chorea, tertiary syphilis, and Pick's disease. In the earliest systemic and pathologic study, Southard (1915) reported on the presence of neuropathologic signs in brains of subjects with schizophrenia, which further pointed to the developmental etiology of this disorder.

Southard, in his careful postmortem analysis of 25 cases of dementia praecox or schizophrenia provides the following important findings: (a) presence of mild brain atrophy in cases with chronic course of illness; (b) predominance of left hemispheric site of brain lesions; (c) high correlation of auditory hallucination with temporal lobe lesions; (d) high correlation of catatonia with parietal lobe lesions; (e) correlation between delusions and frontal lobe disease; and (f) high correlation of large internal hydrocephalus (ventriculomegaly) with catatonic and hallucinatory behavior. The upshot of Southard's neuropathologic findings nearly a century ago was that dementia praecox or schizophrenia was a brain structural disease with neurodevelopmental origins (Southard, 1915).

Thus, based on neurodevelopmental hypothesis of this illness, the genesis of schizophrenia may involve genetic and intrauterine environmental factors, which, when combined, trigger the activation of pathologic neural circuitry during adolescence leading to manifestations of overt disease (Fatemi & Folsom, 2009).

BRAIN PATHOLOGY IN SCHIZOPHRENIA

Historically, Theodor Meynert was the first neuroanatomist and psychiatrist who pointed to frontal lobe pathology in causation of psychosis. Alois Alzheimer working in collaboration with Kraepelin provided the first microscopic observations on disorientation of pyramidal cells and neuronal cell loss in frontal cortex of postmortem brains of patients who suffered from schizophrenia. However, a consistent observation in brain morphology of schizophrenia is the enlargement of the cerebroventricular system. As Southard made this important observation in his classic report (Southard, 1915), later CT and MRI-based studies not only confirmed Southard's observations, but clearly showed that that the abnormalities are present at onset of illness, progress slowly, and are generally unrelated to the duration of disease (Shepherd, Laurens, et al., 2012). Indeed, in a recent meta-analytic review, Shepherd, Laurens, et al. (2012) showed strong evidence supporting an increase in total cerebroventricular volume in chronic (Wright et al., 2000) and first episode schizophrenic subjects (Steen, Mull, McClure, Hamer, & Lieberman, 2006). Cerebroventricular enlargement has been shown to distinguish affected from unaffected discordant monozygotic (MZ) twins (Reveley, Reveley, Clifford, & Murray, 1982). Additionally, gross brain abnormalities have also been identified in several brain regions such as frontal, parietal, temporal, cerebellar, limbic-paralimbic areas (cingulate cortex, insula, parahippocampus, amygdala, hippocampus) and subcortical regions such as basal ganglia and thalamus (Shepherd, Laurens, et al., 2012). Overall, reductions in total volumes of brain were observed in bilateral frontal lobes (Wright et al., 2000; Davidson & Heinrichs, 2003) and grey matter in left inferior and medial frontal gyri (Honea, Crow, Passingham, & Mackay, 2005). The reductions in volume of frontal cortex were observed in both chronic and first episode subjects with schizophrenia (Shepherd, Laurens et al., 2012). In parietal lobe, reduced grey matter volume was observed in post-central gyrus in several studies (Chan, Di, McAlonan, & Gong, 2011; Fornito, Yucel, Patti, Wood, & Pantelis, 2009; Shepherd, Laurens, et al., 2012) of subjects with chronic schizophrenia and at least one study of first episode patients (Chan et al., 2011). Multiple further studies showed volume reductions in grey matter of both left medial and bilateral superior temporal gyri (Honea et al., 2005; Sun, Maller, Guo, & Fitzgerald, 2009; Shepherd, Laurens, et al., 2012). Although some investigators reported volume reduction to be limited to left fusiform (temporo-occipital) gyrus of chronic patients (Fornito et al., 2009), other investigators reported volume reductions in transerve gyrus of both first episode and chronic patients (Chan et al., 2011; Shepherd, Laurens, et al., 2012). In the cingulate cortex, decreases in grey matter volume have been reported mostly in left anterior cingulate as well as left posterior and bilateral regions of cingulate cortex (Baiano et al., 2007; Chan et al., 2011; Fornito et al., 2009; Shepherd, Laurens, et al., 2012). Bilateral volume reductions have also been reported both in hippocampus and amygdalar structures (Chan et al., 2011; Davidson & Heinrichs, 2003; Wright et al., 2000). A recent meta-analysis performed by Shepherd, Matheson, et al (2012) demonstrated reductions of bilateral insula, which were not influenced by illness stage, or sex. In the basal ganglia, several studies reported bilateral increases in volume in chronic patients when compared to controls (Wright et al., 2000). Finally, volume reductions were observed in bilateral thalamus in both first episode and chronic patients with schizophrenia (Adriano, Spoletini, Caltagione, & Spalleta, 2010; Chan et al., 2011; Wright et al., 2000).

Accordingly, the meta-analytic report by Shepherd, Laurens, et al. (2012) indicated reductions in white matter density in frontal and temporal lobes, including corpus callosum, cingulum bundle, and internal capsule as well as reductions in total white matter-volume and disruption in white-matter tracts in frontal, parietal, and temporal lobes in subjects with schizophrenia compared to controls (Konrad & Winterer, 2008; Shepherd, Laurens, et al., 2012).

Two important factors that impact the alterations in brain regional volumes are duration of illness and antipsychotic treatment over the course of patient's lifetime. In general, unsurprisingly, more widespread brain alterations occur in patients who experience schizophrenia chronically, especially in the fusiform gyrus, the amygdala, the parahippocampus, and the posterior cingulate cortex (Shepherd, Laurens, et al., 2012). However, in some brain areas, such as the frontal cortex or the anterior cingulate cortex and the insula, duration of illness either does not appear to have an effect or the current data are inconclusive (Shepherd, Laurens, et al., 2012). As for impact of antipsychotic treatment, medications appear to influence brain volumes especially in basal ganglia (caudate), as well as thalamus and other cortical areas (Shepherd, Laurens, et al., 2012). Interestingly, presence of some of these brain abnormalities have also been identified in individuals at high risk for development of schizophrenia, such as first degree relatives of subjects with schizophrenia who have not been exposed to antipsychotic medications (Chan et al., 2011; Wright et al., 2000).

Above and beyond gross abnormalities of brain described earlier, numerous reports have documented cytologic abnormalities of the brain in schizophrenia. One of the earliest and pioneering series of studies performed by Akbarian et al. (1993) showed presence of abnormal migration of nitric-oxide positive cells (NADPH-diaphorase-positive cells) in the frontal and hippocampal cortices of subjects with schizophrenia. Additional immunocytochemical studies showed reductions in density of Reelin positive cells in the frontal and hippocampal areas of brain in subjects with schizophrenia and mood disorders (Guidotti et al., 2000; Fatemi, Earle, & McMenomy, 2000).

Histologic studies indicate that decreased cortical volume is most likely secondary to reduced neuropil and neuronal size and structural abnormalities in synaptic, dendritic, and axonal composition of the brain (Harrison, 1999). Emerging molecular, biochemical, and immunocytochemical studies of the postmortem brain in schizophrenia (Table 12.1) over the last two decades, indicate involvement of a large number of brain proteins whose expression are dysregulated either early during the development of the brain or later before puberty when overt symptoms of schizophrenia develop. Finally, although evidence for gliosis is generally absent, microglial activation in white matter of the brain reflects immune abnormalities in schizophrenic brain (Najjar & Pearlman, 2015).

ANIMAL MODELS OF SCHIZOPHRENIA

A major focus of schizophrenia research has been to elucidate its etiopathogenic mechanisms as a means of providing treatment opportunities to optimize patient functioning. Most pharmacologic interventions to date focus on treating positive symptoms, while treatments for negative or cognitive symptoms of schizophrenia have lagged. Human postmortem and structural studies have informed our understanding of the pathophysiology of schizophrenia. Animal models provide a unique opportunity to examine and manipulate various systems implicated in the genesis of schizophrenia and test hypotheses and interventions in a timely fashion in a way that is not currently available in clinical studies. Animal models that are used to replicate the neurobiological, pathophysiologic basis of a heterogeneous illness like schizophrenia need to meet face validity (i.e., reproduce schizophrenia symptomatology), construct validity (i.e., produce neurochemical

TABLE 12.1 Neurodevelopmental markers and schizophrenia

Neurodevelopmental Event	Molecule	Findings in Schizophrenia
Cell migration	PSA-NCAM	↓ in dentate hilar area
	Reelin	↓ in mRNA and protein of neocortex, hippocampus and cerebellum
Synaptogenesis and axonal growth	SNAP-25	↓ in hippocampus and frontal cortex
	GAP-43	↑ in prefrontal and inferior temporal cortex; ↓ dentate gyrus
	Synaptophysin	↓ in prefrontal cortex and hippocampus
	Synapsin	↓ in hippocampus
Survival of connections	BDNF	↓ in hippocampus
Neuronal cytoskeletal proteins	MAP-2	↓ in subiculum and entorhinal cortex
	MAP-5	↓ in subiculum
Synaptic plasticity	NRG1	Nrg1 type I ↑ significantly in dorsolateral prefrontal cortex
Regulation of neurotransmitter signaling	RGS4	↓ in prefrontal cortex, motor cortex and visual cortex
Glutamatergic transmission	G72	Association of polymorphisms with early onset and male schizophrenia
	DAAO	4 intronic SNPs associated with schizophrenia in a French Canadian sample
	DTNBP1	Family association studies in Germany and Israel; DTNBP1 haplotype associated with schizophrenia in Chinese and Swedish samples
	GAD67	↓ in lateral cerebellum, PFC, and temporal neocortex
Cognition	COMT	Location in region 22q11 deleted in VCFS; variations in COMT associated with schizophrenia
Production of glutamate and GABA	PRODH	Location in region 22q11.2 deleted in VCFS; complex pattern of association with schizophrenia
	GAD1	↓ in lateral cerebellum
	GAD2	in lateral cerebellum
GABAergic transmission	GABRα2	↑ in lateral cerebellum
	GABRβ1	↓ in lateral cerebellum
	GABRε	↑ in lateral cerebellum
	GABRθ	↓ in lateral cerebellum and PFC
	GABBR1	↓ in lateral cerebellum
	GABBR2	↓ in lateral cerebellum

↑, increase; ↓, decrease

Adapted and modified from Table 4 in Fatemi, S.H. (2008). *Schizophrenia*. In: S. H. Fatemi and P. J. Clayton (Eds), *The medical basis of psychiatry* (3rd ed., p. 92). New York, NY: Springer Science+Business Media.

and structural changes identified in patients with schizophrenia), and be of predictive validity (i.e., respond to interventions with antipsychotic and other adjunct medications; Jones, Watson, & Fone, 2011).

Although it is not possible to evaluate core behavioral symptoms of schizophrenia including positive (hallucinations, delusions), negative (avolition, asociality, alogia, autism) or cognitive/disorganization symptoms (thought disorder, executive function abnormalities, catatonia) using rodent models, other behavioral, molecular, and neuroanatomic phenotypes similar in humans and rodents can be employed to gauge fidelity of animal models in replicating a human disease such as schizophrenia. For example, a number of behavioral measures have been employed that are considered valid translational paradigms in rodent models of schizophrenia (Koenig & colleagues from the Maryland Psychiatric Research Center, 2014). These include: (a) dopamine-related behaviors such as hyperactivity, enhanced response to amphetamine, MK-801 (a noncompetitive antagonist of the NMDA glutamate receptor), and to novel open field, reduction in anxiety, reduction in prefrontal level of dopamine, reduced spontaneous activity, enhanced levels of mesolimbic dopamine; (b) abnormal sensory gating as reflected by either disruption or inhibition of two phenomena known as prepulse inhibition and latent inhibition (Amann et al., 2010). Prepulse inhibition (PPI) is a neurologic event in which a weaker prestimulus (prepulse) inhibits the reaction of an organism (human or rodent) to a subsequent strong startling stimulus (pulse). Here, the stimuli are acoustic and the PPI is deficient in subjects with schizophrenia (Amann et al., 2010) who cannot filter out the unnecessary information. Latent inhibition (LI) refers to the observation that a familiar stimulus takes longer to acquire meaning (either as a signal or a conditioned stimulus) than a new stimulus (Amann et al., 2010). The latent effect (LI) connotes poor learning, and decreased LI is generally associated with high levels of dopamine in the ventral tegmental area of the brain. Impairment in LI is observed in subjects with schizophrenia. (c) Abnormalities in cognition such as impaired memory and abnormal executive function as reflective of hippocampal or frontal lobe dysfunction in schizophrenia, which can be measured by various tests in rodents known as Morris Water Maze learning, social recognition, and Radial Arm Maze performance (Amann et al., 2010). (d) Impaired social discrimination or social interaction seen in subjects with schizophrenia, which can be easily tested in rodents. (e) Molecular/neuroanatomic signatures of schizophrenia such as decreased levels of Reelin protein in brain, increased density of pyramidal cells, and decreases in neuronal cell size, etc. (f) Response to antipsychotic medications, which help reduce hallucinations or delusions and tend to correct certain behaviors in rodents.

In the current review, we will examine several examples of rodent models of relevance to schizophrenia that can be categorized in several groups: (a) neurodevelopmental;

(b) genetic; (c) based on interactions between genes and environment; (d) lesion-based; and (e) drug-induced. For the interested reader, we recommend consulting with Schizophrenia Research Forum website where a total of 136 animal models have been tabulated and described (Koenig et al., 2014).

Neurodevelopmental Models

Epidemiological studies have provided abundant evidence that exposure to environmental insults during the neonatal or perinatal periods increases the risk of developing schizophrenia (Kneeland & Fatemi, 2013; Meyer, 2014). A genetically predisposed individual affected by an adverse event/environmental factor at a critical juncture of development may subsequently develop schizophrenia. The timing of the insult (Figure 12.1) may be as crucial as the nature of the insult itself in influencing the subsequent development of schizophrenia (Fatemi & Folsom, 2009; Jones et al., 2011; Kneeland & Fatemi, 2013). In rodents, embryonic days E0 to E19–21 consist of trimesters 1 and 2, with postnatal days 0–7 reflecting the third trimester (Figure 12.1). As seen in Figure 12.1, the timing of important neurodevelopmental events such as proliferation and migration of neuronal cells (E9-P15), differentiation and synaptogenesis (E11 onwards), apoptosis (E9 to approximately P20), gliogenesis (E9 onward), and myelination (approximately E18

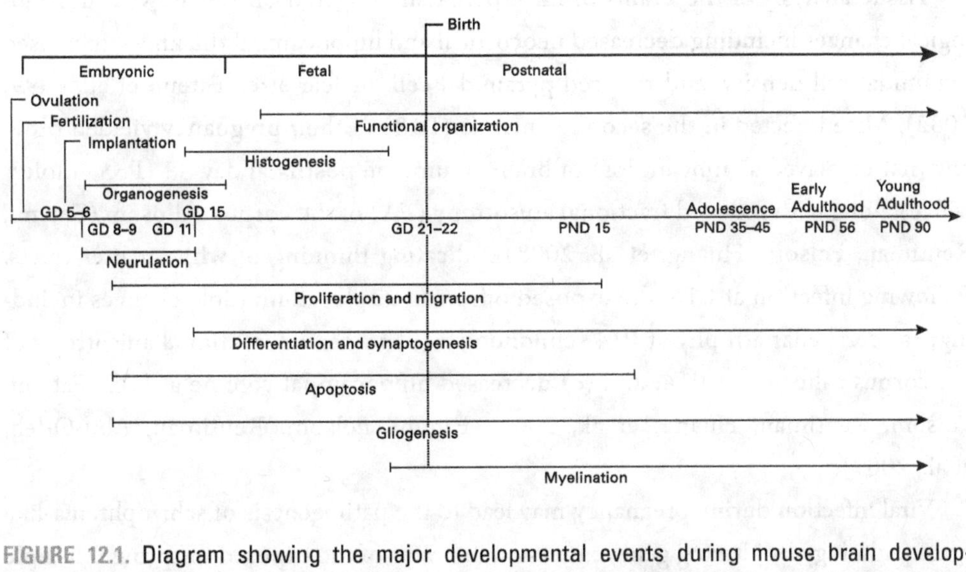

FIGURE 12.1. Diagram showing the major developmental events during mouse brain development and the corresponding prenatal and postnatal ages. Modified from figure 1 in Vorhees CV, Principles of Behavioral Teratology, in Riley EP, Vorhees CV (Eds), Handbook of Behavioral Teratology, New York: Plenum Press and Springer Science+Business Media, copyright (1986), p. 25, with kind permission of Springer Science+Business Media.

onward) have been determined and can be generally correlated to human developmental time table. Experimentally, this allows for the precise timing of environmental insults to determine possible developmental outcomes on the offspring. Various environmental risk factors that have been identified as affecting normal development have been studied in neurodevelopmental animal models (Fatemi, Reutiman, Folsom, Huang, et al., 2008, Fatemi, Folsom, Reutiman, & Sidwell, 2008;, Fatemi, Folsom, Reutiman, Huang, et al., 2009; Fatemi, Folsom, Reutiman, Abu-Odeh, et al., 2009;, Fatemi et al., 2012; Kneeland & Fatemi, 2013; Shi, Fatemi, Sidwell, & Patterson, 2003).

Prenatal Human Influenza Viral Infection Model

Prenatal human influenza virus infection of mice on embryonic day 9 (E9) has been shown to result in behavioral abnormalities akin to those observed in subjects with schizophrenia (Shi et al., 2003). Fatemi's animal model of prenatal viral infection has shown constructive and predictive validity for schizophrenia (Shi et al., 2003). These exposed offspring displayed abnormal exploratory behaviors when compared with controls, suggesting anxiety (Shi et al., 2003). Furthermore, they showed impaired social interactions as evidenced by infrequent contact with other mice (Shi et al., 2003). Finally, PPI deficits similar to those observed in subjects with schizophrenia were similarly observed in the exposed offspring (Shi et al., 2003). PPI deficits were resolved following use of chlorpromazine or clozapine (Shi et al., 2003).

Tissue analysis of the brains of mice prenatally infected on E9 showed morphological changes including decreased neocortical and hippocampal thickness, increased pyramidal cell density, and reduced pyramidal cell nuclear size (Fatemi et al., 1999; 2002). Mice infected in the second trimester (E18) of their pregnancy yielded progeny that displayed significant loss of brain volume on postnatal day 35 (P35; adolescence) along with reduced fractional anisotropy (FA) of the corpus callosum (Fatemi, Reutiman, Folsom, Huang, et al., 2008) indicating thinning of white-matter tracts. Following infection at E16, the exposed offspring displayed multiple changes including: (a) cerebellar atrophy at P14 (childhood); (b) increased fractional anisotropy of the corpus callosum at P14; and (c) decreased hippocampal volume at P35 (Fatemi, Folsom, Reutiman, Huang, et al., 2009,; Fatemi, Folsom, Reutiman, Abu-Odeh, et al., 2009).

Viral infection during pregnancy may lead to the pathogenesis of schizophrenia-like brain pathology by altering gene expression in brains of the exposed offspring. Multiple genes were observed to be altered in the frontal, hippocampal, and cerebellar regions of the offspring of mice infected during specific prenatal timepoints (Fatemi, Pearce, Brooks, & Sidwell, 2005; Fatemi, Reutiman, Folsom, Huang 2008; Fatemi, Folsom, et al., 2008; Fatemi, Reutiman, Folsom, & Sidwell, 2008; Fatemi, Folsom, Reutiman, Huang, et al., 2009; Fatemi, Folsom, Reutiman, Abu-Odeh, 2009; Fatemi et al., 2012). The altered expression of these genes persist into adulthood including multiple genes that have been implicated in schizophrenia such as myelin basic protein (MBP), neurotensin (NTS), neuronal cell adhesion molecule (NCAM), and regulator of G-protein signaling 4 (RGS4) (Fatemi et al., 2005; Fatemi, Reutiman, Folsom, Huang et al., 2008; Fatemi, Folsom Reutiman, & Sidwell, 2008; Fatemi, Reutiman, Folsom, & Sidwell, 2008;, Fatemi, Folsom, Reutiman, Huang, et al., 2009; Fatemi, Folsom, Reutiman, Abu-Odeh et al., 2009).

Poly I:C Administration to Rodents

Poly I:C is a synthetic form of double-stranded DNA that mimics viral infection and activates the immune response in pregnant mice. Poly I:C injection into pregnant mice has been shown to reduce Reelin levels, parvalbumin (PV) positive interneurons, and GABA content in the prefrontal cortices of the offspring in adulthood (Meyer, 2014). Poly I:C treatment also produces behavioral phenotypes similar to what has been observed in subjects with schizophrenia. Shi et al. (2003) found that the offspring of mice exposed to Poly I:C on E9 displayed deficits in PPI, exploratory behavior, and social interaction. The PPI deficit was resolved through the use of clozapine or chlorpromazine. A similar study also found that exposure at E9 (but not E17) resulted in PPI deficits in adulthood (Li et al., 2009). Treatment with Poly I:C at a later gestational date (E17) produced offspring that displayed behavioral inflexibility, LI deficits, anhedonic behavior, impaired social interactions, and increased locomotor activity in response to treatment with apomorphine (Meyer, 2014). Treatment with clozapine has been shown to reverse LI deficits in this model (Zuckerman &Weiner, 2005). Additionally, Zuckerman and Weiner (2005) found increased activity following treatment with MK-801 in the exposed offspring, indicating presence of abnormal dopamine-related behavior (Carpenter & Koenig, 2008).

Brain morphological changes consistent with schizophrenia have also been identified in the offspring of Poly I:C exposed mice. Treatment with Poly I:C on E9 (but not E17) resulted in enlarged ventricles in the offspring in adulthood (Li et al., 2009). Piontkewitz, Arad, and Weiner (2011) found that treatment with Poly I:C at E15 produced morphological changes at P90 including enlarged lateral ventricles and reduced hippocampal size, which are consistent with patients with schizophrenia. Treatment with risperidone during adolescence prevented these brain structural abnormalities from occurring and also prevented deficits in LI and hyperactivity in response to amphetamine treatment (Carpenter & Koenig, 2008; Piontkewitz et al., 2011).

Lipopolysaccharide Rodent and Primate Models

Prenatal administration of lipopolysaccharide (LPS), a bacterial toxin, has also been used in animal models to investigate the role of bacterial infections in causation of schizophrenia. Prenatal LPS exposure has also been demonstrated to have a negative impact on brain development (Cui, Ashdown, Luheshi, & Boksa, 2009; Willette et al., 2011). Treatment of pregnant mice with LPS on embryonic days E15 or E16 resulted in reduced cell proliferation in the hippocampal dentate gyrus of exposed offspring at postnatal day P14, whereas treatment at E18 or E19 resulted in reduced cell survival in the same region at P14 (Cui et al., 2009). However, by P60 (early adulthood), there were no differences in proliferation or survival (Cui et al., 2009). LPS exposure for two consecutive days, six weeks prior to term in pregnant rhesus monkeys was associated with an 8.8 percent increase in global white matter at one year of age in the offspring (Willette et al., 2011).

PPI deficits have been observed in the offspring of LPS-infected rhesus monkey mothers (Willette et al., 2011). PPI deficits have also been observed in the offspring of rats exposed to LPS at E15-E16 and E18-E19 (Fortier, Luheshi, & Boksa, 2007). Chronic administration of LPS from E1-E22 in rats produced offspring with PPI deficits six months following birth (Romero et al., 2007). Moreover, these rats displayed increased levels of dopamine in the nucleus accumbens and dopamine's metabolite 3,4-dihydroxyphenylacetic acid in the striatum at six-months of age (Romero et al., 2007). Treatment with haloperidol ameliorated PPI deficits in exposed offspring and also reduced concentrations of cytokines interleukin-2 (IL-2), IL-6, and tumor necrosis factor alpha (TNF-α) (Romero et al., 2007; Koenig et al., 2014).

Methylazoxymethanol Model

Methylazoxymethanol (MAM) is a naturally occurring antimitotic substance that targets rapidly proliferating neuroblasts without affecting glial cells or peripheral organs. Morphological changes have been observed in the brains of mice exposed in utero to MAM on embryonic days 15 and 17 that are consistent with brains of subjects with schizophrenia. Following MAM exposure at E15, which corresponds with the peak of cortical neurogenesis, there is a reduction in total cortical mass as well as total brain weight (Moore, Jentsch, Ghajarnia, Geyer, & Grace, 2006). MAM exposure at E17 resulted in selective reductions in cortical thickness in the medial prefrontal cortex, hippocampus, and parahippocampal cortices (Moore et al., 2006). The offspring of MAM-treated rats displayed deficits in PPI that emerge only after adolescence, similar to what is observed in subjects with schizophrenia (Moore et al., 2006). MAM exposure at E17 produced rats with LI deficits as well as hyperlocomotion in response to treatment with PCP or MK-801 (Moore et al., 2006). Administration of haloperidol, clozapine, or risperidone significantly reduced hyperlocomotion in response to MK-801 or PCP treatment (Le Pen, Jay, & Krebs, 2011). Finally, MAM-exposed mice displayed perseverative behavior (Moore et al., 2006), similar to what is observed in subjects with schizophrenia.

Rat Placental Insufficiency/Birth Insults

Increased frequency of schizophrenia has been reported in the progeny of mothers who suffered obstetric complications such as cesarean-section (c-section), hypoxia, and placental insufficiency. These complications are believed to affect fetal brain development and thus, increase the risk for schizophrenia in the offspring. Neonatal rats subjected to mild chronic hypoxia from P4-P8 displayed locomotor deficits at P86, P120 (adulthood), and P150 and PPI deficits at P120 and P150, but it had no effect on social recognition or social interaction (Fendt, Lex, Falkai, Henn, & Schmitt, 2008). Animals treated from P86–P120 with clozapine showed reduced PPI deficit but it had no effect on the locomotor deficit (Fendt et al., 2008). Wakuda et al. (2008) using a model of perinatal asphyxia in which offspring were exposed to 15 minutes of anoxia during c-section birth displayed an elevation in methamphetamine-induced locomotion at 12 weeks postnatally. Moreover, at 12 weeks, the hippocampus of exposed offspring displayed a reduced number of hippocampal dentate granule cells (Wakuda et al., 2008). Anoxia during c-section birth has also been shown to reduce dendritic spine density in the prefrontal cortex and increase dendritic spine density in the hippocampus of mice at P35 (Juárez, Gratton, & Flores, 2008). However, spine densities were normal by P70 in both brain regions (Juárez et al., 2008).

Postweaning Social Isolation

Social isolation of rat pups from their littermates early on induces stress that affects brain development and behavior that persists into adult life. Reintegration later in life may not alter these deficits. Rats raised in social isolation exhibited spontaneous locomotor hyperactivity that reflects mesolimbic hyperactivity and enhanced response to new situations. Rats raised in isolation that display induced hyperactivity have been observed to respond to antipsychotic medication and also the NMDA receptor antagonist L-serine proving it to be a model with high predictive validity (Powell, 2010; Watson, Marsden, Millan, & Fone, 2012). Other observed changes using this model include: (a) sensorimotor gating deficits as shown by impaired acoustic startle response when compared to controls that can be partially reversed by antipsychotic medications; (b) cognitive impairments in some executive tasks related to attentional shifting; and (c) decreased dendritic spine density and morphology (Carpenter & Koenig, 2008; Powell, 2010; Koenig et al., 2014).

Genetic Models

Although inheritance of schizophrenia does not follow Mendelian rules, there is a preponderance of evidence by way of twin studies that highlight the role of genetics in the etiopathogensis of schizophrenia (Table 12.2). Although there are a multitude of genes that are implicated in the pathogenesis of schizophrenia, no single gene has been identified to be the causal agent for this illness. Candidate genes that have been associated with schizophrenia code for proteins that play a vital role in neuronal plasticity, synaptogenesis, dopamine and glutaminergic function, cell growth and migration, signal transduction, myelination, and regulation of presynaptic membrane function (Tables 12.1 and 12.2). Recent genome-wide association study (GWAS) arrays have identified loci that are associated with schizophrenia, which code genes such as calcium channel, voltage dependent, L-type, alpha 1-C subunit (CACNA1C), N-acetylase/N-sulfotransferse 3 (NDST3), ankyrin 3 (ANK3), vaccina-related kinase 2 (VRK2), and transcription factor 4 (TCF4), metabotropic glutamate receptor 3 (GRM3), ionotropic glutamate receptor AMPA 1 (GRIA1), and ionotropic glutamate receptor NMDA subunit 2A (GRIN2A) (Schizophrenia Working Group of the Psychiatric Genomics Consortium, 2014). A majority of genetic animal models have been developed on the basis of replicating the abnormalities in expression of mRNA and proteins that are observed in schizophrenia (Carpenter & Koenig, 2008; Koenig et al., 2014). We will discuss six of these models next.

Alpha-amino-3-hydroxy-5-methyl-4-isoxazole Propionate (AMPA) Glutamate Receptor 1 (GluR1) Knockout (KO) Mouse Model

AMPA GluR1 receptor is involved in mediating synaptic plasticity and cognition, and it has been shown to be significantly reduced in medial temporal lobe and frontal cortex of subjects with schizophrenia. Wiedholz et al. (2008) found that GluR1 KO mice displayed numerous behavioral deficits consistent with those experienced by subjects with schizophrenia including hyperlocomotion during the open field test, impaired PPI, and abnormal social interactions when compared to wild type. GluR1 KO mice also displayed dopaminergic dysfunction as shown by reduced dopamine clearance in the striatum (Wiedholz et al., 2008). Treatment with haloperidol reversed hyperlocomotion during the open field test (Carpenter & Koenig, 2008; Koenig et al., 2014; Wiedholz et al., 2008).

Beta-site Amyloid Precursor Protein-cleaving Enzyme 1 (BACE1) KO Mouse Model

BACE1 is the rate-limiting enzyme that makes the initial cleavage of amyloid precursor protein (APP). BACE1 has other substrates as well and is involved in the

TABLE 12.2 Candidate Genes: Postmortem Studies and Animal Models

Gene	Abbreviation	Postmortem	Animal model
Adenosine A2A receptor	ADORA2A	+	+
Apolipoprotein D	APOD	+	+
CDC42 guanine nucleotide exchange factor 9	ARHGEF9	+	
Cholinergic receptor, muscarinic 1	CHRM1	+	+
Alpha7 nicotinic acetylcholine receptor	CHRNA7	+	+
Complexin 2	CPLX2	+	+
Catecholemine-O-methyltransferase	COMT	+	+
Dopamine and cAMP regulated phosphoprotein 32 kDa	DARPP-32	+	
Distal-less homeobox 1	DLX1	+	
Dopamine receptor D1	DRD1	+	
Dopamine receptor D2	DRD2	+	+
$GABA_A$ receptor, subunit alpha 1	GABRα1	+	
$GABA_A$ receptor, subunit alpha 2	GABRα2	+	
$GABA_A$ receptor, subunit alpha 5	GABRα5	+	+
$GABA_A$ receptor, subunit beta 1	GABRβ1	+	
$GABA_A$ receptor, subunit epsilon	GABRε	+	
$GABA_A$ receptor, subunit theta	GABRθ	+	
$GABA_B$ receptor 1	GABBR1	+	+
$GABA_B$ receptor 2	GABBR2	+	
Glutamic acid decarboxylase 2	GAD2	+	
Glial fibrillary acidic protein	GFAP	+	+
Glutamate receptor, ionotropic, AMPA1	GRIA1	+	
Glutamate receptor, ionotropic, AMPA2	GRIA2	+	
Myelin and lymphocite protein	MAL	+	
Myelin basic protein	MBP	+	+
Neuronal PAS domain protein 1	NPAS1	+	+
N-deacetylase/N-sulfotransferse 3	NDST3	+	
Proteolipid protein 1	PLP1	+	
Reelin	RELN	+	+
Regulator of G protein signaling 4	RGS4	+	+
Serotonin 5-HT-1A receptor	5HTR1A	+	
Serotonin 5-HT-2A receptor	5HTR2A	+	
Short stature homeobox 2	SHOX2	+	
Synapsin 2	SYN2	+	+

Adapted and modified from Table 3 in Fatemi, S. H. (2008). ***Schizophrenia.*** **In S. H. Fatemi and P. J. Clayton (Eds),** ***The medical basis of psychiatry*** **(3rd ed., p. 87). New York, NY: Springer Science+Business Media..**

proteolytic processing of neuregulin 1 (NRG1) (see section on Neuregulin 1 Heteromorph (Transmembrane Domain) Mouse Model). BACE1 KO mice similarly display PPI deficits, novelty-induced hyperactivity, increased locomotor activity in response to treatment with MK-801, impaired social recognition, and impaired working and inhibitory avoidance memory (Savonenko et al., 2008). Deficits in PPI and hyperactivity were ameliorated following treatment with clozapine, whereas clozapine had no effect on working memory deficits (Savonenko et al., 2008).

Dopamine Transporter KO Mouse Model

The dopamine transporter (DAT) takes up dopamine and is a target for some psychostimulants, antidepressants, and neurotoxins. Recently, DAT expression has been shown to be reduced in amygdala of subjects with schizophrenia (Markota, Sin, Pantazopoulos, Jonilionis, & Berretta, 2014). DAT KO mice are hyperactive in the open field and display impaired spatial cognition. DAT KO mice also display increased aggression following mild social contact as well as perseverative patterns of social responses. Hippocampal slices from DAT KO mice show impaired long-term depression, an effect that was reversed following application of haloperidol (Morice et al., 2007). Haloperidol has also been shown to reverse deficits by DAT KO mice in behavioral flexibility during the Morris Water Maze test (Morice et al., 2007).

Heterozygous Reeler Mouse Model

During development, Reelin glycoprotein is involved in brain development including mediating cell migration and proper brain lamination. In the mature brain, Reelin is involved in modulating synaptic function. Reelin expression has been shown to be reduced in multiple brain regions of subjects with schizophrenia (Fatemi et al. 2000; Guidotti et al., 2000). Heterozygous reeler mice (HRM), display an approximately 50 percent reduction in Reelin expression. Cognitive deficits including the acquisition of operant tasks, executive function, fear conditioned learning, olfactory-conditioned learning, neophobic behavior on the elevated plus maze, LI, and anxiety and motor impulsivity have been shown to be impaired in HRM (Carpenter & Koenig, 2008; Koenig et al., 2014; Larson, Hoffman, Guidotti & Costa, 2003; Tueting et al., 1999).

Neuregulin 1 Hypermorph (Transmembrane Domain) Mouse Model

NRG1, through its interaction with v-erb-B avian erythroblastic leukemia viral oncogene (ERBB; also known as epidermal growth factor) receptors induces the growth and differentiation of neuronal cells. NRG1 has been identified as a risk gene for schizophrenia (Stefansson et al., 2002) and NRG1 KO mice display PPI deficits and hyperactivity, the latter being reversed following administration of clozapine (Stefansson et al., 2002).

Nuclear Receptor Related 1 (Nurr1) Heterozygous KO Mouse Model

Nurr1 is a member of the steroid receptor family of genes and plays important roles developmentally in the differentiation and survival of dopaminergic neurons. mRNA for Nurr1 has been shown to be reduced in the prefrontal cortex of subjects with schizophrenia. Nurr1 heterozygous KO mice display a 35–40 percent reduction in Nurr1 gene expression (Rojas, Joodmardi, Hong, Perlman, & Ogren, 2007). These mice display increased locomotor activity in response to novelty and in response to administration of amphetamine or PCP (Rojas et al., 2007). Rojas et al. (2007) found that treatment with haloperidol ameliorated hyperlocomotion in response to amphetamine or PCP administration. Additionally, these mice displayed depressive behavior, and learning deficits (Rojas et al., 2007). Finally, Nurr1 heterozygous KO mice displayed altered levels of dopamine, serotonin, and acetylcholine neurotransmitters (Rojas et al., 2007).

Gene x Environmental Models

A number of animal models that investigate the interaction of schizophrenia candidate genes and specific environmental factors have been developed. One such model investigates the interaction of dominant negative disrupted in schizophrenia 1 gene (DISC1) and neonatal immune activation. Ibi et al. (2010) investigated DN-DISC1 mice that were treated daily with PolyI:C between postnatal (PN) days 2 and 6 for behavioral deficits after 8 weeks of age. The researchers identified cognitive deficits including impaired short-term memory, novel object recognition, and fear conditioned memory (Ibi et al., 2010). DN-DISC1 mice displayed increased hyperactivity in response to MK-801 administration but did not display deficits in PPI (Ibi et al., 2010). In terms of social interactions, the mice displayed shorter interaction times and increased aggression (Ibi et al., 2010). Using the same model, Nagai et al. (2011), found that cognitive impairments in mutant mice were resolved following repeated administration of clozapine, but haloperidol had no effect. Both clozapine and haloperidol ameliorated hyperactivity in response to MK-801 administration, but neither drug corrected for social impairments (Nagai et al., 2011).

Brain Lesion Models

A brain lesion model using the excitotoxin ibotenic acid was developed in the early 1990s to model brain imaging data of increased ventricular enlargement and hippocampal changes from subjects with first-episode schizophrenia (Lipska, 2004). Neonatal lesion to the ventral hippocampus (vHip) of the rat on P7 by local injection of ibotenic acid has been shown to result in disruption of the architectural integrity of developing prefrontal cortex and nucleus accumbens and behavioral abnormalities in post-pubertal animals (Koenig et al., 2014). The timing of the lesion appears to be critical as induction of lesions at P14 or later results in less dramatic changes than at P3 or P7. Behavioral changes as a result of vHip lesions occur progressively with deficits in spatial learning and working memory appearing around P25 (adolescence), deficits in social interactions (reflective of negative symptoms), and aggression emerging at P35, and other behavioral symptoms including locomotor hyperresponsiveness to stress, deficits in PPI and reward, presenting around P56 (Koenig et al., 2014; Lipska, 2004).

Adult rats with vHip lesions display: (a) reduced medial prefrontal cortex (mPFC) GAD67 mRNA levels (Lipska, 2004); (b) increased $GABA_A$ receptor expression; (c) reduced spine density and dendritic length of pyramidal neurons in mPFC and nucleus accumbens. vHip lesioned rats exhibit abnormal spatial working memory tasks as evidenced by impaired acquisition of the T maze alternation and Morris water maze tasks, radial arm maze choice accuracy, and retention of passive avoidance learning, suggesting the disruption of PFC-hippocampal communication as a result of the lesion (Koenig et al., 2014; Lipska, 2004).

Drug-Induced Model

Acute treatment with MK-801 has been shown to result in deficits in PPI one day following administration, but not seven or 28 days after administration (Manahan-Vaughan, von Haebler, Winter, Juckel, & Heinemann, 2008). Similarly, Park et al. (2014) have shown deficits in PPI following acute administration of MK-801, a deficit that was corrected following administration of clozapine or oleanolic acid. Additionally both clozapine and oleanolic acid corrected MK-801-induced deficits in novel object recognition in the same animals (Park et al., 2014). Treatment with risperidone, clozapine, or haloperidol has been shown to reverse locomotor deficits associated with MK-801 treatment (Le Pen et al., 2011; Nagai et al., 2011). Injection of MK-801 into rats has been shown to significantly inhibit social interactions. Thus, MK-801 injection can model both positive and negative symptoms of schizophrenia.

CONCLUSIONS

Schizophrenia is a debilitating neurodevelopmental disorder with both genetic and environmental origins (Fatemi & Folsom, 2009). Structural brain studies have revealed brain abnormalities that may be precipitated both in utero and later during adolescence. Many potentially valid animal models exist, which have been important in revealing mechanisms for causation of schizophrenia and testing new pharmacologic interventions for treatment of schizophrenia.

ACKNOWLEDGMENTS

Grant support by Eunice Kennedy Shriver National Institute of Child Health and Human Development (#5R01HD052074-01A2, 5R01HD046589-05, 3R01HD046589-04S1, and 3R01HD052074-03S1), National Institute of Mental Health (#1R01MH086000-01A2), the Stanley Medical Research Institute, the National Alliance for Research in Schizophrenia and Depression, and the Ewald Bipolar Disease Research Fund to SHF is gratefully acknowledged. S.H. Fatemi is also supported by the Bernstein Endowed Chair in Adult Psychiatry.

REFERENCES

Adriano, F., Spoletini, I., Caltagirone, C., & Spalletta, G. (2010). Updated meta-analyses reveal thalamus volume reduction in patients with first-episode and chronic schizophrenia. *Schizophrenia Research 123*, 1–14.

Akbarian, S., Bunney, W. E., Jr., Potkin, S. G., Wigal, S. B., Hagman, J. O., Sandman, C. A., . . . Jones, E. G.: Altered distribution of nicotinamide—adenine—dinucleotide—phosphate-diaphorase cells in frontal lobe of schizophrenics implies disturbances of cortical development. Arch Gen Psychiatry 1993; 50:169–177.

Amann, L. C., Gandal, M. J., Halene, T. B., Ehrlichman, R. S., White, S. L., McCarren, H. S., . . . Siegel, S. J. (2010).Mouse behavioral endophenotypes for schizophrenia. *Brain Research Bulletin*, 83,147–161.

Baiano, M., David, A., Versace, A., Churchill, R., Balestrieri, M., & Brambilla, P. (2007). Anterior cingulate volumes in schizophrenia: a systematic review and a meta-analysis of MRI studies. *Schizophrenia Research, 93*, 1–12.

Carpenter, W. T., & Koenig, J. I. (2008). The evolution of drug development in schizophrenia: Past issues and future opportunities. *Neuropsychopharmacology 33*, 2061–2079.

Chan, R. C., Di, X., McAlonan, G. M., & Gong, Q.-Y. (2011). Brain anatomical abnormalities in high-risk individuals, first-episode, and chronic schizophrenia: an Activation Likelihood Estimation meta-analysis of illness progression. *Schizophrenia Bulletin, 37*,177–188.

Cui, K., Ashdown, H., Luheshi, G. N., & Boksa, P. (2009). Effects of prenatal immune activation on hippocampal neurogenesis in the rat. *Schizophrenia Research, 113*, 288–297.

Davidson, L. L., & Heinrichs, R.W. (2003). Quantification of frontal and temporal lobe brain-imaging findings in schizophrenia: a meta-analysis. *Psychiatry Research, 122*, 69–87.

Fatemi, S. H., Earle, J., Kanodia, R., Kist, D., Emamian, E. S., Patterson, . . . Sidwell, R. (2002). Prenatal viral infection leads to pyramidal cell atrophy and macrocephaly in adulthood: implications for genesis of autism and schizophrenia. *Cellular & Molecular Neurobiology 22*, 25–33.

Fatemi, S. H., Earle, J. A., & McMenomy, T. (2000). Reduction in Reelin immunoreactivity in hippocampus of subjects with schizophrenia, bipolar disorder, and major depression. *Molecular Psychiatry, 5*, 654–663.

Fatemi, S. H., Emamian, E. S., Kist, D., Sidwell, R. W., Nakajima, K., Akhter, P., . . . Bailey K. (1999).Defective corticogenesis and reduction in Reelin immunoreactivity in cortex and hippocampus of prenatally infected neonatal mice. *Molecular Psychiatry, 4*, 145–154.

Fatemi, S. H., & Folsom, T. D. (2009). The neurodevelopmental model of schizophrenia revisited. *Schrizophrenia Bulletin, 35*, 528–548.

Fatemi, S. H., & Folsom, T. D. (2016). Schizophrenia, In S. H. Fatemi and P. Clayton (Eds.), *The medical basis of psychiatry* (4th ed.), New York, NY: Springer. P. 91–120. .

Fatemi, S. H., Folsom, T. D., Reutiman, T. J., Abu-Odeh, D., Mori, S., Huang, H., . . . Oishi, K. (2009). Abnormal expression of myelination genes and alterations in white matter fractional anisotropy following prenatal viral influenza infection at E16 inmice. *Schizophrenia Research 112*, 46–53.

Fatemi, S. H., Folsom, T. D., Reutiman, T. J., Huang, H. , Oishi, K., & Mori, S. (2009). Prenatal viral infection of mice at E16 causes changes in gene expression in hippocampi of the offspring. *European Neuropsychopharmacology, 19*, 648–653.

Fatemi, S. H., Folsom, T. D., Reutiman, T. J., & Sidwell, R.W. (2008). Viral regulation of aquaporin 4, connexin 43, microcephalin and nucleolin. *Schizophrenia Research, 98*,163–177.

Fatemi, S. H., Folsom, T. D., Rooney, R. J., Mori, S., Kornfield, T. E., Reutiman, T. J., . . . Patel, D.H. (2012). The viral theory of schizophrenia revisited: abnormal placental gene expression and structural changes with lack of evidence for H1N1 viral presence in placentae of infected mice or brains of exposed offspring. *Neuropharmacology, 62*, 1290–1298.

Fatemi, S. H., Pearce, D. A., Brooks, A. I., & Sidwell, R. W. (2005). Prenatal viral infection in mouse causes differential expression of genes in brains of mouse progeny: a potential animal model for schizophrenia and autism. *Synapse, 57*, 91–99.

Fatemi, S. H., Reutiman, T. J., Folsom, T. D., Huang, H., Oishi, K., Mori S, . . . Juckel, G. (2008). Maternal infection leads to abnormal gene regulation and brain atrophy in mouse offspring: implications for genesis of neurodevelopmental disorders. *Schizophrenia Research 99*, 56–70.

Fatemi, S. H., Reutiman, T. J., Folsom, T. D., & Sidwell, R. W.(2008). The role of cerebellar genes in pathology of autism and schizophrenia. *Cerebellum, 7*, 279–294.

Fendt, M., Lex, A., Falkai, P., Henn, F. A., & Schmitt, A. (2008). Behavioural alterations in rats following neonatal hypoxia and effects of clozapine: implications for schizophrenia. *Pharmacopsychiatry, 41*, 138–145.

Fornito, A., Yucel, M., Patti, J., Wood, S. J., & Pantelis, C. (2009). Mapping grey matter reductions in schizophrenia: an anatomical likelihood estimation analysis of voxel-based morphometry studies. Schizophr Res 108:104–113.

Fortier, M., Luheshi, G. N., & Boksa, P. (2007). Effects of prenatal infection on prepulse inhibition in the rat depend on the nature of the infectious agent and the stage of pregnancy. *Behavior and Brain Research, 181*, 270–277.

Guidotti, A., Auta, J., Davis, J. M., Gerevini, V. D., Dwivedi, Y., Grayson, D. R., . . . Cost, E. (2000). Decrease in reelin and glutamic acid decarboxylase(67) (GAD(67)) expression in schizophrenia and bipolar disorder – a postmortem brain study. *Archives of General Psychiatry, 57*, 1061–1066.

Harrison, P. J. (1999). The neuropathology of schizophrenia. *Brain 122*, 593–624.

Honea, R., Crow, T. J., Passingham, D., & Mackay, C. E. (2005). Regional deficits in brain volume in schizophrenia: a meta-analysis of voxel-based morphometry studies. *American Journal of Psychiatry, 162*, 2233–2245.

Ibi, D., Nagai, T., Koike, H., Kitahara, Y., Mizoguchi, H., Niwa, M. . . Yamada, K. (2010). Combined effect of neonatal immune activation and mutant DISC1 on phenotypic changes in adulthood. *Behavior and Brain Research, 206*, 32–37.

Jones, C. A., Watson, D. J., & Fone, K. C. (2011). Animal models of schizophenia. *British Journal of Psychiatry, 164*, 1162–1194.

Juárez, I., Gratton, A., & Flores, G. Ontogeny of altered dendritic morphology in the rat prefrontal cortex, hippocampus, and nucleus accumbens following Cesarean delivery and birth anoxia. J Comp Neurol 2008; 507:1734–1747.

Kneeland, R. D., & Fatemi, S.H. (2013). Viral infection, inflammation, and schizophrenia. Prog *Neuropsychopharmacology and Biological Psychiatry, 42,* 35–48.

Koenig, J. & colleagues from the Maryland Psychiatric Research Center.(2014). Animal models of schizophrenia. http://schizophreniaforum.org/res/models/default.asp

Konrad, A., & Winterer, G. (2008). Disturbed structural connectivity in schizophrenia – primary factor in pathology or epiphenomenon? *Schizophrenia Bulletin,* 34,72–92.

Larson, J., Hoffman, J. S., Guidotti, A., & Costa, E. (2003). Olfactory discrimination learning deficit in heterozygous reeler mice. *Brain Research, 97,* 40–46.

Le Pen, G., Jay, T. M., & Krebs, M. O. (2011). Effect of antipsychotics on spontaneous hyperactivity and hypersensitivity to MK-801-induced hyperactivity in rats prenatally exposed to methylazoxymethanol. *Journal of Psychopharmacology, 25,* 822–835.

Li, Q., Cheung, C., Wei, R., Hui, E. S., Feldon, J., Meyer, U., . . . McAlonan, G.M. (2009). Prenatal immune challenge is an environmental risk factor for brain and behavior change relevant to schizophrenia: evidence from MRI in a mouse model. *PLoS One, 4,* e6354

Lipska, B. K. (2004). Using animal models to test a neurodevelopmental model of schizophrenia. *Journal of Psychiatry Neuroscience, 29,* 282–286.

Manahan-Vaughan, D., von Haebler, D., Winter, C., Juckel, G., & Heinemann, U. (2008). A single application of MK801 causes symptoms of acute psychosis, deficits in spatial memory, and impairment of synaptic plasticity in rats. *Hippocampus, 18,* 125–134.

Markota, M., Sin, J., Pantazopoulos, H., Jonilionis, R., & Berretta, S. (2014). Reduced dopamine transporter expression in the amygdala of subjects diagnosed with schizophrenia. *Schizophrenia Bulletin, 40,* 984–991.

Meyer, U. (2014). Prenatal poly(I:C) exposure and other developmental murine activation models in rodent systems. *Biological Psychiatry, 75,* 307–315.

Moore, H., Jentsch, J. D., Ghajarnia, M., Geyer, M. A., & Grace, A. A. (2006).A neurobehavioral systems analysis of adult rats exposed to methylazoxymethanol acetate on E17: implications for the neuropathology of schizophrenia. *Biological Psychiatry,60,* 253–264.

Morice, E., Billard, J. M., Denis, C., Mathieu, F., Betancur, C., Epelbaum, J., . . . Giros, B. (2007). Nosten-Bertrand M: Parallel loss of LTD and cognitive flexibility in a genetic model of hyperdopaminergia. *Neuropsychopharmacology,* 32, 2108–2116.

Nagai, T., Kitahara, Y., Ibi, D., Nabeshima, T., Sawa, A., & Yamada, K. (2011). Effects of antipsychotics on the behavioral deficits in human dominant-negative DISC1 transgenic mice with neonatal polyI:C treatment. *Behavior and Brain Research, 225,* 305–310.

Najjar, S., & Pearlman, D. M. (2015). Neuroinflammation and white matter pathology in schizophrenia: systematic review. Schizophrenia Research.

Park, S. J., Lee, Y., Oh, H. K., Lee, H. E., Lee, Y., Ko, S. Y., . . . Ryu, J. H. (2014). Oleanolic acid attenuates MK-801 induced schizophrenia-like behaviors in mice. *Neuropharmacology, 86,* 49–56.

Piontkewitz, Y., Arad, M., & Weiner, I. (2011). Risperidone administered during asymptomatic period of adolescence prevents the emergence of brain structural pathology and behavioral abnormalities in an animal model of schizophrenia. *Schizophrenia Bulletin,* 37,1257–1269.

Powell, S. B. (2010). Models of neurodevelopmental abnormalities in schizophrenia. *Current Topics in Behavioral Neuroscience, 4,* 435–481.

Reveley, A. M., Reveley, M. A., Clifford, C. A., & Murray, R. M. (1982). Cerebral ventricular size in twins discordant for schizophrenia. *Lancet, 1,* 540–541.

Rojas, P., Joodmardi, E., Hong, Y., Perlmann, T., & Ogren, S. O. (2007). Adult mice with reduced Nurr1 expression: an animal model for schizophrenia. *Molecular Psychiatry, 12,* 756–766

Romero, E., Ali, C., Molina-Holgado, E., Castellano, B., Guaza, C., & Borrell, J. (2007). Neurobehavioral and immunological consequences of prenatal immune activation in rats. Influence of antipsychotics. *Neuropsychopharmacology,* 32,1791–1804.

Savonenko, A. V., Melnikova, T., Laird, F. M., Stewart, K. A., Price, D. L., & Wong, P. C. (2008). Alteration of BACE1-dependent NRG1/ErbB4 signaling and schizophrenia-like phenotypes in BACE1-null mice. *Proceedings of the National Academy of Science USA, 105*, 5585–5590.

Schizophrenia Working Group of the Psychiatric Genomics Consortium. (2014). Biological insights from 108 schizophrenia-associated genetic loci. Nature, 511, 421–427.

Shepherd, A. M., Laurens, K. R., Matheson, S. L., Carr, V. J., & Green, M. J. (2012a). Systematic meta-review and quality assessment of the structural brain alterations in schizophrenia. *Neuroscience and Behavioral Review, 36*, 1342–1356.

Shepherd, A. M., Matheson, S. L., Laurens, K. R., Carr, V. J., & Green MJ. (2012b). Systematic meta-analysis of insula volume in schizophrenia. *Biological Psychiatry, 72*, 775–784.

Shi, L., Fatemi, S. H., Sidwell, R. W., & Patterson, P. H. (2003). Maternal influenza infection causes marked behavioral and pharmacological changes in the offspring. Journal of *Neuroscience, 23*, 297–302.

Southard, E. E. (1915). On the topographical distribution of cortex lesions and anomalies in dementia praecox, with some account of their functional significance. *American Journal of Insanity 76*, 603–671.

Stefansson, H., Sigurdsson, E., Steinthorsdottir, V., Bjornsdottir, S., Sigmundsson, T., Ghosh, S., . . . Stefansson K. (2002). Neuregulin 1 and susceptibility to schizophrenia. *American Journal of Human Genetics, 71*, 877–892.

Steen, R. G., Mull, C., McClure, R., Hamer, R. M., & Lieberman, J. A. (2006). Brain volume in first-episode schizophrenia: systematic review and meta-analysis of magnetic resonance imaging studies. *British Journal of Psychiatry 188*, 510–518.

Sun, J., Maller, J. J., Guo, L., & Fitzgerald, P. B. (2009). Superior temporal gyrus volume change in schizophrenia: a review on region of interest volumetric studies. *Brain Research Review, 61*, 14–32.

Tueting, P., Costa, E., Dwivedi, Y., Guidotti, A., Impagnatiello, F., Manev, R., . . . Pesold, C. (1999). The phenotypic characteristics of heterozygous reeler mouse. *NeuroReport, 10*, 1327–1334.

Wakuda, T., Matsuzaki, H. Suzuki, K., Iwata, Y., Shinmura, C., Suda, S., . . . Mori, N. (2008).Perinatal asphyxia reduces dentate granule cells and exacerbates methamphetamine-induced hyperlocomotion in adulthood. *PLoS One, 3*, e3648.

Watson, D. J., Marsden, C. A., Millan, M. J., & Fone, K. C. F. (2012). Blockade of dopamine D3 but not D2 receptors reverses the novel object discrimination impairment produced by post-weaning social isolation: implications for schizophrenia and its treatment. *International Journal of Neuropsychopharmacology, 11*, 1105–1122.

Wiedholz, L. M., Owens, W. A., Horton, R. E., Feyder, M., Karlsson, R. M., Hefner, K., . . . Holmes, A. (2008). Mice lacking the AMPA GluR1 receptor exhibit striatal hyperdopaminergia and 'schizophrenia-related' behaviors. *Molecular Psychiatry, 13*, 631–640.

Willette, A. A., Lubach, G. R., Knickmeyer, R. C., Short, S. J., Styner, M., . . . Coe, C. L. (2011). Brain enlargement and increased behavioral and cytokine reactivity in infant monkeys following acute prenatal endotoxemia. *Behavior and Brain Research, 219*, 108–115.

Wright, I. C., Rabe-Hesketh, S., Woodruff, P. W., David, A. S., Murray, R. M., & Bullmore, E. (2000). Meta-analysis of regional brain volumes in schizophrenia. *American Journal of Psychiatry, 157*, 16–25.

Zuckerman, L., & Weiner, I. (2005). Maternal immune activation leads to behavioral and pharmacological changes in the adult offspring. *Journal of Psychiatric Research, 39*, 311–332.

PART III

TREATMENT

/// 13 /// MEDICATION TREATMENT STRATEGIES FOR PSYCHOSIS

PHILIP G. JANICAK and KUMAIL HUSSAIN

INTRODUCTION

Schizophrenia causes impairment in cognitive abilities, social interactions, and sensory perception. It usually occurs earlier in life and often evolves into a chronic and debilitating disorder. It is estimated that about 1 percent of the population suffers from schizophrenia worldwide (Schultz, North, & Shields, 2007). Ongoing research to elucidate its pathology focuses on the interactions between environmental and genetic factors, which may alter brain structure and function. These alterations can disrupt relevant neurocircuits, which communicate through various interrelated neurotransmitter systems (Lisman et al., 2008). Although there is much anticipation that biological markers specific for schizophrenia will soon help to better identify patients at risk and improve response to treatment, none are presently available for routine clinical use.

Despite these problems, decades of research have produced a range of therapeutic options for our patients, including multiple biological and psychological therapies (Janicak, Marder, & Pavuluri, 2011). In particular, antipsychotics play a crucial role to help patients maximize the benefit from psychoeducational, psychosocial, and psychotherapeutic approaches. To appreciate the benefit patients receive from these various treatment modalities, it is important to understand the concepts of response, remission, and recovery (Leucht, 2014). Although definitions vary, *response* implies a meaningful symptomatic improvement; *remission* indicates the patient is free of most symptoms for at least six months; and *recovery* emphasizes improvement in cognitive skills, social functioning, and quality of life, even if residual symptoms persist.

This chapter discusses the various treatment approaches for disorders that fall within a psychosis spectrum, focusing on schizophrenia. In this context, we consider individuals who are at *high risk* for developing psychosis, those with *prodromal* symptoms, *first-episode* psychosis, *early-onset* patients, and those with a history of *multiple episodes*. Despite the variety of strategies to manage psychosis, major challenges include treatment resistance and treatment intolerance. Thus, we discuss ongoing efforts to develop new approaches for patients insufficiently benefited by standard therapies. We also consider the risks associated with the available biological therapies.

TREATMENT OF HIGH RISK THROUGH EARLY-ONSET PSYCHOSIS

There is an increasing effort to identify individuals as early in the course of their illness as possible. Appropriate monitoring of these patients in the early stages, assuring the timely introduction of treatment when necessary and monitoring for adequate adherence can all positively alter the long-term prognosis. Ultimately, such efforts may contribute to recovery by improving cognitive abilities, social skills, functionality, and quality of life (QOL) (Harvey et al., 2008; Marchesi et al., 2014).

In this context, a growing body of research is aimed at identifying and treating high risk and prodromal patients to delay or perhaps even avoid a first episode of psychosis. Although it is estimated that 4–8 percent of the population experiences psychotic-like symptoms, less than 40 percent go on to develop a psychotic disorder. This creates a challenge in identifying and managing patients who are at a high risk, since the majority apparently do not progress to a full episode. For example, in a recent meta-analysis of 2,500 patients considered at high risk for psychosis, the mean transition rate was 22 percent at one year, 29 percent at two years, 32 percent at three years and 36 percent after three years (Fusar-Poli et al., 2013). In an effort to better identify these patients, various criteria are being developed by different centers. For example, the ultra-high risk (UHR) criteria require at least one of the following:

- Attenuated psychotic symptoms.
- Brief, limited, intermittent psychotic episodes.
- Trait vulnerability.
- Indeterminate prodromal symptoms.
- Diminished psychosocial functioning (Fusar-Poli et al., 2013).

To help in this assessment, interview methods are available. These include the Structured Interview for Prodromal Symptoms (SIPS) and the Comprehensive Assessment of At-Risk Mental States (CAARMS) (Miller et al., 2003; Yung et al., 2005).

TREATMENT OF HIGH RISK/PRODROMAL PATIENTS

Several clinical studies have evaluated potential therapeutic strategies for this population (Addington & Heinssen, 2012). The Personal Assessment and Crisis Evaluation (PACE) Clinic in Australia conducted one early trial of ultrahigh-risk individuals (McGorry et al., 2002). This six-month, randomized study (n = 59) found that patients who received cognitive behavioral therapy (CBT) plus low-dose risperidone (mean = 1.3 mg/day) had a lower transition rate to first-episode psychosis versus those who received a needs-based intervention (NBI) (Figure 13.1). A more recent study (n = 115) conducted in the PACE Clinic, however, did not find a difference in the transition rates to psychosis at six months for patients receiving CBT plus risperidone, CBT plus placebo, or supportive therapy

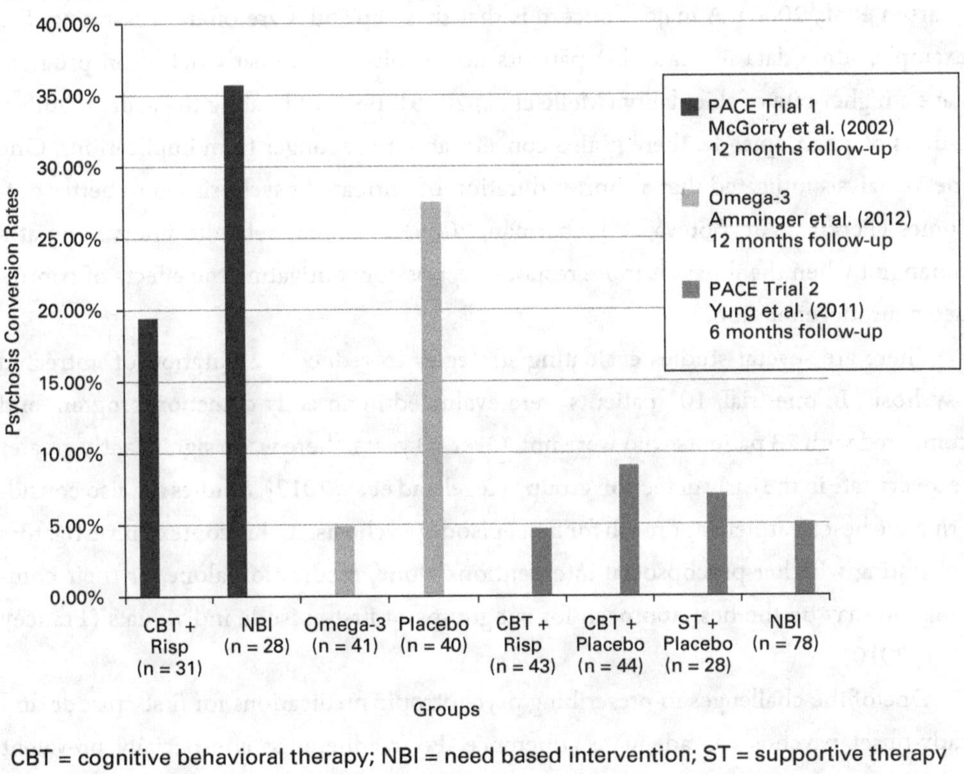

FIGURE 13.1. Trials Evaluating the Psychosis Conversion Rate for High-Risk Patients
CBT = cognitive behavioral therapy; NBI = need based intervention; ST = supportive therapy

plus placebo (Yung et al., 2011). Of note, the low transition rates in all groups may have contributed to this negative outcome.

Given the adverse-effect burden with standard antipsychotics (APs), the use of novel therapies such as omega-3 fatty acids may also benefit these individuals while avoiding AP-related complications (Amminger & McGorry, 2012). This approach stems from the observation that patients with schizophrenia may experience decreased levels of polyunsaturated fatty acids (PUFAs), which are responsible for normal neuronal cell activity. If initial positive findings are replicated in larger, better-designed trials, PUFAs may help prevent a transition to psychosis, benefit first-episode patients, and/or moderate the adverse effects associated with antipsychotics.

TREATMENT OF FIRST EPISODE PATIENTS

Eventually, some high-risk individuals will experience their first episode of psychosis. Unfortunately, although prompt treatment appears to favorably alter the long-term prognosis, many patients go unrecognized and/or untreated for an average of one to two years (Larsen et al., 2006). A major concern is that these episodes are often devastating. For example, some data indicate that patients not involved in an early-detection program have a higher rate of suicidality (Melle et al., 2006). Beyond treating the acute manifestations of a first episode, there is also concern about the longer-term implications. One meta-analysis indicated that a shorter duration of untreated psychosis led to better outcomes (Perkins, Gu, Boteva, & Lieberman, 2005). This may relate to intervening at a timepoint when the illness is more responsive, possibly mitigating the effects of continued neurodegeneration.

There are several studies evaluating strategies to reduce the duration of untreated psychosis. In one trial, 101 patients were evaluated in an early detection program and compared with 73 patients who were not. Over 10 years, there was a significantly greater recovery rate in the early detection group (Hegelstad et al., 2012). Studies are also considering the best treatment approach for first episode psychosis. In this context, investigators are testing whether psychosocial interventions alone, medication alone, or their combination may be the best approach for subgroups of first-episode individuals (Francey et al., 2010).

One of the challenges in prescribing psychotropic medications for first-episode and early-onset psychosis is adequate adherence. Poor adherence is especially prevalent in younger male patients with various complicating issues such as pronounced positive symptoms and/or concurrent substance abuse (Garyfallos, 2007). Although these patients tend to be more responsive to medications, often requiring lower doses of antipsychotics than multi-episode patients, they are also more sensitive to their adverse effects (AEs). In this context, there are several trials that compared first-generation antipsychotics (FGAs) with second-generation antipsychotics (SGAs) for the management of a first episode. One large, double-blind, randomized study (n = 555) assigned patients to risperidone (mean modal dose = 3.3 mg/day) or haloperidol (mean modal dose = 2.9 mg/day). Although both medications significantly improved Clinical Global Impression Improvement (CGI-I) and the Positive and Negative Symptom Scale (PANSS) scores, there was a lower relapse rate and greater median time to relapse in patients on risperidone ($p < 0.04$) (Schooler et al., 2005).

Following acute treatment, the clinician must decide whether patients with remitted first episode psychosis should discontinue their medication, reduce the dose, or receive indefinite maintenance therapy. In one notable trial, a total of 103 patients were followed for seven years. Fifty-two of these patients received maintenance therapy and 51 patients had either a dose reduction or discontinued their medication (Wunderink, Nieboer, Wiersma, Sytema, & Nienhuis, 2013). After seven years, 40.4 percent of the patients who received a dose reduction or discontinued their medication achieved *recovery* versus only 17.6 percent of the patients who received maintenance therapy, even though there was only a minimal difference between the groups for *symptomatic remission.*

TREATMENT OF EARLY-ONSET PSYCHOSIS

Early-onset psychosis usually occurs during adolescence and is associated with a poorer, long-term prognosis. Possible contributing factors are impairment in language, fine motor coordination, and educational abilities (Margari et al., 2008). Most of these patients initially receive SGAs, since they are more prone to the extrapyramidal side effects (EPS) associated with FGAs. In one randomized trial, however, 116 patients with schizophrenia or schizoaffective disorder were assigned to molindone (10–140 mg/day) plus benzotropine (1 mg/day), risperidone (0.5–6 mg/day), or olanzapine (2.5–20 mg/day) (Sikich et al., 2008). There were no significant differences in response rates (i.e., molindone = 50 percent; risperidone = 46 percent; olanzapine = 34 percent) or magnitude of symptom reduction between the groups. Further, patients on risperidone and olanzapine had substantially more weight gain but fewer self-reports of akathisia than those on molindone plus benzotropine. The authors felt these results raise the question of whether the widespread initial use of SGAs in this population is warranted.

TREATMENT OF MULTI-EPISODE PATIENTS

The challenge in treating patients with multiple episodes of psychosis is finding the optimal strategy. It is also important to monitor for adherence, since the highest risk of rehospitalization after an acute psychotic episode is within two months of the initial discharge from the hospital (Markowitz, Karve, Panish, Candrilli, & Alphs, 2013).

Often these patients will present with agitation during an acute exacerbation. If behavioral interventions are not sufficient to manage the episode, various antipsychotic drug formulations (e.g., dissolving tablets, liquid formulations, acute parenteral) can be used for the convenience of the patient or if there is an immediate risk of harm to self or others. Benzodiazepines (e.g., lorazepam) may calm a patient with acute agitation in lieu of using higher doses of an antipsychotic. Haloperidol, aripiprazole, olanzapine, and ziprasidone are also available in acute parenteral formulations as first-line treatments to manage agitation and may be preferred if planning to transition to the oral version for ongoing treatment (Schleifer, 2011).

When managing an acute exacerbation in a multi-episode patient, the clinician should first consider using a previously effective antipsychotic (Parker, 2013). If possible,

TABLE 13.1. Adverse Effects of Antipsychotics*

Drug	Motor	Weight	Anticholinergic	Hematologic	Cardiovascular	Prolactin	Sedation
HPL	IIII	II	0	0	III	III	II
CLZ	0	IIII	IIII	IIII	IIII	I	IIII
RIS	II	III	I	0	II	IIII	II
OLZ	I	IIII	III	0	II	I	IIII
QTP	0	III	I	0	II	I	IIII
ZIP	I	I	I	0	III	I	II
ARP	I	I	0	0	0	0	II
PAL	II	III	I	0	II	IIII	II
ILO	II	II	I	0	I	III	II
ASN	0	II	0	0	0	0	II
LUR	II	I	0	0	I	III	II

*At appropriate doses: 0 = none/minimal risk; IIII = substantial risk

HPL = haloperidol; CLZ = clozapine; RIS = risperidone; OLZ = olanzapine; QTP = quetiapine; ZIP = ziprasidone; ARP =aripiprazole; PAL = paliperidone; ILO = iloperidone; ASN = asenapine; LUR = lurasidone

Adapted from Janicak, P.G.(2014). Pharmacologic treatment of psychosis, . In *Gabbard's treatment of psychiatric disorders*, 5th ed., (pp. 215–229). American Psychiatric Publishing, Washington DC.

the patient should also have a say in the choice of medication. Before choosing a specific agent, other factors that should be assessed include age, medication adverse- effect profile, and any concurrent medical conditions. When patients are initial inadequate responders, options may include adjusting the dose of medication (up or down), augmenting the primary antipsychotic, or switching to an alternate antipsychotic.

MAINTENANCE THERAPY FOR MULTI-EPISODE PATIENTS

Once acute symptoms are adequately stabilized (usually over a six-month period), the focus then shifts to developing an effective maintenance strategy. Additionally, in patients who are insufficiently benefited from oral drugs due to pharmacokinetic issues or have problems with adequate adherence, long-acting injectable (LAI) formulations may be useful. In this context, one meta-analysis of 10 studies found that these agents were associated with a significantly greater reduction in relapse rates compared with oral formulations (Leucht, 2014). The most commonly available antipsychotics in LAI formulations are listed in Table 13.2. Of note, the use of olanzapine pamoate requires careful monitoring for three hours after administration due to a post-injection sedation/delirium reaction in some patients.

At this juncture, psychotherapeutic and psychosocial therapies take on an increasingly important complementary role. Thus, in addition to antipsychotics, various approaches (e.g., cognitive behavioral therapy; cognitive remediation; social-skills training) can facilitate functional recovery (Janicak, Marder, Tandon, & Goldman, 2014). In real-world settings, clinicians often need to try various combinations of medication, psychoeducational, psychosocial, and psychotherapeutic interventions before achieving the optimal results.

TABLE 13.2. Long-Acting Injectable Antipsychotics

Antipsychotic	Dosing Range/Frequency
FGAs	
Haloperidol decanoate	50 to 200 mg/4 weeks
Fluphenazine decanoate	12.5 to 25 mg/2–3 weeks
SGAs	
Olanzapine pamoate	150 to 405 mg/2–4 weeks
Paliperidone palmitate	117 mg/4 weeks
Aripiprazole monohydrate	400 mg/4 weeks
Risperidone microspheres	150 to 405 mg/2–4 weeks

In one small clinical trial, patients were randomized to either an SGA alone (n = 18) or an SGA plus CBT (n = 15) (Pinninti, Rissmiller, & Steer, 2010). Clinical ratings were administered at baseline, at the end of treatment (i.e., 12 weeks) and three months after treatment was completed. Based on the Psychotic Symptom Rating Scale scores, patients who received CBT plus a SGA versus a SGA alone experienced less intense delusions (i.e., final mean scores = 9.57 ± 6.96 and 13 ± 4.84, respectively; $p < 0.05$).

ADVERSE EFFECTS OF ANTIPSYCHOTICS

If medications are used during any stage of the illness, it is critically important to monitor for adverse effects (AEs). The goal is to choose a medication that best facilitates symptomatic and functional recovery in a given patient, while minimizing related safety and tolerability problems. Table 13.1 lists the common AEs associated with the most frequently used FGA, haloperidol, and all available SGAs in the United States.

Motor

Neurological AEs are common but differ in intensity and frequency among the various antipsychotic agents (Janicak & Beedle, 2009). High-potency FGAs such as haloperidol are more likely to cause these problems than SGAs. Common drug-induced movement disorders include akathisia, dystonia, and pseudoparkinsonism. Use of the lowest effective dose, switching medications, and/or the concomitant use of antiparkisonian agents (e.g., benztropine) or beta blockers (e.g., propranolol) can moderate these AEs.

Tardive dyskinesia is a potentially irreversible movement disorder usually associated with more prolonged drug exposure. It is best managed by stopping the antipsychotic or switching to an alternate agent (e.g., from a high-potency FGA to an SGA such as quetiapine or clozapine). Since this is often not clinically feasible, however, there may be limited benefit from trials of clonazepam, ginko biloba, amantadine, or tetrabenazine.

Neuroleptic malignant syndrome (NMS) constitutes a medical emergency, usually presenting with muscle rigidity, delirium, hyperpyrexia, and autonomic dysregulation. It is more likely to occur with high-potency FGAs than with SGAs. If a patient develops NMS, the clinician should immediately stop the agent and initiate appropriate measures such as cooling blankets and hydration. Dopamine agonists, dantrolene, and benzodiazepines may provide benefit as well.

Weight

One of the more common AEs associated with antipsychotics is weight gain. Although this can occur with any agent, clinicians should be aware that certain antipsychotics are more likely to cause this problem; take this into account when choosing a specific agent; be proactive in instituting measures to minimize weight gain (e.g., encourage proper diet and increased exercise); and carefully monitor for and treat complications such as the metabolic syndrome or diabetes mellitus. One meta-analysis of 48 studies considered the associated increase in weight, cholesterol, and glucose with various agents (Rummel-Kluge et al., 2010). Clozapine and olanzapine caused the most elevations; quetiapine, risperidone, and sertindole had intermediate elevations; aripiprazole and amisulpiride had intermediate to low elevations; and ziprasidone the lowest elevations.

Anticholinergic

Anticholinergic adverse effects are prominent with low potency FGAs and certain SGAs (e.g., clozapine; olanzapine). These effects are especially concerning with elderly patients who may be concurrently taking several medications with anticholinergic properties. These adverse effects can be central or peripheral. Central effects may include confusion, memory loss or delirium. Peripheral effects may include constipation, urinary retention, tachycardia and blurred vision. Options are to initially choose agents with a lower propensity to cause these effects; minimize the concomitant use of multiple agents with this property; reduce the dose of the medication when possible; or switch to an agent with less anticholinergic properties (Lieberman, 2004).

Hematologic

Several antipsychotics may cause hematologic problems. These include reductions in platelet count (thrombocytopenia), red blood cell count (anemia) and white blood cell count (leukopenia). Agranulocytosis (i.e., granulocyte count < 500 cells/mm^2) is one of the more serious AEs, primarily associated with clozapine. Therefore, it is mandatory to obtain regular CBC levels as long as a patient is on this agent. With a significant drop in the WBC count, clozapine should be immediately discontinued; white cell stimulating factors (e.g., G-CSF or GM-CSF) introduced; and possibly, the use of IV broad spectrum antibiotics or antifungal agents to prevent serious infections (Flanagan & Dunk, 2008).

Cardiovascular

Patients with schizophrenia have a higher rate of cardiovascular-related morbidity and mortality and a decreased life expectancy compared with the general population. Unfortunately, antipsychotic agents may at times be partially responsible (Mackin, 2008).

One of the more common cardiovascular AEs is orthostatic hypotension. Low potency FGAs (e.g., chlorpromazine; thioridazine) and certain SGAs (e.g., clozapine, olanzapine, risperidone) are more likely to cause this problem. Related complications may be particularly evident in older patients with dementia and associated psychotic symptoms.

QT interval prolongation is another potentially serious AE due to the increased risk of ventricular arrhythmias (e.g., torsade de pointes). Antipsychotics more likely to cause QT prolongation include thioridazine, haloperidol, paliperidone, and ziprasidone. It is important to avoid these agents when possible in patients with preexisting cardiovascular conditions. If they are necessary, monitoring at regular intervals with electrocardiograms (ECGs), using lower doses and avoiding the concurrent use of other agents that also prolong the QT duration may reduce the associated risks.

Prolactin

High-potency FGAs, risperidone, and paliperidone most often induce hyperprolactinemia. Although many patients with increased prolactin levels may be asymptomatic, some can experience problems such as sexual dysfunction, gynecomastia, and amenorrhea. With prolonged prolactin elevations there is an increased risk of osteoporosis and possibly certain cancers (e.g., breast cancer) (Muench & Hamer, 2010). Switching to an agent with less propensity for this complication (e.g., aripiprazole) is the initial strategy. When this is not appropriate, adjunctive aripiprazole in low doses or bromocriptine may ameliorate these symptoms.

Sedation

Sedating properties of an antipsychotic can be beneficial for patients with initial agitation and insomnia. When it persists, however, it can be potentially dangerous (e.g., patients should be cautioned about driving) and is one of the more common reasons for nonadherence. Low-potency FGAs, clozapine and olanzapine are generally more sedating. Steps to reduce any associated risks include minimizing the combination of agents that have this property; lowering the dose when possible; or switching to a less sedating alternative.

TREATMENT-RESISTANT PSYCHOSIS

When patients fail to benefit from standard antipsychotic therapy, several strategies may help to better manage symptoms (Kennedy, Altar, Taylor, Degtiar, & Hornberger, 2014). Clinicians can adjust the dose, try an alternate AP, or augment the primary AP with another agent. Although the focus of most studies in the past was on management of positive symptoms, there is a recent emphasis on improving negative and cognitive symptoms that are more likely to cause persistent functional impairment. The following discussion considers various available and potential approaches to managing treatment resistance. We would note, however, that the real clinical utility of most of these strategies awaits further validation in larger, more rigorously designed trials.

Clozapine

Clozapine should be considered for patients with treatment-resistant psychosis, usually after failing at least two adequate, alternative antipsychotic trials (Kane, 2012). This agent must be used with caution, however, due to its various adverse effects. Some of its important advantages and disadvantages include the following:

Advantages

- Benefits treatment-resistant psychosis.
- Decreases neurological adverse effects.
- Decreases hyperprolactinemia.
- Decreases violent behavior and suicidality.

Disadvantages

- Agranulocytosis.
- Seizures.
- Cardiovascular toxicity (hypotension; myopathy; myocarditis).
- Weight gain.
- Diabetic ketoacidosis.
- Bowel hypomotility.

Antipsychotic Polypharmacy

Since available antipsychotics have varying neuroreceptor profiles, it is postulated by some that combining different agents may "personalize" treatment for a given patient. In a controlled, six-month trial, patients initially on polypharmacy were randomized to a one AP (n = 40) or two AP (n = 48) strategy. After six months, 69 percent of those on monotherapy and 86 percent on polypharmacy remained on that strategy. Additionally, 17 percent initially randomized to a single AP switched back to the combination (Essock et al., 2011). The authors noted, however, that the majority of patients did successfully switch to monotherapy, control of psychotic symptoms did not differ between groups, and more weight gain occurred with polypharmacy. Since clozapine is primarily used for patients who have not responded to other antipsychotics, it is frequently studied in combination strategies when as a monotherapy it also proves insufficient in controlling symptoms. Unfortunately, the results of these studies are mixed, leaving unclear the value of such an approach (Cipriani, Boso, & Barbui, 2009).

Agents Targeting Other Neurotransmitter Receptors

Although all conventional APs modulate dopamine activity (primarily through the D_2 receptor), there is an increased interest in modulating other neurotransmitter receptors to improve efficacy (Kirkpatrick, 2013).

Dopamine

Several studies have explored other DA receptor subtypess (e.g., $DA_{1,3,4,5}$). For example, the D_1 receptor agonist, dihydrexine, can modulate prefrontal dopamine activity, potentially benefiting patients who have hypoactivity in this area (Mu et al., 2007; Snitz et al., 2005). Cariprazine is an antipsychotic currently in development. This agent acts as a partial agonist at the D_2, D_3 and $5HT_{1A}$ receptors and was more effective than placebo for negative and positive symptoms in some, short-term, controlled trials (Caccia, Invernizzi, Nobili, & Pasina, 2013).

Norepinephrine

Norepinephrine (NE) enhances dopamine release in the medial prefrontal cortex and nucleus accumbens, potentially improving cognitive function. Drugs such as guanfacine (an a_{2a} agonist), which is similar to clonidine but with a lower risk of hypotension and sedation, and atomoxetine (a NE reuptake transport inhibitor) may indirectly increase dopaminergic activity in the prefrontal cortex (Friedman, Stewart, & Gorman,

2004). Unfortunately, clinical trials have not clearly demonstrated the benefit of these approaches for schizophrenia (Fitzgerald, 2014).

Serotonin

The serotonin neurotransmitter system has numerous receptors that are implicated in the pathophysiology of schizophrenia, as well as in the mechanism of action of various antipsychotics. In this context, a series of studies have explored the role of the 5-HT_1, 5-HT_2, 5-HT_3, 5-HT_4, 5-HT_6 and 5-HT_7 receptors, including some of their respective subtypes. In particular, the results indicate that 5-HT may play a role in some of the symptom dimensions of schizophrenia (e.g., negative, cognitive); may decrease certain antipsychotic-related AEs (e.g., 5-HT_2 for EPS); but may contribute to other AEs (e.g., 5-HT_{2C} and weight gain) (Meltzer et al., 2012).

Glutamate

Glutamate is the primary excitatory neurotransmitter in the CNS, which works in part through its ionotropic NMDA receptor. Antagonists (e.g., ketamine; PCP) at this receptor can produce symptoms similar to those seen in schizophrenia. Evaluation of glutamate's role in schizophrenia is supported by H-magnetic resonance spectroscopy (H-MRS), which can detect relevant brain metabolite activity. For example, a meta-analysis of 28 studies, including 648 patients and 607 controls, found that medial frontal glutamate levels were decreased and glutamine levels were increased in patients with schizophrenia versus controls (Marsman et al., 2013). Although these studies find glutamate depletion in the prefrontal cortex of patients with schizophrenia, the data is still inconclusive for a potential benefit of treatment with glutamate modulators (Janicak et al., 2014). For example, two large RCTs using lamotrigine (a NMDA receptor modulator) to augment various antipsychotics did not find benefit for this strategy (Goff et al., 2007). In contrast, a meta-analysis did find that lamotrigine augmentation of clozapine was beneficial (Tiihonen, Wahlbeck, & Kiviniemi, 2009).

Glycine is a neurotransmitter that can modulate the effects of glutamate at its NMDA receptor. One example of attempts to capitalize on this is the use of glycine reuptake inhibitors (e.g., bitopertin). In an early controlled trial ($n = 373$), patients were randomized to placebo or bitopertin (10mg, 30mg, or 60mg daily) in addition to their antipsychotic. Patients who received 10 or 30 mg of bitopertin had a greater mean reduction in their negative-symptom factor score on the PANSS in comparison with the placebo group (i.e., $p < 0.05$ and $p < 0.02$, respectively). Another study indicated a potential benefit for N-acetyl-cysteine (NAC), which indirectly impacts the glutamate system by increasing glutathione (GSH) levels. GSH is an antioxidant that is decreased in the medial prefrontal cortex of some individuals with schizophrenia. In a double-blind study (n = 84), patients were randomized to either NAC (2 grams/day) or placebo in addition to their antipsychotic. After four weeks, patients who received NAC had a greater reduction in their total PANSS and CGI–Severity (CGI-S) scores versus placebo (i.e., $p < 0.009$ and $p < 0.004$, respectively) (Umbricht et al., 2014).

GABA

Gamma-aminobutyric acid (GABA) is the primary inhibitory neurotransmitter in the CNS and is implicated in the pathophysiology of schizophrenia (Hasan et al., 2012). Attempts to modulate this system in patients include a six-week, double-blind trial (n = 363) with the GABA agonist BL-1020 (which is also a dopamine antagonist). Patients were randomized to either a placebo, BL-1020 (10 mg/day or 20–30 mg/day) or risperidone (2–8 mg/day). Based on the change scores for the total PANSS, the 20–30 mg/day dose was superior to placebo ($p < 0.02$), had a comparable response rate to risperidone, and produced a significantly greater improvement in cognitive function compared with placebo or risperidone ($p < 0.009$ and $p < 0.019$, respectively) (Geffen, Keefe, Rabinowitz, Anand, & Davidson, 2012).

Acetylcholine

Preclinical studies indicate the activation of muscarinic and nicotinic acetylcholine receptors may enhance cognitive function and alleviate other symptoms associated with schizophrenia.

One study involved the alpha-7 nicotinic receptor partial agonist, TC-5619. Patients on risperidone or quetiapine were randomized to receive either TC-5619 (n = 94) or placebo (n = 91) for 12 weeks (Lieberman et al., 2013). Based on change scores in the Groton Maze Learning Task of the Cogstate Schizophrenia Battery at week 4, the mean difference favored TC-5619 over placebo ($p < 0.036$). There was a similar enhanced benefit for TC-5619 over placebo for negative symptoms ($p < 0.030$) based on the Scale for the Assessment of Negative Symptoms (SANS) scale. Of interest, patients who smoked (46 percent) exhibited a greater benefit with TC-5619 than nontobacco users ($p < 0.028$). The authors concluded that nicotinic partial agonists may have potential cognitive enhancing effects and improve negative symptoms in these patients.

In another small, double-blind, trial (n = 20), patients receiving xanomeline (a M_1 and M_4 receptor agonist) demonstrated a significantly greater improvement on Brief Psychiatric Rating Scale (BPRS) and PANSS scores versus placebo (i.e., $p < 0.05$ and $p < 0.039$, respectively). Further, subjects who received xanomeline had a significantly

TABLE 13.3. Preliminary Positive Results with Novel Therapies

Class of Agents	Potential Benefits
Other Neurotransmitters	
Histamine	Negative symptoms, paranoia
Antidepressants	
Mirtazapine	Negative symptoms, associated depression
Neutraceuticals	
Vitamin D	May reduce risk of developing psychosis
Folate	May reduce risk of developing psychosis
Omega-3-Fatty Acids	Paranoia, auditory hallucinations
N-acetyl-cysteine	Negative Symptoms, cognitive impairment
Hormones	
Estrogen	Positive and negative symptoms
Oxytocin	Positive and negative symptoms
Anti-inflammatory agents	
NSAIDS	May reduce risk of comorbid medical complications
Minocycline	Negative symptoms, cognitive impairment

greater improvement in short-term memory and verbal learning ($p < 0.05$) (Shekhar et al., 2008).

Table 13.3 lists other novel pharmacological strategies that have shown early promise, primarily in proof-of-concept studies.

Therapeutic Neuromodulation

Electroconvulsive therapy (ECT) remains a therapeutic option for some patients with schizophrenia. According to the American Psychiatric Association Guidelines, ECT may be used for those who have previously responded to ECT, those with medication treatment-resistance, or those with catatonic symptoms (Rado & Hernandez, 2014). In a recent meta-analysis of five, randomized, control trials that compared ECT to a sham procedure, patients who received real ECT (with or without antipsychotics) had substantial improvement (RR = 0.76) in their global symptoms versus the sham group (p value not stated) (Tharyan & Adams, 2005). Based on the results of several early trials and decades of clinical experience, most experts agree that ECT remains a viable option for refractory or life-threatening exacerbations of schizophrenia, usually in combination with an antipsychotic.

Transcranial magnetic stimulation (TMS) is a recent therapeutic option for major depression. This device-based treatment delivers intense magnetic pulses to modulate cortical activity. Studies of TMS have also targeted specific symptoms of schizophrenia. One meta-analysis included nine trials (n = 213 subjects), which assessed the benefit of TMS for negative symptoms (Dlabac-de Lange, Knegtering, & Aleman, 2010). The authors concluded that longer duration of treatment and higher frequency of stimulation were associated with larger and more clinically relevant effect sizes. For example, the effect size for studies that used a 10 Hz frequency was (d = 0.63; 95 percent CI = 0.11–1.15) compared with the effect size for all nine studies (d = 0.43; 95 percent CI = 0.05–0.80). In addition, treatment courses that lasted three weeks or more had a greater effect size (d = 0.58; 95 percent CI = 0.19–0.97) versus treatment courses less than three weeks (d = 0.32; 95 percent CI = −0.3 to 0.95). Although other studies suggest that TMS may be a potential therapeutic option for negative, as well as positive and cognitive symptoms associated with schizophrenia, more definitive trials are needed to affirm these promising results.

The potential benefits with TMS and ECT for schizophrenia, open the door for other neuromodulation approaches. One example is transcranial direct cortical stimulation (tDCS), which uses more sustained, low-intensity currents that pass from an anodal to cathodal electrode placed at specific locations on the surface of the head to stimulate or inhibit cortical activity. In one preliminary trial (n = 30), inhibitory tDCS with the cathode placed over the left temporal parietal cortex and the anode over the left DLPFC was more effective for treatment of auditory hallucinations in patients with schizophrenia versus a sham control (i.e., $p<0.001$) (Brunelin et al., 2012). The tDCS course included twice-daily treatments for five weeks using 2mA over 20 minutes with a three-hour break between sessions.

CONCLUSIONS

Schizophrenia often develops into a chronic, debilitating disorder. To more effectively moderate its complications, there is an increasing focus on identifying patients early in the course of their illness. The existing data indicate that timely recognition and appropriate interventions can improve the long-term prognosis. For multi-episode patients, antipsychotics play a crucial role in stabilizing symptoms, so patients may benefit from psychoeducational, psychosocial, and psychotherapeutic interventions. Adverse effects of these agents, however, can pose a significant barrier to achieving the optimal outcome and must be managed effectively.

For the substantial proportion of patients who are insufficiently benefited by standard agents, other approaches are required. Potential strategies include clozapine; antipsychotic polypharmacy; and possibly, novel monotherapy or augmentation approaches. Some of the more promising leads include agents that impact various neurotransmitter systems beyond dopamine, as well as certain neutraceutical, hormonal, and anti-inflammatory agents. Therapeutic neuromodulation (e.g., ECT; TMS) may also represent a potential treatment option for patients with schizophrenia. The optimal strategies to help our patients, however, await the development of biological markers (e.g., genetic; neuroimaging) that will improve diagnosis and provide more targeted treatments. The ultimate goal for our patients is to help them achieve recovery.

CASE DISCUSSION: TREATMENT RESISTANCE

A 20-year-old, African-American male was brought to a psychiatrist by his parents because of increasingly bizarre behavior. The patient had recently dropped out of college and stopped socializing with friends, believing they were transmitting laser beams into his body. The parents also noticed that he appeared to be talking to others when no one else was in the room. Upon confronting him, the patient stated that he was talking to God and that he was Jesus.

The patient was initially started on risperidone (1 mg/day) and eventually titrated up to 6 mg/day for a presumptive diagnosis of schizophrenia. After six weeks, the patient was still only sleeping three hours a night, frequently agitated and constantly hearing voices. He was then switched to quetiapine and titrated up to 600 mg/day. Although the patient's sleep and agitation improved, he continued to experience delusional thoughts and auditory hallucinations. After six months, the patient was switched during a gradual transition from quetiapine to clozapine. The dose of clozapine was adjusted to achieve a serum concentration of 400 ng/ml. Over several weeks, the patient reported less frequent auditory hallucinations, less paranoia, and began attending a support group that he had previously refused. After six months, the psychotic symptoms were substantially reduced and he was able to resume his education at a local college while continuing to live at home.

REFERENCES

Addington, J., & Heinssen, R. (2012). Prediction and prevention of psychosis in youth at clinical high risk. *Annual Review of Clinical Psychology, 8*, 269–289.

Amminger, G. P., & McGorry, P. D. (2012). Update on omega-3 polyunsaturated fatty acids in early-stage psychotic disorders. *Neuropsychopharmacology, 37*(1), 309–310.

Brunelin, J., Mondino, M., Gassab, L., Haesebaert, F., Gaha, L., Suaud-Chagny, M. F., ...Poulet, E.(2012). Examining transcranial direct-current stimulation (tDCS) as a treatment for hallucinations in schizophrenia. *American Journal of Psychiatry, 169*(7), 719–724.

Caccia, S., Invernizzi, R. W., Nobili, A., & Pasina, L. (2013). A new generation of antipsychotics: pharmacology and clinical utility of cariprazine in schizophrenia. *Therapeutics and Clinical Risk Management, 9*, 319–328.

Cipriani, A., Boso, M., & Barbui, C. (2009). Clozapine combined with different antipsychotic drugs for treatment resistant schizophrenia. *Cochrane Database Syst Rev*(3), CD006324.

Dlabac-de Lange, J. J., Knegtering, R., & Aleman, A. (2010). Repetitive transcranial magnetic stimulation for negative symptoms of schizophrenia: review and meta-analysis. *Journal of Clinical Psychiatry, 71*(4), 411–418.

Essock, S. M., Schooler, N. R., Stroup, T. S., McEvoy, J. P., Rojas, I., Jackson, C., & Covell, N. H. (2011). Effectiveness of switching from antipsychotic polypharmacy to monotherapy. *American Journal of Psychiatry, 168*(7), 702–708.

Fitzgerald, P. J. (2014). Is elevated norepinephrine an etiological factor in some cases of schizophrenia? *Psychiatry Research, 215*(3), 497–504.

Flanagan, R. J., & Dunk, L. (2008). Haematological toxicity of drugs used in psychiatry. *Human Psychopharmacology, 23*(Suppl 1), 27–41.

Francey, S. M., Nelson, B., Thompson, A., Parker, A. G., Kerr, M., Macneil, C., . . . McGorry, P. D. (2010). Who needs antipsychotic medication in the earliest stages of psychosis? A reconsideration of benefits, risks, neurobiology and ethics in the era of early intervention. *Schizophrenia Research, 119*(1–3), 1–10.

Friedman, J. I., Stewart, D. G., & Gorman, J. M. (2004). Potential noradrenergic targets for cognitive enhancement in schizophrenia. *CNS Spectrums, 9*(5), 350–355.

Fusar-Poli, P., Borgwardt, S., Bechdolf, A., Addington, J., Riecher-Rossler, A., Schultze-Lutter, F., . . . (2013). The psychosis high-risk state: a comprehensive state-of-the-art review. *JAMA Psychiatry, 70*(1), 107–120.

Garyfallos, G. (2007). [First-episode schizophrenia: Pharmacotherapy and psychosocial interventions]. *Psychiatriki, 18*(1), 29–46.

Geffen, Y., Keefe, R., Rabinowitz, J., Anand, R., & Davidson, M. (2012). Bl-1020, a new gamma-aminobutyric acid-enhanced antipsychotic: results of 6-week, randomized, double-blind, controlled, efficacy and safety study. *Journal of Clinical Psychiatry*, 73(9), e1168–e1174.

Goff, D. C., Keefe, R., Citrome, L., Davy, K., Krystal, J. H., Large, C., ...Webster, E. L. (2007). Lamotrigine as add-on therapy in schizophrenia: results of 2 placebo-controlled trials. *Journal of Clinical Psychopharmacology*, 27(6), 582–589.

Harvey, S. B., Dean, K., Morgan, C., Walsh, E., Demjaha, A., Dazzan, P., ...Murray, R. M. (2008). Self-harm in first-episode psychosis. *British Journal of Psychiatry, 192*(3), 178–184.

Hasan, A., Wobrock, T., Grefkes, C., Labusqa, M., Levold, K., Schneider-Axmann, T. . . . Bechdolf, A.. (2012). Deficient inhibitory cortical networks in antipsychotic-naive subjects at risk of developing first-episode psychosis and first-episode schizophrenia patients: a cross-sectional study. *Biological Psychiatry*, 72, 744–751.

Hegelstad, W. T., Larsen, T. K., Auestad, B., Evensen, J., Haahr, U., Joa, I., ... McGlashan, T. (2012). Long-term follow-up of the TIPS early detection in psychosis study: effects on 10-year outcome. *American Journal of Psychiatry, 169*(4), 374–380.

Janicak, P. G., Marder, S., & Pavuluri, M. (2011). *Principles and practice of psychopharmacotherapy* (5th ed.). Philadelphia, PA: Lippincott, Williams & Wilkins.

Janicak, P. G., Marder, S., Tandon, R., & Goldman, M. (Eds.). (2014). *Schizophrenia: recent advances in diagnosis and treatment*. New York, NY: Springer.

Kane, J. M. (2012). Addressing nonresponse in schizophrenia. *Journal of Clinical Psychiatry*, 73(2), e07.

Kennedy, J. L., Altar, C. A., Taylor, D. L., Degtiar, I., & Hornberger, J. C. (2014). The social and economic burden of treatment-resistant schizophrenia: a systematic literature review. *International Clincali Psychopharmacology, 29*(2), 63–76.

Kirkpatrick, B. (2013). Understanding the physiology of schizophrenia. *Journal of Clinical Psychiatry, 74*(3), e05.

Larsen, T. K., Melle, I., Auestad, B., Friis, S., Haahr, U., Johannessen, J. O., . . . McGlashan, T. (2006). Early detection of first-episode psychosis: the effect on 1-year outcome. *Schizophrenia Bulletin, 32*(4), 758–764.

Leucht, S. (2014). Measurements of response, remission, and recovery in schizophrenia and examples for their clinical application. *Journal of Clinical Psychiatry, 75*(Suppl 1), 8–14.

Lieberman, J. A., 3rd. (2004). Managing anticholinergic side effects. *Prim Care Companion to Journal of Clinical Psychiatry, 6*(Suppl 2), 20–23.

Lieberman, J. A., Dunbar, G., Segreti, A. C., Girgis, R. R., Seoane, F., Beaver, J. S., . . . Hosford, D. A. (2013). A randomized exploratory trial of an alpha-7 nicotinic receptor agonist (TC-5619) for cognitive enhancement in schizophrenia. *Neuropsychopharmacology, 38*(6), 968–975.

Lisman, J. E., Coyle, J. T., Green, R. W., Javitt, D. C., Benes, F. M., Heckers, S., . . . Grace, A. A. (2008). Circuit-based framework for understanding neurotransmitter and risk gene interactions in schizophrenia. *Trends in Neuroscience, 31*(5), 234–242.

Mackin, P. (2008). Cardiac side effects of psychiatric drugs. *Human Psychopharmacology, 23*(Suppl 1), 3–14.

Marchesi, C., Affaticati, A., Monici, A., De Panfilis, C., Ossola, P., & Tonna, M. (2014). Predictors of symptomatic remission in patients with first-episode schizophrenia: a 16years follow-up study. *Comprehensive Psychiatry, 55*(4), 778–784.

Margari, F., Presicci, A., Petruzzelli, M. G., Ventura, P., Di Cuonzo, F., Palma, M., . . . Margari, L. (2008). Very early onset and greater vulnerability in schizophrenia: A clinical and neuroimaging study. *Neuropsychiatric Dieases Treatment, 4*(4), 825–830.

Markowitz, M., Karve, S., Panish, J., Candrilli, S. D., & Alphs, L. (2013). Antipsychotic adherence patterns and health care utilization and costs among patients discharged after a schizophrenia-related hospitalization. *BMC Psychiatry, 13*, 246.

Marsman, A., van den Heuvel, M. P., Klomp, D. W., Kahn, R. S., Luijten, P. R., & Hulshoff Pol, H. E. (2013). Glutamate in schizophrenia: a focused review and meta-analysis of (1)H-MRS studies. *Schizophrenia Bulletin, 39*(1), 120–129.

McGorry, P. D., Yung, A. R., Phillips, L. J., Yuen, H. P., Francey, S., Cosgrave, E. M., . . . Jackson, H. (2002). Randomized controlled trial of interventions designed to reduce the risk of progression to first-episode psychosis in a clinical sample with subthreshold symptoms. *Archives of General Psychiatry, 59*(10), 921–928.

Melle, I., Johannesen, J. O., Friis, S., Haahr, U., Joa, I., Larsen, T. K., ...McGlashan, T. (2006). Early detection of the first episode of schizophrenia and suicidal behavior. *American Journal of Psychiatry, 163*(5), 800–804.

Meltzer, H. Y., Elkis, H., Vanover, K., Weiner, D. M., van Kammen, D. P., Peters, P., . . . Hacksell, U. (2012). Pimavanserin, a selective serotonin (5-HT)2A-inverse agonist, enhances the efficacy and safety of risperidone, 2mg/day, but does not enhance efficacy of haloperidol, 2mg/day: comparison with reference dose risperidone, 6mg/day. *Schizophrenia Research, 141*(2–3), 144–152.

Miller, T. J., McGlashan, T. H., Rosen, J. L., Cadenhead, K., Cannon, T., Ventura, J., . . . Woods, S. W. (2003). Prodromal assessment with the structured interview for prodromal syndromes and the scale of prodromal symptoms: predictive validity, interrater reliability, and training to reliability. *Schizophrenia Bulletin, 29*(4), 703–715.

Mu, Q., Johnson, K., Morgan, P. S., Grenesko, E. L., Molnar, C. E., Anderson, B., . . . George, M. S. (2007). A single 20 mg dose of the full D1 dopamine agonist dihydrexidine (DAR-0100) increases prefrontal perfusion in schizophrenia. *Schizophrenia Research, 94*(1–3), 332–341.

Muench, J., & Hamer, A. M. (2010). Adverse effects of antipsychotic medications. *American Family Physician, 81*(5), 617–622.

Parker, C. (2013). Antipsychotics in the treatment of schizophrenia. *Progress in Neurology and Psychiatry, 13*, 22–30.

Perkins, D. O., Gu, H., Boteva, K., & Lieberman, J. A. (2005). Relationship between duration of untreated psychosis and outcome in first-episode schizophrenia: a critical review and meta-analysis. *American Journal of Psychiatry, 162*(10), 1785–1804.

Pinninti, N. R., Rissmiller, D. J., & Steer, R. A. (2010). Cognitive-behavioral therapy as an adjunct to second-generation antipsychotics in the treatment of schizophrenia. *Psychiatric Service, 61*(9), 940–943.

Rado, J., & Hernandez, E. (2014). Therapeutic neuromodulation for treatment of schizophrenia. In P. Janicak, S. Marder, R. Tandon & M. Goldman (Eds.), *Schizophrenia: Recent Aadvances in diagnosis and treatment.* New York, NY: Springer.

Rummel-Kluge, C., Komossa, K., Schwarz, S., Hunger, H., Schmid, F., Lobos, C. A., . . . Leucht, S. (2010). Head-to-head comparisons of metabolic side effects of second generation antipsychotics in the treatment of schizophrenia: a systematic review and meta-analysis. *Schizophrenia Research, 123*(2–3), 225–233.

Schleifer, J. J. (2011). Management of acute agitation in psychosis: an evidence-based approach in the USA. *Advances in Psychyatry Treatment, 17,* 91–100.

Schooler, N., Rabinowitz, J., Davidson, M., Emsley, R., Harvey, P. D., Kopala, L., . . . De Smedt, G. (2005). Risperidone and haloperidol in first-episode psychosis: a long-term randomized trial. *American Journal of Psychiatry, 162*(5), 947–953.

Schultz, S. H., North, S. W., & Shields, C. G. (2007). Schizophrenia: a review. *American Family Physician, 75*(12), 1821–1829.

Shekhar, A., Potter, W. Z., Lightfoot, J., Lienemann, J., Dube, S., Mallinckrodt, C., . . . Felder, C. C. (2008). Selective muscarinic receptor agonist xanomeline as a novel treatment approach for schizophrenia. *American Journal of Psychiatry, 165*(8), 1033–1039.

Sikich, L., Frazier, J. A., McClellan, J., Findling, R. L., Vitiello, B., Ritz, L., . . . Lieberman, J. A. (2008). Double-blind comparison of first- and second-generation antipsychotics in early-onset schizophrenia and schizo-affective disorder: findings from the treatment of early-onset schizophrenia spectrum disorders (TEOSS) study. *American Journal of Psychiatry, 165*(11), 1420–1431.

Snitz, B. E., MacDonald, A., 3rd, Cohen, J. D., Cho, R. Y., Becker, T., & Carter, C. S. (2005). Lateral and medial hypofrontality in first-episode schizophrenia: functional activity in a medication-naive state and effects of short-term atypical antipsychotic treatment. *American Journal of Psychiatry, 162*(12), 2322–2329.

Tharyan, P., & Adams, C. E. (2005). Electroconvulsive therapy for schizophrenia. *Cochrane Database of Systematic Reviews, 2,* CD000076.

Tiihonen, J., Wahlbeck, K., & Kiviniemi, V. (2009). The efficacy of lamotrigine in clozapine-resistant schizophrenia: a systematic review and meta-analysis. *Schizophrenia Research, 109*(1–3), 10–14.

Umbricht, D., Alberati, D., Martin-Facklam, M., Borroni, E., Youssef, E. A., Ostland, M., . . . Santarelli, L. (2014). Effect of bitopertin, a glycine reuptake inhibitor, on negative symptoms of schizophrenia: a randomized, double-blind, proof-of-concept study. *JAMA Psychiatry, 71*(6), 637–646.

Wunderink, L., Nieboer, R. M., Wiersma, D., Sytema, S., & Nienhuis, F. J. (2013). Recovery in remitted first-episode psychosis at 7 years of follow-up of an early dose reduction/discontinuation or maintenance treatment strategy: long-term follow-up of a 2-year randomized clinical trial. *JAMA Psychiatry, 70*(9), 913–920.

Yung, A. R., Phillips, L. J., Nelson, B., Francey, S. M., PanYuen, H., Simmons, M. B., ... McGorry, P. D. (2011). Randomized controlled trial of interventions for young people at ultra high risk for psychosis: 6-month analysis. *Journal of Clinical Psychiatry, 72*(4), 430–440.

Yung, A. R., Yuen, H. P., McGorry, P. D., Phillips, L. J., Kelly, D., Dell'Olio, M., . . . Buckby, J. (2005). Mapping the onset of psychosis: the Comprehensive Assessment of At-Risk Mental States. *Australian aand New Zealand Journal of Psychiatry, 39*(11–12), 964–971.

/// 14 /// FACTORS INFLUENCING ADHERENCE TO TREATMENT PLANS

DAWN I. VELLIGAN

INTRODUCTION

Adherence to medication is critical for effective illness management. As pointed out by former surgeon general of the United States C. Everett Coop, "drugs don't work in patients who don't take them." Poor adherence to prescribed medication has been called "America's other drug problem" (National Council on Patient Information and Education, 2007).

The recommended treatment for schizophrenia includes maintenance medication to prevent symptom exacerbation. Unfortunately, as many as 60 percent of patients with schizophrenia do not take medication as prescribed (Velligan et al., 2009). Poor adherence to antipsychotic medication has severe consequences including the reemergence or worsening of psychotic symptoms, rehospitalization, and poor functional outcomes. When patients are not taking medication as directed, treatment providers are basing prescribing decisions on poor information. Poor adherence leads to wasted healthcare resources and increases the cost of treatment. Hospitalization costs from nonadherence to antipsychotic medications are estimated to be in the billions of dollars (Sun, Liu, Christensen, & Fu, 2007).

In this chapter, we review the definition of adherence, the scope of the adherence problem for those with schizophrenia, and the consequences of poor adherence for the person seeking treatment, the treatment providers, and society. We describe the many reasons people do not take the medications prescribed and ways a provider can assess and treat problems with medication adherence in this population.

WHAT IS MEDICATION ADHERENCE?

Adherence or *compliance* typically refers to the extent to which a person follows the advice given to him or her by a medical professional. Traditional models of doctor-patient interaction have focused on the expert provider informing the patient about the best course of action for a specific condition. This traditional approach is gradually being replaced with a model of *shared decision making*. Shared decision making is a process involving both the clinician and the person in treatment exchanging information and treatment preferences. In this model, both parties work toward consensus and end with an agreed upon treatment approach (Charles, Gafni, & Whelan, 1997). Thus, the terms *adherence* and *compliance* are giving way to terms such as *medication interest and follow through* or *concordance*. A more patient-centered definition describes adherence or medication follow through as the extent to which a patient follows through on an *agreed upon* treatment plan sufficiently to achieve symptom remission and prevent relapse (Velligan et al., 2009). In this context, the physician takes into account the individual priorities and goals of the person in treatment as a way to determine the optimal medication regimen (i.e., a regimen that is both feasible and effective for that person).

There are many different ways in which people can be considered nonadherent to medication. There are some individuals who completely refuse medication. Although there are a select few who take all the medication prescribed to them, most people with schizophrenia, just like everybody else, take some of their medication some of the time. They may take less than the recommended dose, or take medication intermittently, for example only when they notice that symptoms worsen. This pattern of medication taking is called partial adherence. For an illness like schizophrenia in which insight about being ill tends to fluctuate, it is not clear how much medication needs to be missed before a person may start to believe that she is not ill and does not have to take medication at all. A recent survey of 41 experts in the field revealed that these experts most often defined adherence as taking 80 percent or more of prescribed medication (Velligan et al., 2009).

THE SCOPE OF THE ADHERENCE PROBLEM AND ITS CONSEQUENCES FOR PATIENTS

Adherence to medication treatments is poor across a wide range of physical and psychiatric disorders. This is particularly true for conditions in which medication is taken to prevent the onset or recurrence of symptoms and the consequences of stopping treatment are delayed. For individuals with schizophrenia, this is especially important becase patients do not often experience an immediate worsening of symptoms following missed doses of medication or stopped medication. Symptomatic worsening may not be apparent to someone for days or weeks. This makes it difficult for those with schizophrenia to learn the connection between poor medication adherence and negative consequences such as hospitalization and symptom exacerbation.

In over 35 double-blind trials, which have included more than 3,500 patients, the role of antipsychotic medications in preventing symptom exacerbation and rehospitalization has been firmly established (Davis, Janicak, Singla, & Sharma, 1993). Average rates of relapse for medicated and nonmedicated patients across studies with variable lengths of follow up have been found to be about 20 percent and 55 percent, respectively (Hirsch & Barnes, 1995). Even in first-episode psychosis, the rate of relapse for individuals who are nonadherent to medication is five times greater than for those who consistently take medication following hospitalization (Robinson et al., 1999). Research has shown that as many as 74 percent of patients with schizophrenia become nonadherent with medication within two years after hospital discharge (Weiden et al., 1991). Another report suggested that one in four outpatients was nonadherent between psychiatric visits (Velligan et al., 2009). In a sample of 4,000 people with schizophrenia participating in the California Medicaid program, Weiden et al. also found that medication nonadherence increased the risk for hospitalization (Weiden, Kozma, Grogg, & Locklear, 2004). The number of studies have also documented that poor adherence is related to poor symptom control, poorer functional outcomes, and increased risk for suicide (Velligan et al., 2009).

THE IMPACT OF PROBLEM ADHERENCE ON PROVIDERS

Adherence problems do not just impact the person with schizophrenia but have significant consequences for the prescriber and treatment team. Psychiatrists may have difficulty distinguishing between poor response to medication and poor adherence (Velligan et al., 2007). If a clinician does not know how much medication is being taken, he or she is making treatment decisions based on poor information. He may elect to discontinue a medication, raise a dose, start a new antipsychotic or add a concomitant medication unnecessarily. Moreover, if multiple antipsychotic medications are tried and fail over time due to an individual's poor adherence, that person with schizophrenia may be labeled as "treatment resistant" (Velligan, Lam, Ereshefsky, & Miller, 2003b; Velligan et al., 2007; Velligan et al., 2009).

It is very difficult for a provider to identify all the factors contributing to a person's clinical state during a relatively short medication follow-up appointment, which may occur as infrequently as every three months. During such visits it is difficult to engage the person in building a strong therapeutic alliance. Without a good working alliance with the patient, it may be difficult for him to disclose missed doses or problems with adverse events that may decrease his willingness to follow through with medication.

THE IMPACT OF POOR ADHERENCE ON HEALTHCARE COSTS

Poor adherence increases the direct costs of treatment for patients with schizophrenia by increasing hospitalizations and contact with emergency services. Sun et al. (2007) conducted a review of papers published regarding the economic costs of nonadherence and found that antipsychotic nonadherence was related to an increase in hospitalization rate, hospital days, and hospital costs. Cost for nonadherence in 2005 in the United States was estimated at a staggering $1479 million. In addition, poor adherence increases the indirect costs of schizophrenia by contributing to loss of productivity of the person with the illness as well as family members who have to miss work to assist the person in time of crisis. Other costs associated with poor adherence include the bottles of medication that have been dispensed but not taken.

WHY DON'T PEOPLE TAKE ANTIPSYCHOTIC MEDICATIONS AS PRESCRIBED?

The Treatment Delivery System

There are a host of reasons that medications are not taken as directed (Figure 14.1). Systemic factors such as the availability of prescribers and appointments, waiting time to see the clinician, availability of the physician or other staff between appointments, customer-service philosophy of the agency, location of services, and communication among inpatient and outpatient facilities can either foster or impede medication adherence (Sowers & Rohland, 2004). Poor communication between inpatient and outpatient services can leave patients without appropriate follow-up after discharge leading to a situation in which they have no prescriber to continue medication started on an inpatient unit. If outpatient appointments are rescheduled because physicians are overbooked, patients will have longer gaps between refills. If patients feel unwelcome and like they are burdening physicians by asking questions and taking up their time, medication adherence is likely to be negatively affected.

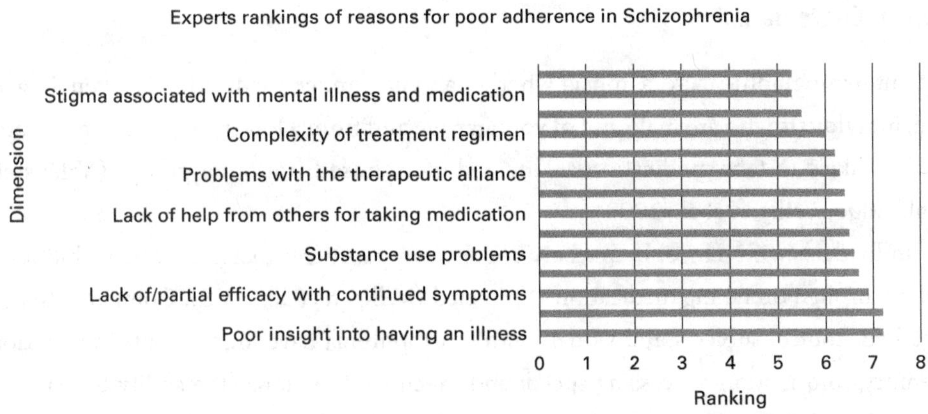

FIGURE 14.1. The expert consensus guidelines for adherence in serious mental illness asked experts to rank the reasons for poor adherence to antipsychotic medications in schizophrenia on a 9-point scale with higher scores indicating greater importance. Here we present the experts mean responses for all reasons rated 5 or greater in order of ranking.

The Medication

Medication factors have also been found to impact an individual's willingness to take medication. Side effects such as weight gain, sleepiness, sexual impairment, restlessness, or involuntary movements can make medication difficult to accept, especially on a long-term basis (Velligan et al., 2009). Some studies have not found medication side effects to be consistent predictors of adherence (Lacro, Dunn, Dolder, Leckband, & Jeste, 2002). Even more than the side effects themselves, the perceived distress caused by specific side effects from the perspective of the individual being treated have been associated with adherence (Velligan et al., 2009). The greater the distress, the less likely the person is to take medication as directed. There is some evidence that timing of medication doses impacts adherence. Medication prescribed multiple times a day in a complicated regimen is less likely to be taken as directed than medication prescribed once a day (Velligan et al., 2009).

If medication is perceived as not being effective in treating a person's symptoms it is less likely to be taken. Sometimes a person's expectations of the medication are not realistic or prescribers may have overpromised efficacy (e.g., medication will stop the voices). When the individual's expectations are not met or the medication initially started has poor efficacy this can decrease his or her willingness to continue with care (Weiden, 2011).

Patient Characteristics

Patient demographic factors impact whether and how much medication is taken. In general, individuals who are male and of younger age and from a lower socioeconomic status are less likely to take medication as directed than those from other groups (Valenstein et al., 2006; Velligan et al., 2009).

Individuals with schizophrenia have cognitive impairments that impact their abilities to follow through on taking medication as directed (Velligan et al., 2008). Compared to age-matched, control subjects, individuals with schizophrenia have impairments in attention, memory, information-processing speed, and executive functions (the ability to plan and carry out goal directed behavior; Green et al., 1997). These impairments make it difficult for individuals to anticipate and solve problems in filling their prescriptions, make it to follow-up appointments, and overcome practical barriers. Even in the absence of formal cognitive impairments, simple forgetting and distraction cause people to miss medication doses. In addition, many individuals with schizophrenia lack a regular daily routine. They have irregular sleep and meal patterns, and chaotic home environments. These factors get in the way of taking medication regularly (Velligan et al., 2008). An intervention developed by Velligan and colleagues (2008) has demonstrated that the use of environmental supports such as calendars, signs, checklists, voice alarms, and specialized pill containers can improve adherence to medication and reduce rates of relapse for individuals with schizophrenia. This suggests that a fair amount of problem adherence in this population is not intentional.

Some individuals with schizophrenia lack insight into their illness and the need for medication (Weiden et al., 1991). Others do not understand the continued need for medications once symptoms of psychosis have subsided. Poor insight may lead to a complete refusal of medication or to more-subtle intermittent patterns of medication taking that are not effective in controlling symptoms. Early in treatment, individuals who have a psychotic illness may not be willing to believe that they have a persistent condition. Some individuals have negative attitudes toward medications in general. These attitudes may be based on general beliefs about health and wellness or on their past experiences with prescribed medications.

Poorer adherence has also been found for individuals with co-occurring substance use disorders (Velligan et al., 2009). Regular assessment of adherence to medication is extremely important in providing optimal treatment for individuals using substances.

The Family

Individuals are more likely to take medication if their families are supportive and stresses to them the need for medication and treatment (Velligan et al., 2009). Some families actively discourage the use of medication. Sometimes this results from a misunderstanding of the illness; family members may not understand the need for continued medication once the patient is doing better. They may confuse illness symptoms with medication effects and blame the medications for "causing" voices or "taking away the individual's personality." At times, family members are just not involved in the individuals' treatments and do not take active roles in their care.

Therapeutic Alliance

Patients' medication compliance is substantially influenced by perceived support from their physician. With increasing pressure from all sides for doctors to perform medication checks, the interpersonal aspects of the doctor–patient relationship are diminished. Optimal therapeutic alliance depends on mutual trust, respect, honesty, openness, and comfort between doctor and patient, all of which take time. Velligan et al., (2009) conducted a survey of 41 experts in adherence to medication in serious mental illness. Problems with the therapeutic alliance were rated among the most important risk factors in predicting problem adherence.

Practical and Environmental Factors

Practical and environmental factors contribute substantially to poor adherence (Figure 14.2). These factors are often underemphasized by clinicians who blame the patient for not following through with prescribed treatment. Transportation, stable housing, and financial concerns are all barriers to good medication adherence. Even for patients with medical insurance, financial concerns often interfere with filling medication prescriptions. A study conducted in the Veterans Administration system by Zeber and colleagues found that even a small increase in the copay from \$2 to \$7 decreased refills of psychiatric medications by 25 percent (Zeber, Grazier, Valenstein, Blow, & Lantz, 2007). Although assistance is often available for those who cannot pay for medications, the forms and process may be too difficult for many people to follow through with on their own. Although many individuals with schizophrenia live in care homes, it is not correct to assume that this means medication is administered by staff. In one study, clinicians found that patients discharged from a state psychiatric hospital to group homes received only 60 percent of their medication during the first 14 days after discharge. Staff members at group homes do not necessarily go and find individuals who do not get in line at medication time.

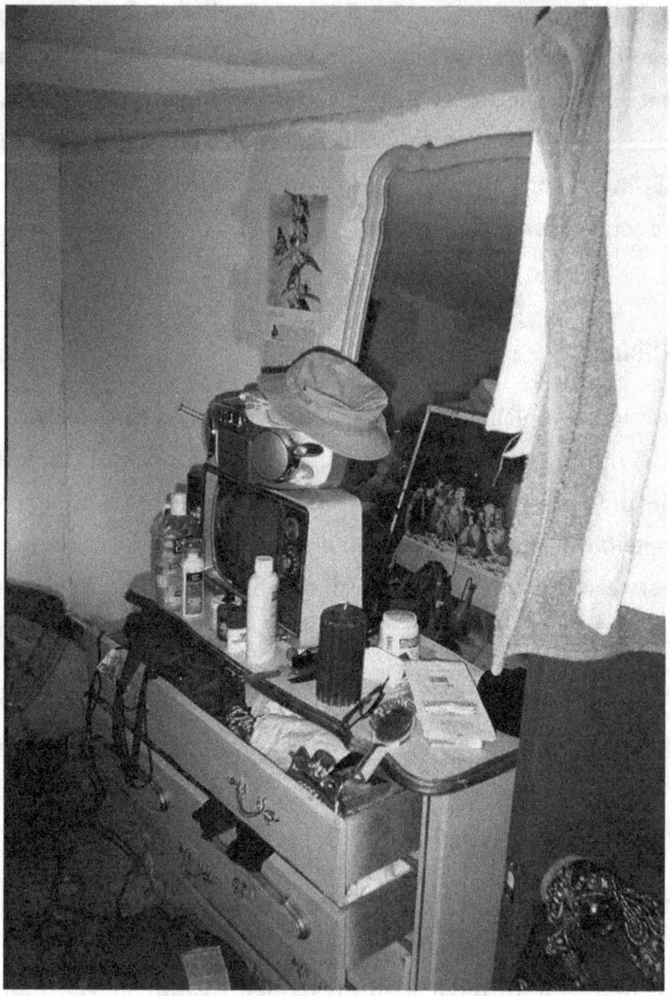

FIGURE 14.2: Actual home environment of a patient taking medications
Imagine finding and taking medication in an environment that is disorganized. Even getting dressed to go to the doctor would be challenging when you can't find what you need. Chaotic and disorganized environments contribute to problem adherence.

WHEN IS POOR ADHERENCE GOOD?

Finally, it is important to remember that not taking medication as prescribed can be a rational response to inappropriate treatment. Doses of medication tend to creep up during periods in which the person has been nonadherent. Concomitant mediations are sometimes added in an attempt to treat symptoms when the problem is that the person is not taking the medication. One hundred percent adherence in such a scenario may lead to increased side-effect burden and may not be best for the patient.

ASSESSING MEDICATION ADHERENCE

There is a host of ways to assess adherence to medication. Most of these do not tell you how much medication is really getting into the person. Subjective methods of assessing adherence include using the report of the patient or caregiver or using the impression of the patient's adherence formed by the physician during the visit. These are the most common ways of assessing adherence in a clinical encounter. Other, more objective measures of adherence include the use of pharmacy refill records, pill counts, electronic monitors, and blood plasma levels. These methods are more commonly used in research studies to assess adherence (Velligan et al., 2006). However, with healthcare moving more toward a pay for performance model, the use of objective measures of medication adherence may become more commonplace in clinical settings as a way of improving patient outcomes.

Self-report and Caregiver Report

Self-report is the simplest way to obtain information about the amount of medication a person is taking. This method is not particularly intrusive and takes little time on the part of the clinician or the person seeking treatment. Unfortunately, this method is also the least reliable (Velligan et al., 2006). Although individuals who say they miss doses or admit nonadherence are usually nonadherent, the majority of patients have been found to overestimate the extent to which they adhere to a treatment regimen. In a recent study comparing multiple measures of medication adherence, self-report identified only 16 percent of patients who were identified as nonadherent based upon electronic monitoring (Velligan et al., 2007). Self-report is impacted by a variety of factors including memory and social desirability. People who generally accept medication and agree that it is important often remember taking medication when they have actually not taken it. In these situations, the intention to take medication is confused with the actual behavior.

Caregivers can also report on adherence. The accuracy of caregiver reports depends on the amount and extent of contact the caregiver has with the patient.

New ways to obtain self-report of medication adherence may make the method more reliable. For example text messages or electronic phone reminders can ask people whether they have taken their medication *today*. Electronic pill containers can ask patients whether the medication is being taken when the container is opened. These technologies produce self-report data that correlates more strongly with objective measures of adherence than self-report based on recall over longer periods of time (Velligan, 2013).

Another common way to assess adherence to medication is by asking the prescriber to make a judgment. Providers often base their assessment of adherence on the report of the patient or on assessment of the patient's clinical state (Velligan et al., 2006). If patients are doing well, it is assumed that they must be taking their medication, and if they are not doing well—it is assumed that they may be missing doses). Unfortunately, a good deal of research has demonstrated that providers are poor judges of medication adherence (Velligan et al., 2007). In multiple studies, the correlations among provider- estimated adherence and objective measures such as pill counts or electronic monitoring were very low (Byerly et al., 2005; Velligan et al., 2007). One recent study reported that providers identified only 40 percent of nonadherent patients who were classified based upon electronic monitoring. In fact, providers were completely unable to identify patients who had or had not taken at least 80 percent of their medication (Velligan et al., 2007). Despite the evidence, providers continue to believe that a majority of their own patients are adherent to medication (Velligan et al., 2009).

Objective Measures of Adherence

A number of objective measures of medication adherence exist, but these are rarely used in clinical settings. Pill counts are one example. Providers can either ask individuals to bring pill bottles into the clinic to be reviewed or case managers can count pills on home visits in cases where these activities can be reimbursed (Velligan et al., 2006). Patients who are the most adherent are also the ones most likely to remember to bring pills in to be counted. Pill counts conducted in the home are moderately correlated with adherence data obtained from electronic monitoring (Velligan et al., 2007). Conducting pill counts in the home can be intrusive and very labor intensive unless patients are part of an assertive community treatment ACT team or are visited in the home at regular intervals by a case manager. However, this method of adherence assessment can provide valuable information. Pill counts are not always accurate. It is possible for some individuals to be perfectly adherent without obtaining a prescription refill for a year because they have so many bottles of unused pills in their home! (Velligan, Lam, Ereshefsky, & Miller, 2003a). Pills can be dumped prior to visits so that the person may appear more adherent than they actually are.

Electronic monitoring is an objective way to assess adherence. Electronic monitors that keep track of when medication bottles are opened can be contained in the bottles' caps (Velligan et al., 2006; Velligan et al., 2008). Information from the cap is downloaded to a computer. The assumption with such devices is that medication is taken when the cap is opened. Problems include that the cap can be left off resulting in no data being recorded. More sophisticated electronic monitors are capable of multiple functions including prompting medication, storing multiple types of medication, asking the patient when the container is opened whether the medication is really being taken, and warning patients when they are taking the wrong medication or taking it at the wrong time (Velligan et al., 2013). These devices are capable of downloading information to secure websites that can be examined by family members or case managers. Moreover, these devices can email case managers or family members if adherence falls below a pre-specified level. This method is somewhat intrusive and labor intensive. The device must be placed in the home by a caseworker and the monitor needs to be filled either by a pharmacy or by the patient with the assistance of a visiting caseworker. In addition, there needs to be a person responsible for intervening if problem adherence is identified. However, patients can press a button indicating that they have taken medication when they have not, which is just one of the problems with this kind of monitoring system However, this type of "in the moment" self-report is moderately to strongly correlated with objective measures of adherence (Velligan, 2013).

Another objective measure of adherence is directly observed behavior. This method is impractical and highly intrusive as the individual either needs to be present at the clinic or someone must go to the home and watch medication ingestion (Velligan et al., 2008). However, smartphones with video talk features can now be used to observe medication-taking behavior, making the method more feasible and fairly easy to use. With this approach, a member of the treatment team must be available to watch the person take medication via video. A potential problem is that an individual could spit the medication out following the call.

Blood levels of psychiatric medications and/or their metabolites can be used to track adherence. Blood levels are fairly intrusive for the patient and are only useful when there is a known relationship between the clinical effects of the drug and blood/serum concentration (Gualtieri & Golden 1984; Morselli & Bianchetti, 1983). Blood levels of antipsychotic medications can tell you whether medication is or is not being taken, but they are unable to provide information on how much medication is being taken (Velligan et al., 2007). Therefore, they are not particularly useful for the vast majority of individuals with schizophrenia who take some of the medication some of the time. Blood levels are impacted by the behavior in the several days before the blood draw. This means that someone could take no medication for the majority of the month and then take medication for several days before the draw and still appear adherent.

Prescription renewals can be used to monitor medication adherence in an unobtrusive way (Velligan et al., 2006; Velligan et al., 2009). Getting feedback from the pharmacy regarding if and when an individual is picking up medication can tell the treatment team if there are any gaps of time during which medication is not available to the patient. The method can be complicated. Patients sometimes get medications from more than one pharmacy, more than one doctor, or from friends or family. This method tends to underestimate actual ingestion of medication. Patients can fill prescriptions and not take them. HMOs and insurance plans may require patients to refill their medication quarterly. Patients may accept unneeded prescriptions because they are embarrassed to admit that they are not taking the medication as prescribed or because they are passive (Rudd et al., 1989). However, in large samples, prescription-refill data has proven a valid indicator of risk for poor outcome. For patients with schizophrenia, gaps as short as 11 days in which medication is not available for the patient to take have been found to increase the risk of hospitalization (Valenstein et al., 2002).

A more recent advance for objectively assessing adherence to medication is the "smart pill." In 2010, the FDA approved a tiny digestible microchip that is placed on medication tablets. The microchip communicates with a watch sensor worn by the patient that can identify when medication has been taken. Noningestion of medication can prompt the sensor to send messages to the patient, care workers, or family. The use of such technologies may be the future of adherence assessment (Velligan & Kamil, 2014).

An important strategy for assessing adherence is the use of long-acting injections (Weiden, 2011). Although patients may or may not be more adherent to medication delivered by injection, nonadherence is immediately apparent when the person does not show up for their shot (Velligan et al., 2011). Using long-acting injectable antipsychotic medication can help the clinician disentangle lack of efficacy from poor adherence to medication (Velligan et al., 2009). If a person is getting an injection regularly and symptoms are poorly controlled, the prescriber can be more confident that the medication is either at the wrong dose or is not the best medication for the individual. Injectable medication allows the prescriber to make treatment recommendations based on good-quality data about adherence.

Assessing Medication Adherence in a Clinical Interview

Weiden (2011) recommends assessing attitudes toward medication, and adherence behavior during initial and follow-up medication appointments. Prior to discussing adherence, it is helpful to normalize the fact that everybody misses medication sometimes. He also points out that the clinician should avoid projecting irritation or disappointment about adherence behavior if he or she wants to know the truth. Asking questions about whether there are any logistical or practical problems with obtaining or taking the medication, inquiring about substance use, and problems remembering to take medication or getting refills can give the prescriber a better idea of the challenges faced by the patient.

It is important not to blame the patients for nonadherence, but to attempt to understand their perspective about taking medication.

WHAT TO DO ABOUT PROBLEM ADHERENCE

The first step in addressing adherence problems is to prevent them. Shared decision making is particularly important in prescribing medications for schizophrenia and related disorders. A focus on understanding the preferences and values of the patient is central to both treatment outcomes and medication adherence in situations in which there is no clear "best" treatment and there are many choices with variable sideeffect profiles (Joosten et al., 2008; Mahar, 2007; Roe, Goldblatt, Baloush-Klienman, Swarbrick, & Davidson, 2009). This is exactly the case in treating schizophrenia, with large differences in side-effect profiles among antipsychotic medications but little difference in efficacy (other than clozapine for treatment refractory schizophrenia) (Lieberman & Stroup, 2011). Research has demonstrated that consumers with serious mental illnesses want more input into decisions regarding their treatment and want treatment decisions to be derived in a shared manner (Adams, Drake, & Wolford, 2007; Curtis et al., 2010; Klein, Rosenberg, & Rosenberg, 2007).

The therapeutic approach to dealing with adherence problems when they arise depends to a great extent on the reasons for problem adherence (Velligan et al., 2009). When there is little insight into having an illness or needing medication, adherence can be challenging. After all, why should individuals take medication if there is nothing wrong with them? Research has demonstrated that insisting that someone accept a psychiatric diagnosis or educating him or her about the diagnosis in this situation is counterproductive (Weiden, 2011). Instead, approaches based on Cognitive Behavior Therapy (CBT) can be helpful. CBT focuses on the patient's perspective of their medication treatment. In treatment, patients tell their stories about the kinds of treatment they have had and what approaches were and were not helpful. Treatment techniques in CBT include normalizing the desire not to take medication, rolling with resistance (understanding it and not engaging in argument), avoiding giving advice, and using a series of guided questions to help the patient associate meeting their personal goals with taking medication. CBT interventions have been found to improve adherence in schizophrenia (Julius, Novitsky, & Dubin, 2009; Scott & Tacchi, 2002; Turkington, Dudley, Warman, & Beck, 2004; Turkington, Kingdon, & Weiden, 2006).

One of the reasons that individuals with serious mental illnesses such as schizophrenia are treated in community outpatient clinics is that case managers are available in these settings to help patients overcome practical issues that interfere with adherence.

Case managers who make home visits can do a lot to improve adherence (Velligan et al., 2008).

Environmental supports such as signs, checklists, clocks, calendars, pill containers and the organization of belongings are highly effective techniques for improving adherence to medication (Figure 14.3). In a series of studies, a systemized approach to using environmental supports to bypass impairments in cognitive function was found to improve adherence and decrease rates of relapse for patients with schizophrenia (Velligan et al., 2013; Velligan et al., 2008). Common interventions include the following: a sign placed on the back of the front door to remind the person to take medication before leaving

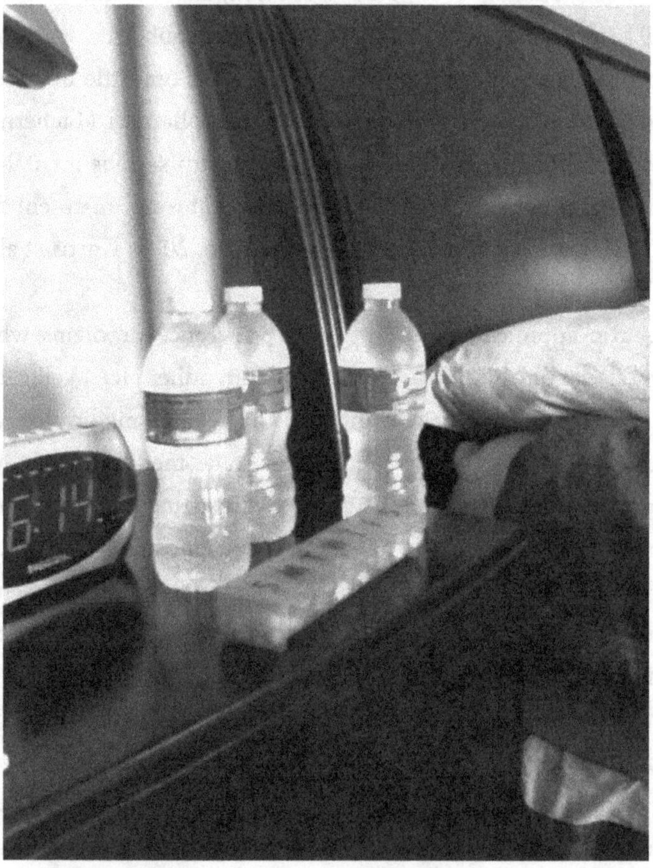

FIGURE 14.3: Environmental supports to make medication easier to take
This is one example of an environmental support that can improve adherence. Medication and medication bottles are placed on the night stand right by the person's bed so that if the person forgets to take night doses, he or she does not have to go all the way into the kitchen to find their medication and get some water. This intervention is maintained on weekly home visits.

home, a checklist used for daily activities including taking pills, medications placed in specialized pill containers, and use of a voice alarm with a personal message recorded by the patient to remind him or her to take medication and why it's important (e.g. "it's time to take medication. I want to take medication so I can work on getting a job"). In a more recent study, these environmental supports were compared to the use of an electronic pill container that was designed to remind patients to take medication. When problem adherence was identified, a brief telephone intervention was used to address reasons for the problem. Adherence in both of these active treatments was 90 percent compared to treatment as usual where medication adherence was 70 percent (Velligan et al., 2008).

Other technologies such as the use of test messaging are increasingly being used to improve adherence in medical illness. Granholm and colleagues found that it was feasible to deliver simple reminders to take medication via cell phone to patients with schizophrenia (Granholm, Ben-Zeev, Link, Bradshaw, & Holden, 2012).

Finally, interventions for providers can also be helpful. Training physicians in using CBT techniques to ensure that the patient's perspective regarding medications is addressed can be helpful. In addition, physicians can be trained to spot individuals who are not receiving optimal benefit from medications. For example, people on more than one antipsychotic medication at the same time, people for whom a prescriber has tried several antipsychotic medications over the course of the past year, people who are not happy with the amount of symptom control they have, people who abuse substances, and people who say they miss medication doses may all be candidates for long-acting injection, because poor response may be related to problem adherence. Simple checklists can be used in the clinic setting to identify individuals who are having a less-than-optimal response and for whom the physician may want to consider long-acting injection (Velligan, 2013).

CONCLUSIONS

In sum, adherence is a complex problem with multiple risk factors. Identification and treatment of adherence problems is one of the most pressing public health issues for schizophrenia and many other illnesses.

REFERENCES

Adams, J. R., Drake, R. E., & Wolford, G. L. (2007). Shared decision making preferences of people with severe mental illness. *Psychiatric Services, 58*(9), 1219–1221.

Byerly, M., Fisher, R., Whatley, K., Holland, R., Varghese, F., Carmody, T., . . . Rush, A. J. (2005). A comparison of electronic monitoring vs. clinician rating of antipsychotic adherence in outpatients with schizophrenia. *Psychiatry Research, 133*(2–3), 129–133.

Charles, C., Gafni, A., & Whelan, T. (1997). Shared decision-making in the medical encounter: What does it mean? (or it takes at least two to tango. *Social Science and Medicine, 44*, 681–692.

Curtis, L. C., Wells, S. M., Penney, D. J., Ghose, S. S., Mistler, L. A., Mahone, I. H., . . . Lesko, S. (2010). Pushing the envelope: Shared decision making in mental health. *Psychiatric Rehabilitation Journal, 31*(1), 14–22.

Davis, J. M., Janicak, P. G., Singla, A., & Sharma, R. P. (1993). Maintenance antipsychotic medication. In T. R. E. Barnes (Ed.), *Antipsychotic drugs and their side effects* (pp. 183–203). New York, NY: Academic Press.

Granholm, E., Ben-Zeev, D., Link, P. C., Bradshaw, K. R., & Holden, J. L. (2012). Mobile Assessment and Treatment for Schizophrenia (MATS): A pilot trial of an interactive text-messaging intervention for medication adherence, socialization, and auditory hallucinations. *Schizophrenia Bulletin, 38*(3), 414–425. doi: 10.1093/schbul/sbr115

Green, M. F., Marshall, B. D., Wirshing, W. C., Ames, D., Marder, S. R., McGurk, S., . . . Mintz, J.. (1997). Does risperidone improve verbal working memory in treatment-resistant schizophrenia? *American Journal of Psychiatry, 154*(6), 799–804.

Gualtieri, C. T., & Golden, R. N. (1984). Blood level measurement of psychoactive drugs in pediatric psychiatry. *Therapeutic Drug Monitoring 6*, 127–141.

Hirsch, S. R., & Barnes, T. R. E. (1995). The clinical treatment of schizophrenia with antipsychotic medications. In S. R. Hirsch & D. R. Weinberger (Eds.), *Schizophrenia.* Oxford, England: Blackwell Science.

Joosten, E. A. G., Defuentes-Merillas, L., De Weert, G. H., Sensky, T., van der Staak, C. P. F., & De Johng, C. A. J. (2008). Systematic review of the effects of shared decision making on patient satisfaction, treatment adherence and health status. *Psychotherapy and Psychosomatics* 77(4), 219–226.

Julius, R. J., Novitsky, M. A., & Dubin, W. R. (2009). Medication adherence: A review of the literature and implications for clinical practice. *Journal of Psychiatric Practice, 15*, 34–44.

Klein, E., Rosenberg, I., & Rosenberg, S. (2007). Whose treatment is it anyway? The role of consumer preferences in mental health care. *American Journal of Psychiatric Rehabilitation, 10*, 65–80.

Lacro, J. P., Dunn, L. B., Dolder, C. R., Leckband, S. G., & Jeste, Dilip V. (2002). Prevalence of and risk factors for medication nonadherence in patients with schizophrenia: a comprehensive review of recent literature. *Journal of Clinical Psychiatry, 63*(10), 892–909.

Lieberman, J. A., & Stroup, T. S. (2011). The NIMH-CATIE schizophrenia study: What did we learn? *American Journal of Psychiatry, 168*, 770–775.

Mahar, M. (2007). Braveheart: Jack Wennberg. *Dartmouth Medicine, 32*, 31–68.

Morselli, P. L., & Bianchetti, G. (1983). Therapeutic drug monitoring of psychotropic drugs in children. *Pediatric Pharmacology 3*, 149–156.

National Council on Patient Information and Education. (2007). Educate before you medicate. Enhancing prescription medicine adherence: A National Action Plan. URL: http://www.talkaboutrx.org/documents/enhancing_prescription_medicine_adherence.pdf. Rockville (MD).

Robinson, D., Woerner, M. G., Alvir, J. M., Bilder, R. M., Goldman, R., Geisler, S., . . . Lieberman, J. A. (1999). Predictors of relapse following response from a first episode of schizophrenia or schizoaffective disorder. *Archives of General Psychiatry, 56*(3), 241–247.

Roe, D., Goldblatt, H., Baloush-Klienman, V., Swarbrick, M., & Davidson, L.. (2009). Why and how people decide to stop taking prescribed psychiatric medication. Exploring the subjective process of choice. *Psychiatric Rehabilitation Journal 33*, 366–374.

Rudd, P., Byyny, R. L., Zachary, V., LoVerde, M. E., Titus, C., Mitchell, W. D., & Mrshall, G. (1989). The natural history of medication compliance in a drug trial: limitations of pill counts. *Clinical Pharmacology and Therapeutics 46*, 169–176.

Scott, Jan, & Tacchi, M. J. (2002). A pilot study of concordance therapy for individuals with bipolar disorders who are non-adherent with lithium prophylaxis. *Bipolar Disorders, 4*(6), 386–392.

Sowers, W. S., & Rohland, B. (2004). American Association of Community Psychiaatrists' principles for managing transitions in behavioral health services. *Psychiatric Services, 155*, 1271–1275.

Sun, S. X., Liu, G. G , Christensen, D. B., & Fu, A. Z. (2007). Review and analysis of hospitalization costs associated with antipsychotic nonadherence in the treatment of schizophrenia in the United States. *Current Medical Research and Opinion, 23*(10), 1205–1212.

Turkington, D., Dudley, R., Warman, D. M, & Beck, A. T. (2004). Cognitive-behavioral therapy for schizophrenia: A review. *Journal of Psychiatric Practice, 10*(1), 5–16.

Turkington, D., Kingdon, D., & Weiden, P. J. (2006). Cognitive behavior therapy for schizophrenia. *American Journal of Psychiatry, 163*, 365–373.

Valenstein, M., Copeland, L. A., Blow, F. C., McCarthy, J. F., Zeber, John E., Gillon, L., . . . Stavenger, T. (2002). Pharmacy data identify poorly adherent patients with schizophrenia at increased risk for admission. *Medical Care, 40*(8), 630–639.

Valenstein, M., Ganoczy, D., McCarthy, J.F., Kim, H. M., Lee, T. A., & Blow, F. C. (2006). Antipsychotic adherence over time among patients receiving treatment for schizoprhenia: A retrospective review. *Journal of Clinical Psychiatry, 67*(10), 1542–1550.

Velligan, D. I. (2013). *Developing methodologies for tracking and improving adherence*. Paper presented at the 53rd Annual NCDEU Meeting, Hollywood, FL.

Velligan, D. I., Diamond, P. M., Mintz, J., Maples, N., Li, X., Zeber, J., . . . Miller, A. L. (2008). The use of individually tailored environmental supports to improve medication adherence and outcomes in schizophrenia. *Schizophrenia Bulletin, 34*(3), 483–493. doi: 10.1093/schbul/sbm111

Velligan, D. I., & Kamil, S. H. (2014). Enhancing patient adherence: Introducing smart pill devices. *Therapeutic Delivery* 5(6), 611–613.

Velligan, D. I., Lam, F., Ereshefsky, L., & Miller, A. L. (2003a). Obstacles in assessing adherence to oral antipsychotic medications. *Psychiatric Services, 54*(5), 665–667.

Velligan, D. I., Lam, F., Ereshefsky, L., & Miller, A. L. (2003b). Psychopharmacology: Perspectives on medication adherence and atypical antipsychotic medications. *Psychiatric Services, 54*(5), 665–667.

Velligan, D. I., Lam, Y. W., Glahn, D. C., Barrett, J. A., Maples, N. J., Ereshefsky, L., & Miller, A. L. (2006). Defining and assessing adherence to oral antipsychotics: A review of the literature. *Schizophrenia Bulletin, 32*(4), 724–742. doi: 10.1093/schbul/sbj075

Velligan, D. I., Medellin, E., Draper, M., Maples, N., Dassori, A., Moore, T. A., & Lopez, L. (2011). Barriers to, and strategies for, starting a long acting injection clinic in a community mental health center. *Community Mental Health Journal*. doi: 10.1007/s10597-011-9389-6

Velligan, D. I., Mintz, J., Maples, N., Li, X., Gajewski, S., Carr, H., & Sierra, C. (2013). A randomized trial comparing in person and electronic interventions for improving adherence to oral medication in schizophernia. *Schizophrenia Bulletin, 39*(5), 999–1007. doi: 10.1093/schbul/sbs116

Velligan, D. I., Wang, M., Diamond, P., Glahn, D. C., Castillo, D., Bendle, S., . . . Miller, A. L. (2007). Relationships among subjective and objective measures of adherence to oral antipsychotic medications. *Psychiatric Services, 58*(9), 1187–1192. doi: 58/9/1187 [pii] 10.1176/appi.ps.58.9.1187

Velligan, D. I., Weiden, P. J., Sajatovic, M., Scott, J., Carpenter, D., Ross, R., & Docherty, J. P. (2009). The expert consensus guideline series: adherence problems in patients with serious and persistent mental illness. *Journal of Clinical Psychiatry, 70*(Suppl 4), 1–46; quiz 47–48. doi: v70s0401 [pii]

Weiden, P., Dixon, L., Frances, A., Appelbaum, P., Haas, G., & Rapkin, B. (1991). Neuroleptic noncompliance in schizophrenia. In C. A. Tamminga & S. C. Schutz (Eds.), *Advance in neuropsychiatry and psychopharmacology* (pp. 285–296). New York, NY: Raven Press.

Weiden, P. J. (2011). The adherence interview: Better information, better alliance. *Psychiatric Annals, 4*(5), 279–285.

Weiden, P. J., Kozma, C., Grogg, A., & Locklear, J. (2004). Partial compliance and risk of rehospitalization among California Medicaid patients with schizophrenia. *Psychiatric Services, 55*(8), 886–891.

Zeber, J. E., Grazier, K. L., Valenstein, M., Blow, F. C., & Lantz, P. (2007). Effect of a medication copayment increase in veterans with schizophrenia. *American Journal of Managed Care, 13*(6 part 2), 335–346.

/// 15 ///

OVERVIEW OF COGNITIVE REMEDIATION IN SCHIZOPHRENIA

IAN S. RAMSAY, TASHA M. NIENOW, and ANGUS W. MACDONALD III

INTRODUCTION

The cognitive impairments observed in schizophrenia are broad and pervasive (Heinrichs & Zakzanis, 1998) and are associated with functional disability (Green, Kern, & Heaton, 2004). This recognition has spurred interest among researchers and clinicians alike in the development of interventions that target this aspect of the illness. Though numerous clinical trials have been conducted to test the efficacy of medications as cognitive enhancing agents, only modest improvements in cognitive status have been observed as the result of pharmacotherapy (Choi, Wykes, & Kurtz, 2013). At present, cognitive remediation training (CRT), a behavioral-training approach, is emerging as a promising class of interventions. This chapter will synthesize findings from intervention studies, cognitive neuroscience, and psychopathology to describe the nature and scope of these interventions, to review evidence of efficacy with regard to cognitive, psychosocial, and biological outcomes, and to unpack our current understanding of the factors that may influence response to the intervention.

DEVELOPMENT OF COGNITIVE REMEDIATION TRAINING IN SCHIZOPHRENIA

CRT refers to various efforts to improve the cognitive symptoms of schizophrenia, such as impaired attention, problem solving, and memory, using behavioral learning strategies (Keefe et al., 2011). The development of modern cognitive training interventions for people with schizophrenia began in the 1960s and 1970s. As an understanding emerged of the cognitive difficulties faced by people with schizophrenia, so did efforts to improve cognitive faculties in areas of attentional control, concept formation, and reinforcement learning. Many early intervention studies borrowed techniques from previously successful studies with stroke and traumatic brain injury (TBI) patients and offered either a repeated practice or a strategy-based intervention (Kurtz Moberg, Gur, & Gur, 2001). Typically, these studies targeted a specific cognitive domain such as attention or memory, and change in performance on the training task was used to assess improvement in cognitive performance. The majority of these studies lacked the methodological rigor of a randomized clinical trial, however they demonstrated that people with schizophrenia could learn new skills and showed that cognitive impairments in schizophrenia were modifiable. These studies were followed by small-scale experimental and naturalistic studies in which participants received relatively focused training in a cognitive domain, and change was assessed with neuropsychological measures of the same and related cognitive domains. Although findings from these studies were mixed, enough support was found to support the emergence of full-scale clinical trials in the 2000s (for review, see Twamley, Jeste, & Bellack, 2003).

In the last 15 years, there has been tremendous growth in the development of CRT, with a number of clinical investigators developing variants. The dimensions along which CRT interventions differ will be summarized later. However, regardless of the scope of the intervention and the training techniques, all CRT interventions assume that people with schizophrenia are able to recover or compensate for cognitive functions lost to the ravages of the disease.

DIMENSIONS OF COGNITIVE REMEDIATION TRAINING

One of the most fundamental ways in which CRT interventions differ is in the choice of training techniques employed. Historically, approaches have utilized either drill and practice training or strategy-based coaching. These approaches are not mutually exclusive, and many CRT interventions incorporate both to some extent. Drill and practice approaches, which are arguably more prominent, typically rely on computers to deliver adaptive cognitive training. Task difficulty is modified based on participant performance, and training programs offer concentrated practice with cognitive skills during the course of a session (Saperstein & Kurtz, 2013). In contrast, strategy coaching provides practice that applies techniques such as mnemonics, chunking, goal setting, and self-monitoring to performance on cognitive tasks of graded difficulty (Wykes & van der Gaag, 2001). The focus of the training approach reflects theoretical differences about hypothesized treatment mechanisms. Drill and practice approaches are based on the underlying assumption that intensive training can change the brain circuitry supporting impaired cognitive processes. In contrast, those who rely more heavily on strategy-based coaching assume that the aim of training is to teach compensatory strategies with preserved abilities so that the individual is better able to circumvent existing deficits. The goal of strategy coaching is to provide patients with skills they can use to organize and simplify information processing demands. In practice, these approaches are often used in a complimentary manner, with the prominence of training techniques varying by intervention.

When restorative drill and practice approaches integrate aspects of strategy coaching, this is often accomplished through the provision of a bridging group that compliments the computerized training (Medalia & Saperstein, 2013). The purpose of the group is to address barriers to applying cognitive gains made through computer-based training to real-world situations. The transfer of cognitive training gains to application in everyday life is a process called generalization. To promote this process, the bridging groups provide education about compensatory strategies, encourage practice of cognitive skills outside the training environment, identify the relevance of cognitive training to participant life goals, and address psychological barriers such as performance anxiety and lack of confidence. The content of bridging groups varies considerably among interventions but may include group discussion, performance feedback, and activities to practice cognitive skills in a real-life context.

Another distinction that can be made among restorative drill and practice CRT interventions is with regard to the structure of the cognitive training curriculum: top-down versus bottom-up. In theory, top-down refers to executive abilities such as reasoning, working memory, and attention, whereas bottom-up refers to perceptual processes, although this distinction is loose in practice. The Neuropsychological and Educational Approach to Cognitive Remediation (NEAR) is an example of a top-down approach (Medalia, Revheim, & Herlands, 2009). Proponents of the top-down approach argue that cognitive abilities are used together in everyday life to accomplish tasks and, therefore, training will be most effective if abilities are trained in coordination with one another. The curriculum in top-down training approaches begins with higher-order executive processes with the assumption that foundational abilities such as attention are being trained simultaneously (Medalia & Choi, 2009). In contrast, in a bottom-up curriculum, such as POSIT Science's, cognitive processes are arranged hierarchically and practiced in relative isolation, enabling focused, massed training on each cognitive domain targeted by the intervention (Vinogradov, Fisher, & de Villers-Sidani, 2012). Basic cognitive processes such as attention, motor skills, and perceptual processes are introduced into the curriculum initially, and then higher-order cognitive processes such as memory and executive processes are incorporated into later stages of training. Some clinics have capitalized on the benefits of each approach using a blend in which training relies on a bottom-up presentation of curriculum and then transitions to a top-down administration.

Breadth of training focus is another dimension along which CRT approaches differ. The majority of CRT interventions have been broad-based, meaning that they target multiple cognitive domains. Most typically, attention, verbal and visual memory, and executive functioning are among the trained cognitive domains. The broad focus of most interventions reflects our current understanding of cognition in people with schizophrenia from a neuropsychological perspective. People with schizophrenia have been characterized as having a generalized deficit in cognition, meaning that patients typically often perform one or more standard deviations below their healthy peers across a wide range of cognitive domains (Heinrichs & Zakzanis, 1998). In addition, people with schizophrenia are a heterogeneous population, and there is considerable variability in severity, type, and number of cognitive domains impaired from person to person (Palmer et al., 1997). Without a consistent pattern of cognitive impairment in the patient population or guidance about whether there are specific, potentially rate limiting, cognitive domains that contribute to the range of cognitive and psychosocial deficits observed in schizophrenia, intervention programs often adopt a broad focus. In contrast, a focused approach may target a single cognitive domain. This approach is more likely to be used when the interventionist has a very specific goal. For instance, an intervention may be focused on attentional training, because this ability is deemed necessary before engagement in other types of rehabilitation is possible.

Historically, a therapist who works with patients individually or in small groups has administred CRT. However, as computerized training software has become more sophisticated, investigators explored the feasibility of administering CRT as a self-paced intervention (Fisher et al., 2014; Ventura, Wilson, Wood, & Hellemann, 2012). The promise of self-paced CRT interventions is that they may enable broad-spread use of the intervention. Advocates of self-paced CRT interventions have expressed concern that therapist-guided, and thus, clinic-based interventions are not accessible to many patients given the frequency with which patients attend training sessions and the resources that treatment facilities must provide to offer CRT as a regular clinic service (computer lab, staffing of a small group intervention). At present, only two studies have examined the feasibility of self-paced CRT. They found that 70–75 percent of patients assigned to the self-paced cognitive training were able to follow through with the cognitive training independently. Their results suggest that self-paced training is likely to be feasible for the majority of outpatients with schizophrenia; however, the attrition rates in these studies are slightly higher than those typically reported in therapist-guided, clinic-based studies of CRT, which have ranged between 10–25 percent. Additional research is needed to determine if self-paced interventions can be designed to be user-friendly and engaging enough to motivate patients to sustain independent practice.

Although computer software may enable self-paced practice of cognitive skills, it is less clear whether the programs will be able to provide the other therapeutic components of a therapist-guided, clinic-based intervention. The role of CRT therapists is not only to develop a cognitive training curriculum, but also to engage participants in the process of learning, to enhance self-awareness, to promote personal growth, and to facilitate transfer of learning to application in other settings (Medalia et al., 2009). To accomplish these objectives, therapists actively involve patients in curriculum choices and goal setting and link the classroom training to real-world activities. Throughout the course of the intervention, patient frustration tolerance is closely monitored, and therapists coach patients in the use of adaptive problem solving strategies. Therapist-patient interactions promote and reinforce the use of personal competencies. Therapists reinforce adaptive coping strategies, highlight signs of progress in treatment, and address emotional and learning styles that detract from progress. In theory, the provision of CRT in a clinic setting can support these therapeutic objectives, and the experience of being part of a class can offer individuals emotional support, provide an opportunity to practice interpersonal skills, and offer peer-based learning opportunities such as observation and sharing of learning styles, feedback about personal competencies, and peer-to-peer teaching experiences. As the development of self-paced CRT interventions progresses, the role of therapists in CRT is likely to become more varied. It will be important for research to determine whether self-paced training interventions maintain the integrity of therapist-guided approaches.

ASSESSMENT OF COGNITIVE REMEDIATION TRAINING

With the growth in CRT, there has been a greater need to define what it is and to develop standards for assessing its effectiveness. In 2011, the Cognitive Remediation Experts Workgroup defined CRT as "a behavioral training-based intervention that aims to improve cognitive processes (attention, memory, executive functioning, social cognition, or metacognition) with the ultimate goal of durability and generalization (Keefe et al., 2011)." Two years later, the workgroup updated the definition to "an intervention targeting cognitive deficits using scientific principles of learning with the ultimate goal of improving functional outcomes" (Saperstein & Kurtz, 2013). As the latter definition more explicitly states, the need to reduce the disability associated with the illness drives the development of these interventions.

This concern was also voiced in 2004 when, as part of the Measurement and Treatment Research to Improve Cognition in Schizophrenia (MATRICS) initiative, the U.S. Food and Drug Administration and the National Institute of Mental Health established standards for measuring change in clinical trials of new drugs seeking approval as cognitive enhancers. The guidelines from this process became the standard used to evaluate all cognitively enhancing interventions, pharmacological or behavioral. This group concluded that for a pharmacological agent to be approved as cognitively enhancing, the medication would need to produce change not only on a cognitive battery but also on another measure of change in functioning (Green et al., 2008).

In terms of change on a cognitive battery, the MATRICS Cognitive Consensus Battery (MCCB) was normed specifically for clinical trials of cognitively enhancing interventions for people with schizophrenia (Nuechterlein & Green, 2006). The battery was assembled by selecting from established neuropsychological measures of seven cognitive domains: working memory, attention and vigilance, verbal learning and memory, visual learning and memory, reasoning and problem solving, speed of processing, and social cognition. Currently, the MCCB serves as the measure most commonly used to assess CRT-related change in cognition.

The MATRICS work group specified that the co-primary measure in clinical trials could be a measure of functional capacity or an interview-based assessment of cognition. Presently, measures of functional capacity are much more commonly used in CRT clinical trials. Functional capacity is defined as an individual's ability to complete a skill under optimal conditions (e.g., in a laboratory setting). Functional capacity is assessed with performance-based tools in which participants are asked to demonstrate performance of a skilled activity with the materials provided by the investigator. For instance, the University of California San Diego Performance Skills Assessment (UPSA) is a task that uses this approach to assess five domains of independent living skills (Patterson, Goldman, McKibbin, Hughs, & Jeste, 2001). Functional capacity measures are preferred to measures of functional outcomes (real-world outcomes) in clinical trials, because functional capacity measures are more sensitive to change and are often more easily and reliably administered (Harvey, Velligan & Bellack, 2007). In the next section the impact of CRT of cognitive performance and measures of functioning will be reviewed.

MEASUREMENT AND EFFICACY OF COGNITIVE REMEDIATION

One way of evaluating the efficacy of an intervention is with a statistical procedure called meta-analysis. With this procedure, findings from multiple studies can be combined to derive an estimate of an intervention's strength. Magnitude of change is often reported in terms of effect size. When Cohen's d is used to measure effect size, d = 0.20, 0.50, and 0.80 are considered a small, medium, and, large effect sizes, respectively. The most recent meta-analysis of CRT was conducted in 2011 by Wykes and colleagues, and included a total of 40 studies with 2,104 total participants. Wykes et al. reported that the mean overall effect of CRT on global cognition was d =0.45 and that change on individual cognitive domains ranged from d = 0.25 to 0.65. Only 11 of the studies included in the meta-analysis assessed the stability of intervention-induced cognitive change, but intervention-induced cognitive change was found to be relatively stable in the months post-CRT, d =0.43. A similar level of intervention-induced change was found on measures of functioning, with change in overall functioning reported to be d = 0.42 at postintervention and d = 0.37 at follow-up.

Another way of evaluating the effectiveness of CRT is to examine the specificity of the treatment effect by comparing outcomes from CRT to that of cognitively stimulating comparison groups. In studies that have compared the magnitude of cognitive change with CRT versus a cognitively stimulating condition such as work therapy (Bell, Bryson, Greig, Corcorsn, & Wexler, 2001; McGurk, Mueser, DeRosa, & Wolfe, 2009), skills training (Bowie, McGurk, Mausbach, & Harvey, 2012) enriched supportive therapy (Hogarty, Flesher, Ulrich, et al., 2004), or cognitive behavioral therapy (Penadés et al., 2006), investigators have found significantly greater change on some or all of the indices of cognitive performance included in the study assessment. These results suggest that CRT is offering a benefit not obtained by many other types of stimulating environments.

However, when CRT is compared to another type of computer-based training, the findings regarding the specific benefit of CRT on cognition are less consistent. Three studies have compared CRT to a comparison condition in which participants played video games. A comparison group in which participants play video games controls for time spent on the computer but engages participants in an activity that is not designed to specifically target or train cognitive skills. Two of these studies found that the cognitive training offered by CRT produced significantly greater change than the comparison group on a global measure of cognition as well as verbal memory specifically (Fisher, Holland, Merzenich, & Vinogradov, 2009; Fisher et al., 2014). These studies suggest that the cognitive training offered by CRT is enhancing to cognition in a way that is specific to the intervention. However, two other studies using a computer-based comparison group have not found support for this conclusion. In a third study that compared CRT to a video game comparison group, recipients of CRT were found to demonstrate improved performance on the tasks on which they trained; however, they did not demonstrate any significant improvement on the postintervention assessment of cognition as compared to participants in the video game comparison group (Dickinson et al., 2010). Similarly,

Kurtz, Seltzer, Shagan, Thime, & Wexler (2007) compared CRT to a computer skills class and found that participants in both conditions changed significantly on measures of verbal, spatial, and working memory, processing speed, and executive functioning. Those who received CRT demonstrated significantly greater performance than the computer skills group in only one domain, working memory. The authors concluded that the computer-skills class along with the support of the training environment was sufficient to produce meaningful change in many aspects of cognition, because only one domain, working memory, appeared to benefit from the focused training offered by CRT.

Another domain that has been investigated is the efficacy of CRT when offered as a stand-alone intervention compared to training in the context of a larger psychiatric rehabilitation program. CRT has been paired successfully with work therapy (Bell et al., 2001; Wexler & Bell, 2005), supported employment (McGurk, 2005), supported education (Kidd, Kaur Bajwa, McKenzie, Ganguli, & Haji Khamneh, 2012), training in social skills and social cognition (Hogarty et al., 2004), and functional adaptation-skills training (Bowie et al., 2012). These studies suggest that offering CRT with another type of skills training, either sequentially or concurrently, can reinforce and may potentiate the treatment gains made from either individually. This principle was initially discovered in studies that combined CRT with a form of work therapy. Compared to work therapy alone, patients who received CRT and work therapy were found to make greater improvements in cognitive functioning (McGurk, 2005; Bell et al. 2001) and to obtain higher rates of employment (McGurk, 2005; Bell, Zito, Greig, & Wexler, 2008). Wexler and Bell hypothesized that productivity in the work place may allow patients to use their cognitive skills in a meaningful way, thus supporting long-term maintenance of cognitive gains. Of note, in the Bell et al. (2008) study, it was only in the follow-up period that participants in CRT and work therapy functioned better than those who received work therapy only. Although people in work therapy alone experienced a decline in employed hours after the active intervention period, those who received CRT with work therapy maintained treatment gains, suggesting that CRT may enhance the durability of other types of skills training.

A similar synergy was found in a recent study that examined the independent and additive contribution of CRT and functional adaptation skills training. Bowie et al. (2012) found that participants who received CRT and skills training demonstrated significantly greater change on measures of independent living skills than patients who received only skills training or CRT. In addition, gains in functional skills were maintained through the follow-up period in those who received the combined treatment, whereas those who received skills training declined. Together, the results of these studies suggest a synergistic relationship between CRT and other types of psychiatric rehabilitation. Skills-based psychiatric rehabilitation has facilitated maintenance of cognitive training gains and transfer of cognitive skills to real-world functioning, and CRT has allowed participants in other types of skills training to learn more and maintain gains longer. These findings have been reflected in meta-analyses: functional change was found to be small when CRT was offered as a stand-alone intervention across studies, but became moderate when offered with psychiatric rehabilitation or strategy coaching (McGurk, Twambley, Sizer, Mchugo, & Mueser, 2007).

Taken together, these studies suggest that CRT is more cognitively enhancing than many activities in a person's day-to-day life. However, it is less clear if cognitive training is offering benefit greater than that provided by other types of computer activities that offer a cognitive challenge. CRT may also meet it's objective of improving functional outcomes most efficiently by including elements of psychiatric rehabilitation or strategy coaching that promote the use of cognitive skills in everyday life. Further research is needed to better understand these synergies and the active and specific components of CRT interventions.

BRAIN CHANGES ASSOCIATED WITH COGNITIVE REMEDIATION

Although measures of cognition and psychosocial functioning serve as the primary indices of improvement in response to CRT, changes in neural functioning are thought to underlie these behavioral changes. Translational research has established that neural plasticity, the brain's ability to change in response to new behaviors or environments, is feasible well into adulthood (Buonomano & Merzenich, 1998). CRT has been hypothesized to work through this mechanism and to restore disrupted neural networks through repeated practice of cognitive skills. As we now reviewed, support for this hypothesis has been garnered from studies examining the brain's response to cognitive tasks as well as training-related changes in cortical health.

In recent years, several studies have been conducted to examine whether the cognitive training offered as part of CRT influences the neural function of supporting brain regions. In one of the first studies of this type, Haut , Lim, and MacDonald (2010) used a focused training intervention to target working memory. Haut and colleagues found that patients who received CRT improved more than a psychosocial comparison group on trained and untrained versions of a working memory task (N-back task) and that the change in performance on the working memory task was related to increased activation in brain regions that support working memory functioning. Hooker et al. (2012) found a similar pattern of findings in a study focusing on emotion recognition ability. Participants who were assigned to a CRT intervention focused on both neurocognitive processes and emotion recognition abilities demonstrated greater improvement on an emotion-recognition task than participants in the control group. Improved performance on this task was related to greater brain activation in regions supporting emotion-recognition performance. The results of these studies suggest that the mechanism of CRT is restorative and that it is possible to improve brain function in schizophrenia.

In addition, training-induced neural improvement may predict changes in psychosocial functioning (Subramaniam et al., 2012). Subramaniam and colleagues found that people with schizophrenia who completed 80 hours of CRT showed increased activation in the medial prefrontal cortex and that this improvement in neural functioning predicted psychosocial functioning six months later. Related work has demonstrated that training-induced change in the lateral prefrontal cortex also predicted occupational functioning in six months. If these results are replicated, imaging technology may become another means of measuring ability to respond to the intervention.

Research with neuroimaging techniques also suggests that CRT is enhancing other aspects of cortical functioning and structure. For instance, people with schizophrenia have been found to have poor neural connectivity between regions of the brain (dysconnectivity) that is believed to contribute to poor cognitive performance (Lynall et al., 2010). In a study focused on functional connectivity rather than regional brain activation, patients showed functional connectivity patterns more like those of healthy controls after CRT (Penadés et al., 2013), supporting theories that this type of training may restore healthy neural functioning. Similarly, a study that used imaging techniques to observe brain structure rather than function noted gray matter preservation in the hippocampus, amygdala, and fusiform gyrus as the result of CRT, suggesting that this treatment may confer neuroprotective factors to support improved cognitive functioning (Eack et al., 2010).

PATIENT CHARACTERISTICS PREDICTIVE OF RESPONSE TO CRT

Presently, one of the challenges facing clinicians and CRT developers is a limited understanding of who responds to CRT. As with other types of skills training, variability in response has been observed among recipients. For instance, Kurtz et al. (2007) observed that only 22 percent of recipients in the study sample demonstrated a large response to CRT treatment. A better understanding of who is able to benefit from CRT would enable clinicians to more effectively refer patients to CRT or tailor the intervention to the individual.

Several studies have examined whether patient demographics, illness, or cognitive characteristics are predictive of the amount of change in cognitive performance with

CRT. Few relationships have been reported consistently. With regard to demographics, the impact of age has been of greatest interest. Although age has been unrelated to cognitive improvement in some studies (Fiszdon, Cardenas, Bryson, & Bell, 2005; Medalia & Richardson, 2005, Wykes et al. 2011), others have reported that patients 40 and over have a smaller response to CRT than patients under 40 (Kontis, Huddy, Reeder, Landau, & Wykes, 2012; Wykes, Reeder, Landau, Matthiasson, Haworth, & Hutchinson, 2009). If this age effect is found to be robust, then it will be important for researchers to determine if a larger dose of CRT can lead to greater change in cognition among older adults. Other patient characteristics that have been found to be important include a cooperative attitude (Fiszdon 2005), motivation to complete treatment, and effective work habits (Medalia & Richardson, 2005).

Studies examining the impact of illness characteristics on the efficacy of CRT have focused on diagnosis, chronicity, and symptom severity. Diagnosis (schizophrenia versus schizoaffective disorder) and indicators of illness chronicity (number of previous hospitalizations) have not been predictive of treatment response (Medalia & Richardson, 2005; Scheu et al., 2013). Symptom severity has been found to relate to CRT-induced cognitive change in some (Vita et al. 2013; Wykes , Huddy, Cellard, McGurk, & Czobor, 2011) but not all studies (Medalia & Richardson, 2005; Scheu et al., 2013). When a relationship was found, lower baseline symptom severity was associated with a greater response to CRT. Although illness factors have not been strong predictors of outcome thus far, more research is being done in this area. In particular, there is great interest in determining whether CRT interventions make a greater impact on cognitive and functioning outcomes for individuals in the prodromal or early phase of illness (for review see Fisher, Loewy, Hardy, Schlosser & Vinogradov, 2013).

Research has also looked at whether baseline cognitive characteristics are predictive of response to CRT. Baseline cognitive performance measured by neuropsychological test performance has not been found to be predictive of intervention induced cognitive change (Medalia & Richardson; 2005, Scheu et al., 2013; Vita et al., 2013). However, clinician rating of cognitive difficulties has been predictive of treatment response. People with schizophrenia who were rated as less impaired on the Positive and Negative Syndrome Scale Cognitive Factor, an index reflecting difficulties with disorientation, poor attention and abstract thinking, and conceptual disorganization, were found to be more likely to improve with CRT. Although results appear to differ depending on how cognitive difficulties are assessed, it is encouraging that intervention-induced cognitive improvement is not related to baseline neuropsychological performance, because this may mean that patients can benefit from CRT regardless of their level of illness-related cognitive impairment.

In recent years, a few studies have begun to examine whether patient characteristics at the onset of CRT are predictive of postintervention *functional change.* Age, baseline cognitive performance, and pre-intervention functioning have been found to be predictive of change in functional status. Similar to the research on cognitive change, Vita et al. (2013) reported that patient age was predictive of functional improvement, with younger patients making greater gains with CRT. With regard to baseline cognitive performance, baseline attention and working memory ability have been found to be predictive of change in functional capacity (Kurtz et al. 2007), and a trend has been noted for executive functioning to predict post-CRT functioning in the community (Vita et al., 2013). In both studies higher baseline performance predicted greater functional gains with CRT. In addition, pre-intervention level of functioning is related to functional improvement with CRT (Bell, Choi, Dyer, & Wexler, 2014). In this study, participants were assigned to receive either supported employment or supported employment with CRT. The lower-functioning people with schizophrenia who received supported employment and CRT achieved significantly higher employment rates than individuals in supported employment only. In contrast, among higher-functioning participants, the addition of CRT to supported employment did not enhance outcomes. As additional research is conducted, it will be of interest to clarify the extent to which there are common versus unique predictors of cognitive and functional change with CRT.

TREATMENT CHARACTERISTICS ASSOCIATED WITH RESPONSE TO THE INTERVENTION

Investigators have examined the impact of treatment factors on response to CRT, including medication dose and type, therapist characteristics, and CRT treatment dose. In people with schizophrenia, CRT is intended to be an adjunct to pharmacotherapy. Two recent studies have examined the impact of medication-related factors on response to CRT. Vita et al. (2013) reported that a lower antipsychotic dose at baseline was the strongest predictor of cognitive and functional improvement with CRT. The nature of these relationships cannot be determined from the design of their study. It may be that participants with a milder course of illness were on a smaller dose of medication and also made greater gains from treatment. Alternatively, the relationships may suggest that high doses of antipsychotic medications actually attenuate the benefits of training. Future research is needed to determine if this is an illness or treatment characteristic of interest. A medication-related factor that has been found to influence CRT response is anticholinergic burden. Many medications, including a few of the antipsychotics prescribed to treat schizophrenia and some of the medications prescribed to control antipsychotic-related side effects have anticholinergic properties. Vinogradov et al. (2009) examined the level of serum anticholinergic activity at baseline and found that it negatively predicted CRT-induced improvement on a global measure of cognition, indicating that this medication factor is adversely impacting response to CRT. The results of this study call attention to the need to carefully coordinate CRT with other aspects of an individual's care.

With regard to CRT treatment characteristics that appear to influence outcome, Medalia and Richardson (2005) found that patients were more likely to respond to CRT when a highly trained, doctoral-level therapist provided it, as compared to a clinician with less training. They also found intensity of CRT training to be a significant moderator of treatment response. Individuals who completed the training more efficiently, attending at least two sessions a week, benefited significantly more than individuals who attended sporadically. Surprisingly, the literature currently offers very little guidance regarding the amount and intensity of cognitive training needed for CRT to be effective. In recent clinical trials, intervention dose has ranged from 24 to 100 sessions (McGurk et al., 2009; Fisher et al. 2009). Recently, a panel of experts met to develop recommendations for future studies. They suggested that, at a minimum, programs offer at least two hours of training weekly for a total of 30 to 40 sessions over a three-month period (Keefe et al., 2011). Although this guideline is helpful, several CRT developers have noted that intervention dose is likely to be dependent on treatment goals, with different doses needed to produce short- versus long-term change in cognition or impact other potential treatment targets such as psychosocial functioning or neural systems (Vinogradov et al. 2012; Wykes & Spaulding, 2011). As we gain a better understanding of how and for whom this intervention is effective, additional dosing recommendations are likely to emerge.

CONCLUSIONS AND FUTURE DIRECTIONS

Cognitive remediation is a behavioral training technique to address the cognitive and functional impairments associated with schizophrenia. Randomized clinical trials of the intervention offer modest support for its effect on cognitive and functional outcomes. Although these findings are promising, investigators have voiced concerns that treatment gains have remained relatively stable in the last decade (Vinogradov et al., 2012), suggesting that the intervention is not becoming more effective. One response to this concern has been to more carefully examine individual, illness, and treatment characteristics that might moderate treatment response. Although this is a newly emerging literature, some findings have been replicated, suggesting that it will be possible to identify factors that support or detract from treatment response.

Currently, one barrier to treatment development is our lack of understanding of the critical elements of the intervention and the relative effectiveness of training techniques and approaches (Saperstein & Kurtz, 2013). Although CRT is described as a single intervention, there are multiple dimensions that may distinguish one approach from another, making it difficult to compare results of one study with another. Direct comparisons of cognitive remediation techniques and dismantling studies that identify the active components of an intervention approach are needed. Accomplishment of this task will require carefully designed studies that control for potential confounds and other threats to the study's validity. A second barrier to developing more effective CRT interventions may be the way in which treatment developers have conceptualized cognitive problems in schizophrenia. For instance, Vinogradov and colleagues (2012) have suggested that rather than the historical focus on neuropsychologically based cognitive domains, interventions may be more effective if they are designed to target underlying neural systems, which may impact aspects of multiple cognitive processes. This is an idea that can be directly tested through development and comparison of treatment approaches. Alternatively, treatment developers are also beginning to explore the efficacy of pairing CRT with a range of interventions that may boost treatment gains such as physical activity, neuromodulation techniques, and medications developed with the aim of being cognitively enhancing.

A final challenge for this field is to begin transitioning CRT from an experimental intervention to one incorporated into standard clinical care. Research will be needed to determine how feasibly to implement this intervention while maintaining its critical elements (Saperstein & Kurtz, 2013). CRT holds promise for improving the quality of life of many patients and their families. The challenge now for treatment developers is to determine how to make the intervention most effective and accessible to them.

ACKNOWLEDGMENTS

ISR was supported by National Research Service Award F31MH105080; TMN was supported by a Merit Award D6981R from the Veteran's Affairs Rehabilitation, Research & Development section; AWM was supported by NIMH Grant R01MH084861. AWM has consulted for Astellas Pharma.

REFERENCES

Bell M. D., Bryson G., Greig T., Corcoran C., Wexler B. E. (2001). Neurocognitive enhancement therapy with work therapy: Effects on neurocognitive test performance. *Archives of General Psychiatry, 58*, 763–768.

Bell, M. D., Choi, K.-H., Dyer, C., & Wexler, B. E. (2014). Benefits of cognitive remediation and supported employment for schizophrenia patients with poor community functioning. *Psychiatric Services (Washington, D.C.)*, *65*(4), 469–475. doi:10.1176/appi.ps.201200505

Bell, M. ., Zito, W., Greig, T., & Wexler, B. E. (2008). Neurocognitive enhancement therapy with vocational services: Work outcomes at two-year follow-up. *Schizophrenia Research, 105*, 18–29.

Bowie, C. R., Mcgurk, S. R., Mausbach, B., Patterson, T. L., Harvey, P. D. (2012). Combined cognitive remediation and functional skills training for schizophrenia: Effects on cognition, functional competence, and real-world behavior. *American Journal of Psychiatry, 169*(10), 710–718.

Buonomano, D. V, & Merzenich, M. M. (1998). Cortical plasticity: from synapses to maps. *Annual Review of Neuroscience, 21*, 149–186. doi:10.1146/annurev.neuro.21.1.149

Choi, K.-H., Wykes, T., & Kurtz, M. M. (2013). Adjunctive pharmacotherapy for cognitive deficits in schizophrenia: meta-analytical investigation of efficacy. *British Journal of Psychiatry : The Journal of Mental Science, 203*, 172–178. doi:10.1192/bjp.bp.111.107359

Dickinson, D., Tenhula, S., Morris, S., Brown, C., Peer, J., Spencer, K., . . . Bellack, A.S. (2010). A randomized, controlled trial of computer-assisted cognitive remediation for schizophrenia. *American Journal of Psychiatry, 167*, 170–180.

Eack, S. M., Hogarty, G. E., Cho, R. Y., Prasad, K. M. R., Greenwald, D. P., Hogarty, S. S., & Keshavan, M. S. (2010). Neuroprotective effects of cognitive enhancement therapy against gray matter loss in early schizophrenia: results from a 2-year randomized controlled trial. *Archives of General Psychiatry, 67*, 674–682. doi:10.1001/archgenpsychiatry.2010.63

Fisher, M., Holland, C., Merzenich, M. M., & Vinogradov, S. (2009). Using neuroplasticity-based auditory training to improve verbal memory in schizophrenia. *The American Journal of Psychiatry, 166*(7), 805–811. doi:10.1176/appi.ajp.2009.08050757

Fisher, M., Loewy, R., Carter, C., Lee, A., Ragland, J. D., Niendam, T., . . . Vinogradov, S. (2014). Neuroplasticity-based auditory training via laptop computer improves cognition in young individuals with recent onset schizophrenia. *Schizophrenia Bulletin*, 1–9. doi:10.1093/schbul/sbt232

Fisher, M., Loewy, R., Hardy, K., Schlosser, D., & Vinogradov, S. (2013). Cognitive intervenions targeting brain plasticity in the prodromal and early phases of schizophrenia. *Annual Review of Clinical Psychology, 9*, 435–463.

Fiszdon, J. M., Cardenas, A. S., Bryson, G. J., & Bell, M. D. (2005). Predictors of Remediation Success on a Trained Memory Task. *Journal of Nervous and Mental Disease, 193*(9), 602–608. doi:10.1097/01.nmd.0000177790.23311.ba

Green, M. F., Kern, R. S., & Heaton, R. K. (2004). Longitudinal studies of cognition and functional outcome in schizophrenia: implications for MATRICS. *Schizophrenia Research, 72*(1), 41–51.

Green, M. F., Nuechterlein, K. H., Kern, R. S., Baade, L. E., Fenton, W. S., Gold, J. M., ...Marder, S. R. (2008). Functional co-primary measures for clinical trials in schizophrenia: Results from the MATRICS psychometric and standardization study. *American Journal of Psychiatry, 165*, 221–228.

Harvey, P. D., Velligan, D. I., & Bellack, A. S. (2007). Performance-based measures of functional skills: Usefulness in clinical treatment studies. *Schizophrenia Bulletin*, 33, 1138–1148.

Haut, K. M., Lim, K. O., & MacDonald, A. (2010). Prefrontal cortical changes following cognitive training in patients with chronic schizophrenia: effects of practice, generalization, and specificity. *Neuropsychoph armacology : Official Publication of the American College of Neuropsychopharmacology*, 35(9), 1850–1859. doi:10.1038/npp.2010.52

Heinrichs, R. W., & Zakzanis, K. K. (1998). Neurocognitive deficit in schizophrenia: a quantitative review of the evidence. *Neuropsychology, 12*(3), 426–445.

Hogarty, G.E., Flesher, S., Ulrich, R., Carter, M., Greenwald, D., Pogue-Geile, M., . . . Zoretich, R. (2004). Cognitive enhancement therapy for schizophrenia. Effects of a 2-year randomized trial on cognition and behavior. *Archives of General Psychiatry, 61*, 866–876.

Hooker, C. I., Bruce, L., Fisher, M., Verosky, S. C., Miyakawa, A., & Vinogradov, S. (2012). Neural activity during emotion recognition after combined cognitive plus social cognitive training in schizophrenia. *Schizophrenia Research, 139*, 53–59.

Keefe, R. S. E., Vinogradov, S., Medalia, A., Silverstein, S. M., Bell, M. D., Dickinson, D., . . . Stroup, T. S. (2011). Report from the working group conference on multisite trial design for cognitive remediation in schizophrenia. *Schizophrenia Bulletin, 37*(5), 1057–1065. doi:10.1093/schbul/sbq010

Kidd, S. A., Kaur Bajwa, J., McKenzie, K. J., Ganguli, R., & Haji Khamneh, B. (2012). Cognitive remediation for individuals with psychosis in a supported education setting: A pilot study. *Rehabilitation Research and Practice, 2012*, 715176. http://doi:10.1155/2012/715176

Kontis, D., Huddy, V., Reeder, C., Landau, S., & Wykes, T. (2012). Effects of age and cognitive reserve on cognitive remediation therapy outcome in patients with schizophrenia. *American Journal of Geriatric Psychiatry, 21*, 218–30.

Kurtz, M. M., Moberg, P. J., Gur, R. C., & Gur, R. E. (2001). Approaches to cognitive remediation of neuropsycholgical deficits in schizophrenia: A review and meta-analysis. *Neuropsychology Review, 11*, 197–210.

Kurtz, M. M., Seltzer, J. C., Shagan, D. S., Thime, W. R., & Wexler, B. E. (2007). Computer-assisted cognitive remediation in schizophrenia: What is the active ingredient? *Schizophrenia Research, 89*, 251–260. doi:10.1016/j.schres.2006.09.001

Lynall, M.-E., Bassett, D. S., Kerwin, R., McKenna, P. J., Kitzbichler, M., Muller, U., & Bullmore, E. (2010). Functional connectivity and brain networks in schizophrenia. *The Journal of Neuroscience : The Official Journal of the Society for Neuroscience, 30*(28), 9477–9487. doi:10.1523/JNEUROSCI.0333-10.2010

McGurk, S. R. (2005). Cognitive training and supported employment for persons with severe mental illness: One-year results from a randomized controlled trial. *Schizophrenia Bulletin, 31*(4), 898–909. doi:10.1093/schbul/sbi037

McGurk, S. R., Mueser, K. T., DeRosa, T. J., & Wolfe, R. (2009). Work, recovery, and comorbidity in schizophrenia: A randomized controlled trial of cognitive remediation. *Schizophrenia Bulletin, 35*, 319–335.

McGurk, S. R., Twamley, E. W., Sitzer, D. I., Mchugo, G. J., & Mueser, K. T. (2007). Reviews and overviews A meta-analysis of cognitive remediation in schizophrenia. *Psychiatry: Interpersonal and Biological Processes*, (December), 1791–1802.

Medalia, A., & Choi, J. (2009). Cognitive remediation in schizophrenia. *Neuropsychology Review, 19*(3), 353–364.

Medalia, A., Revheim, N., Herlands, T. (2009). *Cognitive remediation for psychological disorders: Therapist guide*. Los Angeles, CA: MATRICS Assessment, Inc.

Medalia, A., & Richardson, R. (2005). What predicts a good response to cognitive remediation interventions? *Schizophrenia Bulletin, 31*(4), 942–953. doi:10.1093/schbul/sbi045

Medalia, A., & Saperstein, A. M. (2013). Does cognitive remediation for schizophrenia improve functional outcomes? *Current Opinions in Psychiatry, 26*, 151–157. doi:10.1097/YCO.0b013e32835dcbd4

Nuechterlein, K. H., Green, M. F. (2006). *MATRICS Consensus Cognitive Battery*. Los Angeles, CA: MATRICS Assessment.

Palmer, B. W., Heaton, R. K., Paulsen, J. S., Kuck, J., Braff, D. L., Harris, M. J. (1997). Is it possible to be schizophrenic yet neuropsychologically normal? *Neuropsychology, 11*, 437–446.

Patterson, T. L., Goldman, S., McKibbin, C. L., Hughs, T., & Jeste, D. V. (2001). UCSD Performance-based skills assessment: development of a new measure of everyday functioning for severely mentally ill adults. *Schizophrenia Bulletin, 27*, 235–245.

Penadés, R., Catalan, R., Salamero, M., Boget, T., Puig, O., Guarch, J., & Gastó, C. (2006). Cognitive remediation therapy for outpatients with chronic schizophrenia: A controlled and randomized study. *Schizophrenia Research, 87*, 323–331.

Penadés, R., Pujol, N., Catalán, R., Massana, G., Rametti, G., García-Rizo, C., . . . Junqué, C. (2013). Brain effects of cognitive remediation therapy in schizophrenia: a structural and functional neuroimaging study. *Biological Psychiatry, 73*(10), 1015–1023. doi:10.1016/j.biopsych.2013.01.017

Saperstein, A. M. & Kurtz, M. M. (2013). Current trends in the empirical study of cognitive remediation for schizophrenia. *Canadian Journal of Psychiatry, 58*, 311–317.

Scheu, F., Aghotor, J. Pfueller, U., Mortiz, S., Bohen, F., Weisbrod, M., & Roesch-Ely, D. (2013). Predictors of performance improvement within a cognitive remediation program for schizophrenia. *Psychiatry Research, 209*, 375–80.

Subramaniam, K., Luks, T. L., Fisher, M., Simpson, G. V, Nagarajan, S., & Vinogradov, S. (2012). Computerized cognitive training restores neural activity within the reality monitoring network in schizophrenia. *Neuron, 73*(4), 842–853. doi:10.1016/j.neuron.2011.12.024

Twamley, E. W., Jeste, D. V, & Bellack, A. S. (2003). A review of cognitive training in schizophrenia. *Schizophrenia Bulletin, 29*(2), 359–82.

Ventura, J., Wilson, S. A., Wood, R. C., & Hellemann, G. S. (2012). Cognitive training at home in schizophrenia is feasible. *Schizophrenia Research, 143*, 397–398.

Vinogradov, S., Fisher, M., Warm, H. Holland, C., Kirshner, M.A., & Pollock, B.G. (2009). The cognitive cost of anticholinergic burden: Decreased response to cognitive training in schizophrenia. *American Journal of Psychiatry, 166*, 1055–1062.

Vinogradov, S., Fisher, M., & de Villers-Sidani, E. (2012). Cognitive training for impaired neural systems in neuropsychiatric illness. *Neuropsychopharmacology : Official Publication of the American College of Neuropsychopharmacology, 37*(1), 43–76. doi:10.1038/npp.2011.251

Vita, A., Deste, G., De Peri, L., Barlati, S., Poli, R., Cesana, B. M., & Sacchetti, E. (2013). Predictors of cognitive and functional improvement and normalization after cognitive remediation in patients with schizophrenia. *Schizophrenia Research, 150*, 51–57. doi:10.1016/j.schres.2013.08.011

Wexler, B. E., & Bell, M. D. (2005). Cognitive remediation and vocational rehabilitation for schizophrenia. *Schizophrenia Bulletin, 31*(4), 931–941. doi:10.1093/schbul/sbi038

Wykes, T., Huddy, V., Cellard, C., McGurk, S. R., & Czobor, P. (2011). A meta-analysis of cognitive remediation for schizophrenia: methodology and effect sizes. *American Journal of Psychiatry, 168*(5), 472–485. doi:10.1176/appi.ajp.2010.10060855

Wykes, T., Reeder, C., Landau, S., Matthiasson, P., Haworth, E., & Hutchinson, C. (2009). Does age matter? Effects of cognitive rehabilitation across the age span. *Schizophrenia Research, 113*, 252–258.

Wykes, T., & Spaulding, W. D. (2011). Thinking about the future of cognitive remediation therapy – What works and could we do better? *Schizophrenia Bulletin, 37*, S80–S90.

Wykes, T., & van der Gaag, M. (2001). Is it time to develop a new cognitive therapy for psychosis--cognitive remediation therapy (CRT)? *Clinical Psychology Review, 21*(8), 1227–1256.

/// 16 /// FAMILY PSYCHOEDUCATION

ALEX KOPELOWICZ

INTRODUCTION

To many who recognize the biological nature of severe mental illness, it is difficult to imagine that 50 years ago the family was often seen as a causative factor in the development of schizophrenia and related disorders. Notions of the "schizophrenogenic mothers" (Fromm-Reichmann, 1948) and "double binding" families (Bateson , Jackson, Haley, & Weakland, 1956) were all too common in the psychoanalytic literature of the day. Interestingly, in those early years of deinstitutionalization, a few clinicians began to notice the crucial, salutary role that families played in the care and rehabilitation of mentally ill family members. For example, Evans, Bullard, and Solomon (1961) noted that, contrary to the belief that families abandoned their mentally ill relatives, most families maintained involvement with their ill relatives even after long periods of separation. Moreover, not only did families maintain interest, but Freeman and Simmons (1963) wrote that families were the key influence on the patients' ability to function and to remain out of the hospital.

It is in this context that a few clinical research pioneers became increasingly dissatisfied with the refractoriness of schizophrenia to the conventional psychoanalytic approaches of the day. Seeking alternatives to help patients improve their functioning so they could resume their lives in the community, these investigators recognized the practical value of using behavioral learning principles within an educational framework to involve families in providing support for the rehabilitation of patients with mental illness. In contrast to the prevailing zeitgeist, these new approaches viewed family members as potentially positive sources of therapeutic influence for their mentally ill relatives while recognizing their need for knowledge, coping skills, supportiveness, and collaboration with professional caregivers. A variety of terms have been used to describe these interventions, but as a group they are called family psychoeducation.

Family psychoeducational approaches have substantial elements in common. First, they provide structured and clear expectations for participation by family members and the patient. Second, they emphasize outreach and other efforts to connect with the family and provide them with support and guidance. Third, they offer practical education about the nature of schizophrenia and how to cope with it. Fourth, they assist the family's efforts to effectively utilize available treatments and community resources. Fifth, the families are taught stress management techniques as well as better means of communicating and problem solving. Finally, family members are encouraged to pursue their own goals and well-being without becoming emotionally overinvolved with each other (Dixon et al., 2001).

Family psychoeducation models differ in their format (single family versus multiple family), the duration of treatment (ranging from three months to two years), location of sessions (home versus clinic based), and the degree of emphasis on didactic, cognitive-behavioral, and systemic techniques. Overall, family psychoeducation has a compelling evidence base with over 100 randomized controlled trials showing greater reductions in relapse and rehospitalization rates among people with schizophrenia whose families received psychoeducation than among those who received standard mental health services, with differences ranging from 20 to 50 percent over two years (Lyman et al., 2014). Moreover, family psychoeducation has been shown to enhance the well-being of family members, improve the ill relative's participation in vocational rehabilitation, and decrease the cost of mental health care. Taken together, this solid research base has led the Schizophrenia Patient Outcomes Research Team (PORT) to include family psychoeducation among its treatment recommendations since its inception. In its most recent publication, the PORT guidelines recommended that all families who have contact with a relative who has a severe mental illness be offered a family intervention that spans at least nine months and that includes education about mental illness, family support, crisis intervention, and problem solving (Kreyenbuhl, Buchanan, Dickerson, & Dixon, 2010).

This chapter will include a review of the two family psychoeducation approaches that have the most extensive research support; namely, behavioral family therapy and multi-family groups. In addition, a discussion of the importance of cultural factors in working with families will be provided.

BEHAVIORAL FAMILY THERAPY

Efforts to design and evaluate a family intervention that would help individuals with serious mental disorders and their family members better cope with these illnesses dates back to the late 1960s and early 1970s (Liberman 1970, 1972). Out of this work, Falloon and colleagues developed and refined the Behavioral Family Therapy (BFT) model, also known as Behavioral Family Management (Falloon & Liberman, 1983). The BFT model is a clear departure from the focus on abnormal family interaction patterns, instead proposing that the family is the basic unit for the promotion of the healthy functioning of all its members and it is a crucial determinant in the recovery and rehabilitation of those suffering from schizophrenia. The natural care-giving function of families is considered to be the greatest resource available to the mental health services. For this reason, the BFT approach seeks first to evaluate the healthy elements of family communication in solving everyday problems before assisting the family to enhance their problem-solving efficiency.

BFT occurs in five stages, with considerable recycling of each stage throughout the therapy as shown in Box 16.1. The first stage, behavioral assessment, involves an assessment of the strengths and weaknesses of the family as a problem-solving unit. Particular note is made of the precise manner in which members of the family tackle the problems of everyday life together, as well as their responses to significant life events. Life problems include the personal goals of individual family members. Initially, family members are interviewed individually to establish their unique assets and deficits, their personal life goals, and the assistance they obtain from other family members in their attempts to achieve their goals. The second step in the behavioral analysis of a family unit involves an assessment of the relationships between the various goals and problems of individual family members. It is clear that the aspirations of individual family members may conflict at times with the wishes and values of other family members. This analysis of how the family fits together as a system is described as a functional analysis. The third step involves observation of the family having a problem-solving discussion. Families are asked to work on the solution of a "hot issue" that affects all family members for 10 minutes. This time interval is often too brief to allow detailed planning to be achieved but, despite its brevity,

BOX 16.1

COMPONENTS OF BEHAVIORAL FAMILY THERAPY

1. Behavioral assessment.
2. Education about schizophrenia and its care.
3. Communication-skills training.
4. Problem-solving training.
5. Behavioral strategies for special problems

provides surprisingly good insight into the structure and strategies the families employ in their discussions. Once these steps have been undertaken, the BFT clinician is in a position to formulate a management plan that is uniquely structured to enhance the problem-solving efficiency of each family unit.

The second stage in BFT is providing education about schizophrenia. Although the mutual sharing of information about the nature, course, and treatment of schizophrenia is a continuous process, two sessions at the onset of BFT are devoted to discussion about the diagnosis, etiology, management, course, and medication and psychosocial treatment of the disorder. These initial sessions provide a rationale for the subsequent family therapy and for the continuing medication treatment that is carefully monitored throughout the intervention. The individuals with schizophrenia play a crucial role in this education as they are encouraged to describe their own experiences of schizophrenia and its management to their families. Usually, this is the first occasion on which the nature of the patient's symptoms has been discussed among the family members. The person assumes the "expert" role, although at times other family members may report similar episodes of symptoms in the past or even the present.

The third stage of BFT is communication training. At times of crisis, ineffective patterns of communication substantially impede coping efforts and contribute to the stress that may trigger exacerbations of schizophrenia. Effective communication is the basis for efficient problem solving. The major components of family communication that are assessed involve the ability to listen empathically to one another when discussion problem issues, mutual communication of positive and negative feelings, and making constructive requests for behavior change. The nonverbal and verbal components of interpersonal communication are addressed, particularly where major deficits detract from the clarity of such expression. Improved communication is shaped through skills training procedures, whereby brief segments of interaction are rehearsed repeatedly with instructions, modeling, social reinforcement, and performance feedback from the BFT clinician and family members.

The fourth stage of BFT is formal training in problem-solving techniques. Families are encouraged to adopt a structured approach to their problem-solving discussions. This involves arranging specific times when the whole family can meet, free of distractions, to discuss important issues. The frequency of such family meetings, their duration, and the choice of topic for discussion is left to the discretion of the family. However, they are advised to meet at least once a week, to limit the time spent, and to choose relatively straightforward problem issues for their initial meetings. The family therapy sessions examine the progress of their family discussions and provide a workshop for enhancing their effectiveness. A six-step model of problem solving is advocated as a guide for the family meetings. The six steps are listed and briefly described in Box 16.2.

The final stage of the BFT approach is developing behavioral strategies for specific problems. Few families have an adequate repertoire of coping behaviors to manage all the problems that arise in the course of schizophrenia. Although the problem-solving structure helps facilitate creative resolution of difficult problems, there are times when additional professional assistance may be employed. Behavioral strategies that have been validated in research studies to assist with a variety of psychiatric symptoms (such as anxiety, depression, persistent hallucinations, and delusions) are taught within the family problem-solving context. In addition to teaching methods of dealing more efficiently with symptomatic states, families may learn a broad range of general management skills, such as operant reinforcement strategies, contingency contracting, role-playing limit setting, and skill training.

By specifically defining the essential components of BFT and writing the first treatment manual for the application of BFT to families with a member diagnosed with

BOX 16.2.

SIX-STEP PROBLEM SOLVING STRATEGY

1. *Identify a specific problem.* This step entails active listening to each person's description of the problem, seeking clarification when necessary, and avoiding giving premature advice or reassurance.
2. *List alternative solutions.* Once the problem has been specified, a brain-storming approach is used to generate a list of potential solutions. Discussion about the relative merits of each solution is postponed, and both good and bad ideas are recorded.
3. *Discuss merits of each solution.* Each solution is discussed in turn. The advantages and disadvantages of each are highlighted.
4. *Choose the optimal solution.* The family chooses that solution (or combination of solutions) that best fits the needs of the problem and the resources of the family.
5. *Plan how to implement the solution.* Detailed plans are made to map out the steps through which the solution will be implemented. Strategies for ensuring that the solution is implemented smoothly are devised. Major roadblocks are anticipated and ways of coping with these and other important consequences are discussed.
6. *Review all efforts.* Any genuine attempt to implement the plan is acknowledged and praised, even if a successful outcome was not achieved. The family is encouraged to review their efforts and to use all knowledge gained to construct a more effective plan.

schizophrenia (Falloon, Boyd, & McGill, 1984), this work set the stage for the first randomized controlled outcome study of a family intervention for schizophrenia. Individuals with schizophrenia discharged from psychiatric facilities to stressful home environments were randomly assigned to either nine months of home-based behavioral family management or equally intensive individual therapy. After nine months and at the two year follow-up, those who received the family treatment had fewer hospitalizations, spent less time in the hospital, experienced fewer major exacerbations of psychotic symptoms, and required fewer emergency crisis sessions than those who received individual therapy and no family intervention. Subjects who received the family intervention also improved more in their social and vocational adjustment, and were prescribed lower doses of antipsychotic medication to control their symptoms than their counterparts who received individual supportive therapy (Falloon et al., 1985).

Rehabilitation programs of skills development for family management of schizophrenia were replicated with similar results in the United Kingdom (Leff, Kuipers, Berkowitz, Eberlein-Vries, & Sturgeon, 1982; Tarrier et al., 1989) and the United States (Hogarty et al., 1986; Randolph et al., 1994). For example, in one study at the West Los Angeles Veterans Affairs Medical Center, BFT was added to customary antipsychotic medication and clinic care. The BFT group had a 5 percent rate of relapses after one year, whereas the customary care group had a 30 percent rate (Randolph et al., 1994).

More recent international studies have shown similar results. In Italy, Magliano, Fiorello, Malangone, DeRosa, and Maj (2006) randomized 71 people with schizophrenia and their families to BFT or a wait list. They found significant improvements in the social functioning and self-care of the person with schizophrenia, as well as better social contacts and perceptions of professional support for the family members. In India, Kulhara and colleagues randomized 76 subjects with schizophrenia and their key relative to either nine months of BFT or usual outpatient care. The BFT participants showed significantly more improvement in psychopathology, disability, caregiver satisfaction with treatment, and perceptions of social support. The authors also reported that the program was practical to implement and not expensive (Kulhara, Chakrabarti, Avasthi, Sharma, & Sharma, 2009).

In the past decade, several reviews of the literature have addressed the efficacy of BFT as part of an overall assessment of family psychoeducational approaches (Murray-Swank & Dixon, 2004; Rummel-Kluge & Kissling, 2008; Lucksted, McFarlane, Downing, Dixon, & Adams, 2012; Lyman et al., 2014). These reviews all come to similar conclusions: BFT as a clinical intervention for schizophrenia is an effective practice for reducing relapse and hospitalizations, and for several functional outcomes, especially in conjunction with effective psychiatric medication. Moreover, studies conducted in community-based clinics show results comparable to those in experimental settings (Mueser & Glynn, 1999).

MULTIFAMILY GROUPS

By 1990, it was apparent from multiple published studies that a new psychosocial treatment for schizophrenia had been developed, one that significantly improved outcome beyond that of medication alone, and an outcome that could not be achieved without fully involving the family in treatment and rehabilitation. Although these approaches all involved training families in coping skills and interactional styles that were specific to the needs of people with schizophrenia, they were different from past efforts in that they included families as partners in the treatment; that is, the family members were seen as agents of positive change who could participate as an effective part of the treatment team. William McFarlane and his colleagues expanded on the therapeutic advantages of involving family members as active participants by experimenting with an intervention that included multiple families (McFarlane, Stastny & Deakins, 1992). He found that people with schizophrenia and their families provided direct emotional support to each other by trading ideas, empathizing with burdens, and suggesting and fostering behaviors that promoted recuperation. Importantly, the group allowed a framework in which a family could more clearly establish a balance between the needs of an individual and those of the family (McFarlane, 2002).

Over the ensuing 25 years, McFarlane's now well-validated and widely used multifamily group (MFG) approach has been implemented in many states and over a dozen countries. It is estimated that several thousand sites are presently using MFG for schizophrenia and other severe mental disorders. Tens of thousands of people have participated in MFGs (McFarlane, 2002) and it remains one of the few psychosocial interventions to be recognized by the National Registry of Evidence-based Programs and Practices, a prestigious designation made by the Substance Abuse and Mental Health Services Administration (United States Department of Health and Human Services, 2009).

The practitioner uses structured exercises for engaging the family and the person with a mental illness in the educational process. Interventions for reducing the family's emotional burden include ways to broaden their social support network. Training is accomplished by the mental health professional using a trainer's manual, with the family member and individual with a mental illness following a consumer's guide and a demonstration video that employs real family members achieving the learning objectives set for each session.

MFG consists of three components: Engagement or "joining" sessions, an educational workshop, and longer-term multiple family group sessions. The first phase is designed to engage patients and family members in the treatment enterprise. These three initial "joining" sessions are conducted with each of the families separately. These sessions are also used to assess the special needs, strengths, and problems of each family unit. They take place while the patient is separately undergoing treatment of acute psychotic symptoms followed by orientation to the purposes of the MFG therapy in which the patient will subsequently participate.

The three joining sessions offer each family an individualized approach designed to facilitate the process of engaging in treatment. The sessions are designed to familiarize the family with the therapists who will be conducting the ongoing multiple family sessions, and to educate them about the need for ongoing treatment. The sessions also help the family identify and overcome the obstacles to pursuing outpatient treatment. Typically, during the initial joining period, three meetings occur at short intervals. These meetings have a flexible schedule, occurring generally once per week and lasting approximately one hour. The patient is not included in these sessions but instead participates in separate sessions with the clinician at this time, also with the intent to foster a treatment alliance.

The structure for the meetings is straightforward. All family members with whom the patient has frequent interactions are contacted by the clinician, who invites them to meet at a convenient time. Special attention is paid to ensure that those most frequently involved with the patient attend. Before each meeting, the clinician ensures that he or she has communicated with other staff engaged in treating the patient in order to be aware of the latest clinical status of the patient. The assessment with the family can be conceived as a triad: (1) evaluating the present crisis; (2) eliciting family reactions to the illness; and (3) evaluating the family and social system. The overall goal of this phase is to create a collaborative treatment system in which family members become engaged as partners with their ill relative and the clinician.

The second component of the MFG enterprise is an educational workshop, in which the clinicians present information and describe key behavioral guidelines didactically. Typically, the workshop is a six-hour educational experience held on a single day with all families that will be involved in the continuing MFG therapy. The workshop is primarily didactic with open discussion of the information provided by lecture and videotape about the etiology, biology, genetics, symptoms, and treatment of serious mental illness. A list of topics covered in the workshop is presented in Box 16.3.

Workshops are not therapy sessions; this is immediately communicated and is an important reason for a dramatically different format. A formal classroom setting is used for informal lecture and discussion sessions. Extensive use is made of audiovisual aids

BOX 16.3

TOPICS COVERED IN FAMILY EDUCATION WORKSHOP

1. Translation of mental illness as problems in living.
2. Determinants of illness behaviors, symptoms, and impairments: The central nervous system ("the world inside") and the environment ("the world outside").
3. Social learning principles: The ABCs of behavioral modification (learning through imitation and reinforcement).
4. Reinforcing small steps in the desired direction (shaping).
5. The power of social reinforcement: Shaping behavior, especially the amount and content of conversation.
6. Family contracting: Giving and getting needs and rewards through negotiated exchanges.
7. Description of social psychiatric programs at the day hospital: Educational workshops, personal effectiveness training.
8. Recognizing the early warning signs of relapse.

to illustrate concepts of brain function, medication effects, and signs and symptoms of mental illness. Scientific information about schizophrenia is presented in a manner that is professional but understandable to the group. To assure comprehension of the material, the presenter allows plenty of time for questions and discussions. Information about the way in which the MFG clinician and the family will work together is also presented. This includes guidelines for managing the symptoms of schizophrenia (see Box 16.4). These behavioral instructions for the family members integrate the biological, psychological, and social aspects of the disorder, along with recommended responses aimed at helping maintain a home environment that minimizes relapse-inducing stress. During breaks and over lunch, there is ample opportunity for informal social contact between families, as well as between families and clinicians. The opportunity to interact with other families in similar circumstances enhances the power of this phase of the intervention.

Following the workshop, the third component of MFG begins, in which a group of between five to seven families meets twice monthly for at least nine months. Depending on the needs and progress of each family and patient unit, some families can participate in family therapy for up to two years. All sessions are co-led by the clinicians who conducted the joining sessions and the educational workshop. Each group session is structured in the following manner: a brief caring and sharing period followed by group discussion that includes questions and answers related to each family unit's concerns and problems. Therapists encourage the families to share their personal experiences, describe

BOX 16.4

FAMILY GUIDELINES

1. *Go slow.* Recovery takes time. Things will improve but only at their own pace. Rest is important for all family members.
2. *Keep it cool.* Enthusiasm is normal. Tone it down. Disagreement is normal. Tone it down, also.
3. *Give them space.* It is okay to offer something; it is also okay to refuse the offer. Nerves get frayed on occasion and a time-out is important for everyone.
4. *Set limits.* A few good, consistent rules keep things clear. Everyone needs to know the rules and agree to follow them.
5. *Ignore what you cannot change.* Some things are better to let slide. However, do not ignore violence.
6. *Keep things simple.* Good communication starts with being clear, calm, and positive.
7. *Follow doctor's orders.* Take medications as prescribed. Take only medications prescribed.
8. *No street drugs or alcohol are allowed.* They make symptoms worse. Family members affect one another so no one is exempt.
9. *Pick up on early signs.* Note changes. Consult with your family clinician.
10. *Carry on business as usual.* Stay in touch with extended family and friends. Reestablish family routines as quickly as possible.
11. *Solve problems step by step.* Work on one thing at a time. Changes that last often occur on a steady, gradual course.
12. *Start at the beginning and build.* Lower expectations, temporarily. Use a personal yardstick. Compare this month to last rather than this person to another person.

their coping strategies for dealing with family and patient problems, and provide group support for one another. The principal technique used in the ongoing family sessions is teaching coping and problem-solving skills with families serving as the role models for one another as they describe their own experiences using these skills in their home environments. The problem-solving method utilized is very similar to the six-step approach described earlier in the section on Behavioral Family Therapy except that members of all families are encouraged to contribute potential solutions. Finally, each MFG session ends with reviews of the gains made by family members that week.

A large number of controlled and comparative clinical trials have demonstrated markedly decreased relapse and rehospitalization rates among individuals with schizophrenia whose families participated in MFGs compared to those who received standard services (see Jewell, Downing, & McFarlane, 2009 for a thorough review of the literature). Overall, the relapse rates for MFG participants is about 15 percent per year compared to a consistent 30–40 percent for customary care in a community mental health center. Moreover, the reduction in relapse rates has been shown to persist for up to four years (McFarlane, Link , Dushay, Marchal, & Crilly, 1995).

Other MFG studies have focused on outcomes other than relapse rates. For example, a Washington state team of researchers randomized 97 adults with schizophrenia and their families to two years of MFG against standard care. In addition to reductions in relapse rates, the MFG participants had decreased negative symptoms and the family members reported less caregiver burden and distress (Dyck et al., 2000; Dyck et al., 2002). Moreover, studies in which MFG has been combined with vocational services have found increased employment rates and improved quality of life when compared to vocational services alone (McFarlane et al., 2000).

Although the consensus of reviews of single-family approaches (such as BFT) and multiple-family formats are that they are equally effective treatments, three groups have directly compared these interventions (Leff et al., 1989; McFarlane, Lukens et al., 1995; Schooler et al., 1997). Across the three studies, the rates of relapse at the end of the study were similar (approximately 25–30 percent). However, in the one large multisite study conducted in community-based agencies (as opposed to research institutions), MFG participants had lower relapse rates in five of the six sites (McFarlane, Lukens et al., 1995). This study was also informative in that it identified a subgroup for which the single-family format was more effective—patients with unusually good response to medication during the index hospitalization (McFarlane, 2002). In contrast, first-episode patients did substantially better in the MFGs compared to the single-family format (McFarlane, 2002).

CULTURAL ADAPTATIONS OF FAMILY INTERVENTIONS

Over the past 10 years, family psychoeducation efforts have been extended to a variety of cultural groups. For example, Kopelowicz and colleagues adapted the MFG approach for their work with Mexican-Americans with schizophrenia living in Los Angeles. Incorporating family members into the treatment process was particularly relevant in this population given that over 80 percent of Latinos with schizophrenia live with their families (Guarnaccia & Parra, 1996). To appropriately adapt the intervention for this group, focus groups were conducted with a representative sample of family members whose ill relatives were receiving treatment for schizophrenia at a community mental health center serving a large Mexican American population. The family members met in groups with two facilitators who conducted the meetings in Spanish. The facilitators asked the family members to identify their concerns related to the treatment of their ill relatives.

A predominant theme raised by the family members was adherence to antipsychotic medications. Families often felt frustrated that their ill relatives seemed to do well on these medications only to stop them once they felt better and thereby begin a cycle of relapse and rehospitalization (Kopelowicz et al., 2007).

Based on the results of the focus groups, the MFG approach was chosen as the framework for working with these families. The reasons for this selection included: (a) its emphasis on problem-solving skills rather than the more culturally mediated communication-skills training, which was found to be ineffective for low-acculturated Mexican Americans with schizophrenia (Telles et al., 1995); (b) its focus on psychoeducational presentations by mental health professionals, which was found to be the preferred type of support group identified by Mexican Americans (Medvene, Mendoza, Lin, Harris, & Miller, 1995); (c) its central premise of enlarging families' social-support network, which is congruent with a fundamental aspect of Mexican-American culture (Vega et al., 2007); (d) its documented efficacy in improving medication adherence rates in individuals with schizophrenia (Zygmunt, Olfson, Boyer, & Mechanic, 2002); and, (e) its structural flexibility, which enables investigators to incorporate specific content that addresses issues germane to the treatment population (McFarlane, 2002).

In addition, the principles of the Theory of Planned Behavior (TPB; Ajzen, 1991) were used to guide the procedures used in the group. The TPB, a well-researched social psychology theory, has been used to improve adherence to treatment in various health-related interventions such as the treatment for individuals with coronary artery disease, hypertension and HIV (Armitrage & Conner, 2001). Specifically, the TPB proposes that people engage in a *behavior* based on their *intention* to perform the behavior, which is a function of a person's *attitude toward the behavior, subjective norms,* and *perceived behavioral control* (see Figure 16.1). The person's attitudes toward the behavior are composed of *beliefs* about the advantages and disadvantages of performing a particular behavior, in this case, taking or not taking medication. Subjective norms are a function of a person's *beliefs* about what significant others' think regarding the behavior (e.g., "My family thinks the pills turn me into a zombie") and his or her motivation to comply with the wishes of these others. Perceived behavioral control refers to the individual's belief that he or she has the resources and opportunities required to perform a particular behavior and can overcome the obstacles that stand in the way of doing it, for example, sufficient funds to purchase the medication. In summary, individuals will try to perform a behavior if they believe that the benefits of success outweigh the risks of failure, if they feel that significant others (with whom they want to comply) believe that they should perform the behavior, and if they believe they have the resources and capabilities to perform the behavior. We first gathered individualized information about participants' beliefs along these three

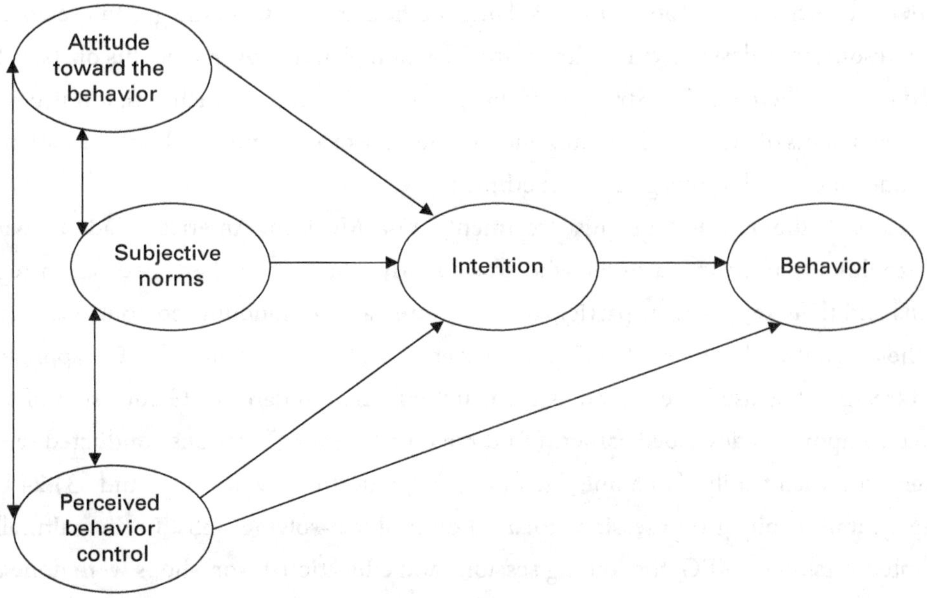

FIGURE 16.1. The Theory of Planned Behavior

TPB constructs and then incorporated it into individualized interventions within the MFG sessions.

Although MFG has features compatible with a cultural perspective (e.g., families define the problem focus, not the therapist; Lopez, Kopelowicz, & Canive, 2002), incorporating the TPB conceptual framework is consistent with a process-oriented approach to cultural adaptation that allows for cultural themes of this largely immigrant, low-income, Mexican-origin community to be integrated throughout treatment. In contrast to cultural adaptations that apply a treatment modification based on ethnic categories (for a review, see Kopelowicz, Zarate, Gonzalez Smith, Mintz, & Liberman, 2003; Lau, 2006), a process-oriented approach encourages therapists to learn from their clients what about culture matters for the individual patients and families (Lakes, Lopez, & Garro, 2006). Given that treatment adherence is embedded in a rich sociocultural network of beliefs, attitudes, and resources available to each person and family, carrying out a systematic assessment of the TPB constructs with each patient/family enabled us to capture significant cultural elements. For example, many of the patients who did not have or were ineligible for medical benefits did not take their medications because they could not afford to purchase them. This reflects a socio-cultural belief shared by some persons of low socio-economic status. These patients and families did not realize they could receive antipsychotic medications at no cost through an indigent medication program available at the mental health center. After identifying the perceived lack of resources, the

MFG-A clinicians used the problem-solving method and drew on the group's sociocultural resources to design a culturally informed action plan that overcame this obstacle to medication adherence. The strength of this process-oriented approach is that it is based on assessments of individual patients and does not make assumptions about the patient's attitudes and social norms given their ethnicity.

To test the efficacy of this treatment, 174 Mexican Americans adults with schizophrenia-spectrum disorder who were poorly adherent to their medication regimens and their key relatives participated in a three-armed, randomized controlled trial of the culturally adapted MFG (Kopelowicz et al., 2012). The standard MFG approach and treatment as usual were used as comparators. The standard MFG consisted of the three components described earlier: (1) three initial "joining" sessions conducted separately with each family; (2) a one-day (six-hour) educational workshop; and (3) 24 bi-weekly, multifamily group sessions focused on problem-solving skills. In the culturally adapted version of MFG, the joining sessions and educational workshops were done as in the standard MFG approach. However, the bi-weekly sessions were focused on specific obstacles to maintaining medication adherence. These obstacles were identified through individualized TPB-focused interviews with each person with schizophrenia and his or her key relative that occurred prior to the MFG session.

The results of this study indicated that the year-long culturally adapted MFG was associated with greater medication adherence and more positive clinical outcomes compared with standard MFG treatment and treatment as usual over a 2-year follow-up. In addition, this study found that medication adherence accounted for a significant proportion of the variability in positive outcomes. Given that this study was carried out with a hard-to-reach community of Spanish-speaking Mexican Americans, the results extend the efficacy of family psychoeducation approaches for culturally diverse individuals with schizophrenia and their families.

CONCLUSIONS

As the focus of treatment for serious psychiatric illness has changed dramatically in the past 50 years, it is now clear that long-term family intervention in combination with antipsychotic medication is a very effective treatment for schizophrenia. Through its emphasis on teaching family members the requisite information about psychiatric disorders and improving their communication and problem-solving skills using behavioral-learning principles and social-learning methods, family psychoeducation has been amply documented to enhance outcomes in a variety of clinical and social domains. Moreover, the family psychoeducational approaches described in this chapter, Behavioral Family

Therapy and Multifamily Groups, are not difficult to learn or practice, if adequate training and supervision are available. Although mastery of the technical aspects of the treatments are important to achieve successful outcomes, it is important to realize that what the families who participate in these approaches appreciate is the empathic support of mental health professionals as they struggle with helping their ill relative cope with the burden of schizophrenia.

CASE ILLUSTRATION

When Howard first came to the mental health center with his parents, he was unwilling to talk much about his problems. He was 27 years old, a Jewish white male, single, and unemployed. He looked sad, yet frightened, when asked direct questions by the therapist. He became visibly upset when his parents tried to coax him into answering. Finally, he responded to the question "What is your most distressing symptom?" Although he had been in treatment with numerous therapists since age 17, he stated that no one had ever asked what troubled him. Instead, he said, "They only want to know about the voices." He spoke quietly and hesitated often, but said that what really upset him was that his breath could influence and even endanger people, so much so that he would go to great lengths to avoid contact with others. The power of his breath gave him a sense of overwhelming responsibility, sometimes making him feel "like God." Howard preferred to stay in his room at his parents' house, rarely coming out except for occasional meals, bathroom visits, and to go to synagogue on Friday evenings. He restricted his activities in this way because he believed he could not protect his "power" from malevolent forces.

Howard provided the following account of his beliefs and their development. Shortly after graduating high school, he realized that something strange was happening. He began to feel that people were physically and emotionally affected by him, even if he did not say anything to them. He tested this by going into restaurants and observing the patrons. He noticed that if he looked at someone long enough, he could *make* them rub their eye or scratch their nose. At first, he had to be within close range to have an effect, but as time went on, he could project this ability over great distances. Then, he felt that he could get characters on television programs to move in ways that they ordinarily would not. Gradually, he became convinced that not only people, but inanimate objects like traffic signals and automobiles responded to his nonverbal influence.

At first, he was not sure how he controlled people and things. He did not think it was purely by thought, because the effect on others would occur even if he was not thinking about them. In a flash of insight, Howard suddenly came to believe that he, like God, had a "life-force" in his breath. Soon he began to hear the voices of God's angels telling him that he had been chosen to be the next Messiah. He also became increasingly aware that people were talking about him behind his back, which he presumed meant that they knew about his "power." These feelings persisted for many months, during which Howard became increasingly withdrawn and isolative. He began to use greater and greater amounts of marijuana, because, he said, "It reduces the oxygen in the breath and that reduces its effect." His psychosis increased to the point of incoherence, and soon afterward he had the first of a series of psychiatric hospitalizations. He received the diagnosis of *schizophrenia, paranoid type*.

Over the years, Howard had been placed on numerous psychiatric medications, with intermittent compliance. At the time of the first interview, he had not worked in several years, had one friend (whom he thought was immune to his breath's effect) and usually interacted only with his immediate family and the rabbi at the local synagogue. When he did associate with his one friend, it was to smoke marijuana. His only responsibility was to make his own bed, which he did, though with some prompting from his mother.

In the first visit, he admitted to the therapist that he continued to hear voices and harbor fears that others were talking about him. He tried to understand his situation by immersing himself in biblical study, looking for signs that he indeed was chosen for a special mission. He began to spend more and more time at this endeavor, and it was this preoccupation that led his parents to make the appointment at the mental health center.

Although initially skeptical about seeing another in a long line of therapists, Howard was grateful when the therapist was interested in his religious convictions. He felt that the therapist could help him explain to his parents why his recent biblical studies were his own business and not "craziness." At this point in the session, Howard asked if he could talk to the therapist alone. Howard's parents willingly left the room.

After his parents left, Howard's demeanor changed dramatically. He became more assertive in his statements, matter-of-factly giving a detailed psychiatric and social history. He explained that he was the third of four brothers, each of them successful in business or a profession. Throughout childhood, he and his younger brother were the better students of the four, and as such, received most of the attention from their parents. However, Howard changed radically toward the end of high school, when his father was diagnosed with cancer. Howard's performance in school began to suffer, as he began to spend a lot of time praying for his father's cure. He believed that his father's eventual recovery was a result of his prayer, and subsequently felt that this was the first sign of his "power."

When Howard had finished his "presentation," the therapist asked permission to speak to his parents. He agreed, but did not want to be present. The therapist verified Howard's story with his parents, although they added that Howard's maternal grandmother had spent the last 20 years of her life in a psychiatric hospital in Mexico. They also emphasized that their relationship with Howard had become increasingly strained, which they attributed to his frequent use of marijuana.

To successfully engage Howard and his parents, the clinician realized the need to build a *collaborative relationship* with them that would require that all parties recognize the agenda of each and seek some common ground in developing a comprehensive treatment plan. For example, in response to the clinician's question about what he hoped to accomplish in treatment, Howard said, "To stop my breath from affecting other people." The clinician did not assume that the patient's failure to continue on maintenance antipsychotic medication derived from a lack of motivation or an inability to develop insight into his illness but, rather, from inadequate education about medication benefits.

The task for the clinician in the first few sessions was to educate Howard and his family about the symptoms of schizophrenia, the psychobiological causes and socio-environmental risk factors for the initial development and future recurrences of the disorder, the currently available treatment options, and the long-term prognosis. Over the course of several sessions, the clinician carefully explained to Howard how his effect on people may be related to his illness, and may improve with a trial of medication. Howard agreed to a trial of medication, but reserved the right to discontinue taking the medication if he noticed no change in his breath's effect within four weeks. The family agreed to this arrangement, but his mother asked if she could monitor Howard's medications. Howard grudgingly agreed to allow his father to watch him take the medications prior to bedtime. By mobilizing the patient's assets and resources (including the family) in this way, the clinician facilitated the process of sharing responsibility for adherence to mutually agreed upon treatment prescriptions.

Over time, Howard and his parents wanted to expand on the gains they had made around medication adherence to other aspects of their relationship. The clinician offered Howard and his parents weekly family therapy sessions using the Behavioral Family Management approach. In the first two sessions, Howard and his parents participated in a *behavioral assessment*. The therapist observed the family's interactions, paying particular attention to the number of overly critical, hostile, and intrusive statements made by the family members. For example, Howard's father frequently referred to his son as "lazy" and "good for nothing." Several times, Howard's mother interrupted Howard in mid-sentence, leading to a progressively louder conversation, which eventually degenerated into a shouting match. These interactions demonstrated high levels of expressed emotion, a factor that is known to contribute to high rates of relapse and rehospitalization and that was addressed in later therapy sessions.

The next four sessions were focused on *education*. All parties received both written and verbal information about schizophrenia, including the functional limitations and cognitive deficits of the disorder. In one of these sessions, the family watched a videotape demonstrating the difficulty many patients with schizophrenia have performing routine activities. The therapist noted a look of amazement in both parents' faces. After the videotape, both parents acknowledged their surprise that these deficits, which they attributed to their son's willful lack of motivation, were part and parcel of the illness. Moreover, they expressed concern that their efforts to "encourage" their son to "just get over it" may have been harmful. The family was cautioned not to overreact to this realization with guilt or remorse, but to take this new knowledge and use it productively in future sessions.

This knowledge came in handy in the very next session, which signaled the start of the next stage, *communication-skills training*. Similar to modular skills training, this training focused on the skills needed for expressing emotions positively and obtaining desires effectively. Because of the high number of negative statements made during the assessment stage, the therapist chose to train the skill, "acknowledging positive actions in others." Each person in the family group was given a chance to practice—under the direct supervision of the therapist—the correct use of verbal and nonverbal elements in the communication. For example, Howard was coached to make better eye contact and to say with more vocal emphasis, "Dad, when you let me watch my favorite television show last night, I really felt good. Thanks a lot." During the next few weeks, Howard and his parents practiced this communication skill daily through a homework assignment called, "Catch a Person Pleasing You." A diary was maintained to record all the instances of the successful practice of this skill. This was repeated for other communication skills, including "expressing negative feelings constructively" and "making positive requests of others." Over the course of six to eight sessions, the family members gradually became more adept and natural when using these communication skills.

The final set of tasks in behavioral family management is ***learning problem-solving skills***. Howard and his family presented his tendency to stay in his room as the problem they wished to work on. Howard described how he would spend hours reading the bible in his room to avoid his parents' dissension and arguments. He avoided these arguments because he would invariably be drawn into the conflict, which would heighten his stress and exacerbate his symptoms. Howard's mother and father conceded that there was a lot of hostility in the home, but felt much of it was due to Howard's incessant bible reading. All family members were given a chance to reflect on the problem and to contribute to its clarity and specificity. The therapist then asked Howard to serve as scribe and the family began to generate alternatives for solving the problem.

Howard's mother suggested that he come down for meals three times a day; his father suggested that he could leave the table if he felt anxious or otherwise uncomfortable. Howard countered with the idea that they could go out to dinner once a week, because he felt his parents were less likely to fight in public. He also thought that if he could invite some of his new friends over for dinner, he would enjoy the experience better. Howard's parents welcomed this idea, as they had been encouraging him to become more sociable. Several other possibilities were presented before the family evaluated each alternative. A consensus was reached on several fronts. It was agreed that Howard would eat dinner with his parents every night, provided one night a week they would go to dinner at a local restaurant, and one night a week he could invite a friend to join his family for dinner at the house. Howard even volunteered to help cook and clean up on the night his friend was coming to dinner.

REFERENCES

Ajzen, I. (1991). The theory of planned behavior. *Organizational Behavior and Human Decision Processes, 50,* 179–211.

Armitrage, C. J., Conner, M. (2001). Efficacy of the theory of planned behavior: A meta-analytic review. *British Journal of Social Psychology, 40,* 471–499.

Bateson, G., Jackson, D. D., Haley, J., Weakland, J. (1956). Toward a theory of schizophrenia. *Behavioral Science, 1,* 251–264.

Dixon, L. B., McFarlane, W. R., Lefley, H., Lucksted, A., Cohen, M., Falloon, I., . . . (2001). Evidence-based practices for services to families of people with psychiatric disabilities. *Psychiatric Services,* 52, 903–910.

Dyck, D. G., Short, R. A., Hendryx, M. S., Norell, D., Myers, M., Patterson, T., . . . (2000). Management of negative symptoms among patients with schizophrenia attending multiple-family groups. *Psychiatric Services, 51,* 513–519.

Dyck, D. G., Short, R. A. Voss, W., Hendryx, M. S., Hanken, M., Vitaliano, P., . . . (2002). Service use among patients with schizophrenia in psychoeducational multi-family group treatment. *Psychiatric Services,* 53, 749–754.

Evans, A., Bullard, D., Solomon, M. (1961). The family as a potential resource in the rehabilitation of the chronic schizophrenic patient: A study of 60 patients and their families. *American Journal of Psychology, 117,* 1075–1083.

Falloon, I. R. H., Boyd, J. L., McGill, C. (1984). Family Care of Schizophrenia. New York, NY: Guilford.

Falloon, I. R. H., Boyd, J. L., McGill, C. W., Williamson, M., Razani, J., Moss, H.B., . . . (1985). Family management in the prevention of morbidity of schizophrenia. *Archives of General Psychiatry, 42,* 887–896.

Falloon, I. R. H., Liberman, R. P. (1983). Behavioral family interventions in the management of chronic schizophrenia. In W. R. McFarlane (Ed.), *Family therapy in schizophrenia* (pp 117–140). New York, NY: Guilford.

Freeman, H., Simmons, O. (1963). The Mental Patient Comes Home. New York: Wiley.

Fromm-Reichmann, F. (1948). Notes on the development of treatment of schizophrenics by psychoanalytic psychotherapy. *Psychiatry, 11,* 263–273.

Guarnaccia, P. J., Parra, P. (1996). Ethnicity, social status, and families' experiences of caring for a mentally ill family member. *Community Mental Health Journal,* 32, 243–260.

Hogarty, G. E., Anderson, C., Reiss, D. J., Kornblith, S. J., Greenwald, D. P., Ulrich, R. F., . . . (1986). Family psychoeducation, social skills training, and maintenance chemotherapy in the aftercare treatment of schizophrenia. *Archives of General Psychiatry, 43*, 633–642.

Jewell, T. C., Downing, D., McFarlane, W. R. (2009). Partnering with families: Multiple family group psychoeducation for schizophrenia. *Journal of Clinical Psychology, 65*, 868–878.

Kopelowicz, A., Wallace, C. J., Liberman, R. P., Aguirre, F., Zarate, R., Mintz, J. (2007). The use of the theory of planned behavior to predict medication adherence in schizophrenia. *Clinical Schizophrenia & Related Psychoses, 1*, 227–242.

Kopelowicz, A., Zarate, R., Gonzalez Smith, V., Mintz, J., Liberman, R. P. (2003). Disease management in Latinos with schizophrenia: a family-assisted, skills training approach. *Schizophrenia Bulletin, 29*, 211–227.

Kopelowicz, A., Zarate, R., Wallace, C. J., Liberman, R. P., Lopez, S. R., Mintz, J. (2012).The impact of multifamily groups to improve treatment adherence in Mexican Americans with schizophrenia. *Archives of General Psychiatry, 69*, 265–273.

Kreyenbuhl, J., Buchanan, R.W., Dickerson, F.B., Dixon, L.B. (2010). The Schizophrenia Patient Outcomes Research Team (PORT): Updated Treatment Recommendations 2009. *Schizophrenia Bulletin, 36*, 94–103.

Kulhara, P., Chakrabarti, S., Avasthi, A., Sharma, A., Sharma, S. (2009). Psychoeducational intervention for caregivers of Indian patients with schizophrenia: A randomized-controlled trial. *Acta Psychiatricia Scandinavica, 119*, 472–483.

Lakes, K., Lopez, S. R., & Garro, L. (2006). Cultural competence and psychotherapy: Applying anthropologically informed conceptions of culture. *Psychotherapy: Theory, Research, Practice and Training, 43*, 380–396.

Lau, A. (2006). Making the case for selective and directed cultural adaptations of evidence-based treatments: Examples from parent training. *Clinical Psychology: Science and Practice, 13*, 295–310.

Leff, J., Kuipers, L., Berkowitz, R., Eberlein-Vries, R., Sturgeon, D. (1982). A controlled trial of social intervention in the families of schizophrenia patients. *British Journal of Psychiatry, 141*, 121–134.

Leff, J., Berkowitz, R., Shavit, N., Strachan, A., Glass, I., Vaughn, C. (1989). A trial of family therapy vs. a relatives group for schizophrenia. *British Journal of Psychiatry, 154*, 58–66.

Liberman, R. P. (1970). Behavioral approaches to family and couple therapy. *American Journal of Orthopsychiatry, 40*, 106–118.

Liberman, R. P. (1972). Behavioral methods in group and family therapy. *Semi Psychiatry, 4*, 145–156.

Lopez, S. R., Kopelowicz, A., Canive, J. (2002). Strategies in developing culturally congruent family interventions for schizophrenia: The case of Hispanics. In Lefley, H.P., Johnson, D.L. (Eds.), *Family interventions in mental illness: International perspectives* (pp. 61–92). Westport, CT: Praeger.

Lucksted, A., McFarlane, W. R., Downing, D., Dixon, L., Adams, C. (2012). Recent developments in family psychoeducation as an evidence-based practice. *Journal of Marital & Family Therapy, 38*, 101–121.

Lyman, D. R., Braude, L., George, P., Dougherty, R. H., Daniels, A. S., Ghose, S. S., Delphin-Ritttmon, M. E. (2014). Consumer and family psychoeducation: Assessing the evidence. *Psychiatric Services, 65*, 416–428.

Magliano, L., Fiorillo, A., Malangone, C., DeRosa, C., Maj, M. (2006). Patient functioning and family burden in a controlled, real-world trial of family psychoeducation for schizophrenia. *Psychiatric Services, 57*, 1784–1791.

McFarlane, W. R. (2002). Multifamily Groups in the Treatment of Severe Psychiatric Disorders. New York, NY: Guilford.

McFarlane, W. R., Dushay, R. A., Deakins, S. M., Stastny, P., Lukens, E. P., Toran, J., . . . (2000). Employment outcomes in family-aided assertive community treatment. *American Journal of Orthopsychiatry, 70*, 203–214.

McFarlane, W. R., Link, B., Dushay, R., Marchal, J., Crilly, J. (1995). Psychoeducational multifamily groups: Four-year relapse outcome in schizophrenia. *Family Process, 34*, 127–144.

McFarlane, W. R., Lukens, E., Link, B., Dushay, R. A., Deakins, S. M., Newmark, M.,. . . (1995). Multiple family groups and psychoeducation in the treatment of schizophrenia. *Archives of General Psychiatry,* 52,679–687.

McFarlane, W. R., Statsny, P., Deakins, S. (1992). Family-aided assertive community treatment: A comprehensive rehabilitation and intensive case management approach for persons with schizophrenic disorders. *New Directions for Mental Health Services,* 53, 43–54.

Medvene, L. J., Mendoza, R., Lin, K.M., Harris, N., Miller, M. (1995). Increasing Mexican-American attendance of support groups for parents of the mentally ill: Organizational and psychological factors. *Journal of Community Psychology, 23,* 307–325.

Mueser, K. T., Glynn, S. M. (1999). Behavioral Family Therapy for Psychiatric Disorders (2nded.). Oakland, CA: New Harbinger Publications.

Murray-Swank, A. B., Dixon, L. (2004). Family psychoeducation as an evidence-based practice. *The International Journal of Neuropsychiatric Medicine, 9,* 905–912.

Randolph, E. T., Eth, S., Glynn, S. M., Paz, G. G., Leong, G. B., Shaner, A. L., . . . (1994). Behavioral family management in schizophrenia: Outcome of a clinic-based intervention. *British Journal of Psychiatry, 164,* 501–506.

Rummel-Kluge, C., Kissling, W. (2008). Psychoeducation in schizophrenia: New developments and approaches in the field. *Current Opinion in Psychiatry, 21,* 168–172.

Schooler, N. R., Keith, S. J., Severe, J. B., Matthews, S. M., Bellack, A. S., Glick, I. D., . . . (1997). Relapse and rehospitalization during maintenance treatment of schizophrenia: The effects of dose reduction and family treatment. *Archives of General Psychiatry, 54,* 453–463.

Tarrier, N., Barrowclough, C., Vaughn, C., Bamrah, J., Porceddu, K., Watts, S., . . . (1989). The community management of schizophrenia. A two year follow-up of a behavioral intervention with families. *British Journal of Psychiatry, 154,* 625–628.

Telles, C., Karno, M., Mintz, J., Paz, G., Arias, M., Tucker, D., Lopez, S.R. (1995). Immigrant families coping with schizophrenia: Behavioral family intervention vs. case management with a low-income Spanish-speaking population. *British Journal of Psychiatry, 167,* 473–479.

United States Department of Health and Human Services: Substance Abuse and Mental Health Services Administration. (2009). Family psychoeducation: How to use the evidence-based practice KITS. HHS Pub. No. SMA-09-4422. Rockville, MD: Center for Mental Health Services.

Vega, W. A., Karno, M., Alegria, M., Alvidrez, J., Bernal, G., Escamilla, M., . . . Loue, S. (2007). Research issues for improving treatment of U.S. Hispanics with persistent mental disorders. *Psychiatric Services, 58,* 385–394.

Zygmunt, A., Olfson, M., Boyer, C.A., Mechanic, D. (2002). Interventions to improve medication adherence in schizophrenia. *American Journal of Psychiatry, 159,* 1644–1653.

/// 17 /// SUICIDE AND NONSUICIDAL SELF-INJURY

RYAN COON and S. CHARLES SCHULZ

INTRODUCTION

A certain mystique exists about mental health practitioners. The public may suspect, or even hope, that powers of foresight, fortune telling, or mind reading exist. Hope is central to these beliefs—hope that psychiatrists can predict and prevent all suicides or identify all individuals who would go onto harm others.

Unfortunately, the ability to prevent all suicides or homicides does not exist. But like any medical provider, psychiatrists use the power of prediction. Physicians constantly make predictions when evaluating patients. They weigh protective factors and risk factors to inform predictions. For instance, if Elizabeth, an 18-year-old previously healthy female and John, a 75-year-old male, smoker, with coronary artery disease present to the emergency room describing identical chest pain, one would predict John is more likely having a heart attack. As healthcare providers, we know advanced age, male gender, smoking, and history of coronary artery disease place John at greater risk. Although this risk assessment will guide John's diagnostic work-up and treatment, it cannot guarantee that John is having a heart attack.

Similarly, we use the power of prediction in mental health to guide diagnostic work-up and evaluate the risk of suicide. However, predictions are only as strong as one's knowledge base. Take a moment and visualize which patients are at greatest risk of committing suicide. At first thought, people with depression come to mind. It is also common to think of individuals who have financial challenges or have recently lost a job or a loved one. Risk factors may also pop into mind like access to weapons, chemical dependency, or a history of suicide attempts.

However, healthcare providers are less likely to recognize that psychotic patients are at high risk of completing suicide. Individuals with psychosis may experience unrelenting hallucinations, commanding them to suicide or even to harm others. In other cases, patients harbor delusions that they are persistently followed or endangered, to a point where suicide appears the only option. Hopelessness may also develop after realizing schizophrenia is a lifelong and incurable illness.

In fact, half of all patients with schizophrenia attempt suicide in their lifetime and 10 percent of psychotic patients die by suicide. These high rates of suicide contribute to the, on average, 15-year shorter life expectancy of patients with schizophrenia compared to the general population (Drake & Cotton, 1986; Falcone & Timmons-Mitchell, 2013).

Fortunately, researchers have uncovered a unique set of suicide risk factors for individuals with psychotic illnesses. Tools are available to help stratify the risk of suicide. It is also heartening that evidenced-based interventions to treat suicidality exist.

As mental health practitioners, it is essential to understand these risks and how to treat suicidality in schizophrenic patients. An objective of this chapter is to teach practitioners how to conduct a suicide assessment, learn how to treat suicidality, and know where to refer patients.

HISTORICAL PERSPECTIVES

Suicide has not always been a primary killer of patients with psychosis. Before antibiotics and modern sanitation, systemic tuberculosis and neurosyphilis were both primary causes of psychosis and killers of afflicted individuals. Antibiotics did not become available to civilians until after World War II. Up until the mid-1900s, infectious diseases, as opposed to suicide, were leading causes of death among psychotic patients.

Healy and colleagues compared causes of mortality among psychotic individuals between 1875–1924 and between 1994–2010 in North Wales (Healy et al., 2012). In the modern patient sample, over half of patients who died, did so by suicide. None of the patients in the modern sample died from tuberculosis or syphilis. However, in the historical sample, disseminated tuberculosis was the leading cause of death (37 percent) and less than one percent of patients in the historical sample completed suicide. Healy's findings underscore two remarkable trends:

1. Antibiotics and modern sanitation revolutionized worldwide morbidity and mortality.
2. The modern day risk of suicide has increased substantially in patients with psychosis.

The etiology of increased suicide rates among individuals with schizophrenia is not entirely clear. However, researchers postulate the emptying of asylums in the twentieth century created a void in the psychosocial support system. The development of antipsychotics may have improved insight to the illness, resulting in despair and thoughts of death. Another possible explanation is that stigma attached to suicide was sufficiently strong to decrease reporting rates. Whatever the reason, the mental health community must acknowledge the suffering of our patients and dedicate resources to prevent suicide.

SUICIDE RISK ASSESSMENT

Most discussions of suicide occur outside the walls of psychiatrists' offices. All healthcare providers care for patients experiencing hopelessness, despair, and thoughts of suicide. These encounters occur in the ICU following a near fatal overdose, between a patient and his or her trusted family physician. Discussions of suicide also occur in the offices of specialists, from oncology to cardiology, when caring for terminally ill patients with cancer or heart disease.

It is a critical moment when a patient shares this suffering. A key part of healthcare training is learning to recognize these moments and skillfully explore a patient's suffering. Sometimes inaccurate beliefs about suicide dissuade physicians from asking about suicide. For instance, some providers believe inquiring about suicide puts ideas into their patient's head. Research has found this untrue. Providers may also think assessing suicide is not part of their scope of practice and a mental health referral is adequate. In reality, it is critical to discuss suicide immediately, because delay may be fatal. Lastly, physicians sometimes think patients who commit suicide will simply do it, rather than discuss their thoughts. This is also untrue because most patients who suicide previously shares these thoughts with others.

The next sections explore how to conduct a thorough suicide risk assessment and provide practical questions to ask patients (Box 17.1). When initially learning to talk about suicide, it can feel difficult or even unsettling. But with practice and a few tools, one can be skillful and confident in these conversations.

Step 1. Gentle Question

In mental health settings, providers routinely inquire about mood, stressors, and loss. However, it is also important for general practitioners to inquire further if patients disclose losses, hopelessness, sadness, or worries about health.

BOX 17.1
SUICIDE RISK—ASSESSMENT ELEMENTS

Gentle question.
Assess current suicidal ideation.
Historical risk factors.
Evaluate for depression.
Mobilize protective factors.

Because stigma exists about mental illness, patients first need to know they are in a safe space where they will not be judged or feel ashamed. A statement that recognizes their pain and suffering can put patients at ease, encourage sharing, and decrease isolation. An example statement is, "This is a safe space for you to share your thoughts and feelings. Many people who are confronted with [specific stressor] would be in a dark place. What has your experience been?"

It is also important to ask directly about thoughts of suicide. To start this conversation, it is often easier to first ask about passive suicidal thoughts before active ones. One could inquire, "Are there times when you feel so horrible you might wish you were dead?" When patients disclose thoughts of suicide, it is critical to investigate warning signs that indicate suicide is imminent. The goal of identifying patients at greatest risk is to provide them critical resources and prevent suicide.

Step 2. Assessing Current Suicidal Ideation

The American Association of Suicidology (AAS) published consensus guidelines that identified warning signs that indicate a suicide attempt may be imminent (Rudd et al., 2006):

Threatening to hurt or kill self.
Looking for ways to kill self; seeking access to pills, weapons, or other means.
Talking or writing about death, dying, or suicide.

The AAS also noted the following thoughts and emotions precipitate suicide attempts: hopelessness, anger, impulsivity, feeling trapped, anxiety, agitation, trouble sleeping, or finding no reason to live. Although these factors should be assessed in all individuals who have suicidal ideation, there are additional factors to consider when evaluating individuals with psychosis.

Fortunately, a group of researchers, The International Suicide Prevention Trial (InterSePT) developed a tool to assist clinicians when evaluating suicidality in this population (Lindenmayer et al., 2003)[1]. The ISST (InterSePT Scale for Suicidal Thinking) is a reliable and validated scale designed to evaluate the risk of suicide in patients who are psychotic (Preston & Hansen, 2005).

The ISST evaluates 12 facets of suicidal ideation and can be used as a template for completing a thorough suicide-risk assessment (Lindenmayer et al., 2003). The scores are computed into different categories, ranging from no suicidality to high suicidality. The ISST scale differs from suicide scales used for nonpsychotic individuals. For instance, the ISST includes questions about delusions and hallucinations that may command individuals with psychosis to harm themselves or to suicide. These types of hallucinations have been shown to increase the risk of suicide in other studies as well. Table 17.1 provides the list of items on the ISST and practical questions one can use to conduct a risk assessment (Table 17.1).

Two other key principles in a suicide-risk assessment include the gentle assumption and denial of the specific. For instance, if a patient discloses passive thoughts of death, a follow-up question that includes a gentle assumption is, "What ways of ending your life have crossed your mind?" instead of "Have you thought of specific ways to kill yourself." The first question makes the assumption that the patient has already experienced these thoughts, and directs them to disclose critical information about suicide planning. However, the second question allows an ambivalent patient to simply answer in the negative and shut down dialogue.

The second principle, denial of the specific, encourages providers to also ask specific follow-up questions. This is particularly helpful when assessing how far a patient is in the planning stages of suicide. Examples include, "Have you had thoughts of hanging yourself? Using a gun, or knife? Taking an overdose?" Direct follow-up questions can help uncover whether someone has taken steps to suicide, "Do you have a stockpile of pills? Have you selected a rope?"

Step 3. Historical Risk Factors

In addition to evaluating immediate warning signs, it is important to recognize longitudinal risk factors that put patients at risk of suicide. One of the most alarming and saddening risk factors is that 10 percent of patients with schizophrenia will die by suicide. The diagnosis alone confers significant risk.

TABLE 17.1 ISST Assessment items and inquiring questions

Item	Question
Wish to die	Tell me about these wishes to be dead. How strong have these wishes become?
Reason for living	Tell me about about your reasons to live?
Suicide intent	Reflect on how strongly you feel about killing yourself?
Passive suicidal desire	Would you take steps to avoid death or avoid steps to maintain life?
Frequency of thoughts	How often are you having thoughts of killing yourself?
Attitude toward ideation	Are your thoughts of suicide unwanted and disturbing or welcome and relieving?
Control over suicide	Is there are part of you that can repel the thoughts of suicide and resist death? How are you able to do this?
Deterrents	What prevents you from completing suicide? Who are the people or animals with whom you are connected? How does suicide intersect with your religious and spiritual beliefs?
Reasons for suicide	What current stressors are intensifying these thoughts of death? When exactly did the thoughts start and what was happening at that time?
Method	How would you go about killing yourself? Have you taken steps to suicide? Have you thought about overdosing? Hanging yourself? Using a gun? Or carbon monoxide?
Expectancy	When do you anticipate the suicide attempt would happen?
Command hallucinations	Have you ever experienced voices or visions telling you to harm yourself or others? In the last week, how often are you having experiences like that?

Items adapted from Lindenmayer, J. P., Czobor, P., Alphs, L., Nathan, A. M., Anand, R., Islam, Z., . . . Chou, J. C. (2003)

Among individuals with psychosis, the risk of suicide is greatest following symptom onset. In fact, researchers have found up to 50 percent of all suicides occur within the first two years of illness onset (Tandon & Jibson, 2003). Adolescents with newly diagnosed schizophrenia adolescents are seventy times more likely to attempt suicide relative to their peers (Kelleher et al., 2013). A major mental health initiative is to reduce the time between the onset of psychotic symptoms and first contact with mental health providers. This period of time is termed the "duration of untreated illness" or DUP. The average DUP is between one and two years in the United States (McGlashan, 1999). This prolonged duration of untreated illness is concerning because patients are at the greatest risk of suicide during these early years. Long DUPs portend other poor outcomes including more severe positive and negative symptoms, as well as,poorer psychosocial functioning (Nordentoft, Jeppesen, Petersen, Bertelsen, & Thorup, 2009).

Researchers, including The International Suicide Prevention Trial (InterSePT), have provided vital information about suicide risk factors and how to treat suicidality in patients with schizophrenia. The InterSePT study was a multicenter prospective cohort study involving 980 patients in 11 different countries. Patients had diagnoses of schizophrenia or schizoaffective disorder and were considered high risk for completing suicide. Patients were randomized to treatment with olanzapine or clozapine and monitored for two years. The primary outcomes were suicide attempts and hospitalizations to prevent suicide. The team identified a number of risk factors associated with suicide attempts and hospitalizations (Potkin et al., 2003). Patients with schizoaffective disorder were 41.7 percent more likely than patients with schizophrenia to have a suicide related outcome. Diagnoses of alcohol use disorder or current cigarette use also increased risk. Each lifetime suicide attempt increased likelihood of another attempt by 3.2 percent. Also, each previous hospitalization increased the likelihood of a subsequent hospitalization by 25 percent.

These risk factors have been confirmed and expanded by other researchers. Among individuals with schizophrenia, comorbid depression is consistently found to increase the risk of suicide. Other factors that increase include the lethality and intent of past attempts, comorbid medical conditions such as malignancies, diabetes, stroke, traumatic brain injury, epilepsy or movement disorders (Sadock, Sadock, & Ruiz, 2009). When crafting a suicide-risk assessment, it is key to uncover patients' past psychiatric and medical histories. An easy-to-use checklist is crafted in Table 17.2 and lists these key suicide risk factors.

TABLE 17.2 Demographic risk factor for suicide among individuals with psychosis

Present	Risk Factors
☐	Schizoaffective disorder
☐	Alcohol use
☐	Cigarette smoking
☐	Depression
☐	Medical comorbidity (HIV, CNS disease, diabetes, cancer)
☐	Past suicide attempts (high intent or high lethality)
☐	Recent psychosis diagnosis (within the last two years)
☐	Anxiety
☐	Male gender
☐	Age 20–39

Step 4. Evaluate for Depression

Traditionally, it was thought depression and schizophrenia did not occur in the same individuals. However, it is now clear that depression is common among individuals with schizophrenia. The estimated rate of depression among individuals with schizophrenia varies considerably across studies (7–75 percent) though the modal rate of depression is around 25 percent. In addition, Siris et al. found that 43 percent of outpatients with schizophrenia were prescribed antidepressants medications (Siris et al., 2001). Depression is also critical to detect because research has consistently shown that depression is a major risk factor for suicide in individuals with schizophrenia (Kasckow, Felmet, & Zidook, 2011; Siris, 2000).

However, in clinical practice, it can be difficult to distinguish depression from other symptoms in schizophrenia. When healthcare professionals think about patients with schizophrenia, the "positive symptoms," symptoms that are added most often come to mind. Positive symptoms include hallucinations and delusions or fixed, false beliefs.

However, schizophrenia also causes cognitive symptoms and "negative symptoms" or things taken away. Negative symptoms include loss of motivation, poverty of speech, loss of affect, and restricted range of interests. Negative symptoms can lead to social withdrawal, poor self-hygiene, and even an absence of facial expressions or emotions. Cognitive symptoms such as thought blocking or disorganized thoughts may appear like slowed or difficult-to-follow speech.

There is considerable overlap among symptoms of depression and the negative and cognitive symptoms in schizophrenia (Table 17.3). Many people with depression also withdraw socially, have a flattening of affect or lack motivation to maintain personal hygiene. It is important to make the distinction because antidepressant agents are more likely to help the person with major depression than with negative psychotic symptoms.

Fortunately, tools like the Calgary Depression Scale (CDS) for Schizophrenia, are available online and free to use for clinicians and students (Addington, Addington, & Schissel,

TABLE 17.3 Similarities between Negative Psychotic Symptoms and Depression

Negative Symptoms	Depression
Apathy, lack of motivation	Anhedonia, absence of pleasure
Thought blocking	Psychomotor slowing
Loss of affect/Parkinsonism	Restricted affect
Delusions of guilt	Guilt and hopelessness
Social isolation	Social isolation
Disorganized thoughts	Impaired concentration

1990). The CDS is comprised of nine questions evaluating the following: frequency of depression, hopelessness, worthlessness, guilty ideas of reference, sense of guilt, morning depression, early awakenings, thoughts of suicide, and clinician observed depression. Because of significant overlap between depression and the negative symptoms of schizophrenia, the CDS does not inquire about psychomotor slowing, anhedonia, or impairments in concentration or energy. The CDS has been shown to have strong reliability and has been translated into a number of other languages. In addition, the instrument has demonstrated validity for predicting suicide-related outcomes. In the InterSePT study, every point increase in the CDS was associated with a 4 percent increased risk of a suicide-related outcome.

Step 5. Mobilize Protective Factors

When evaluating patients who are demoralized or even suicidal, we must mobilize patients' resilience. Griffith and Gaby identify seven existential postures that capture the dichotomy between vulnerability and resilience (Griffith & Gaby, 2005). Connection with others versus isolation is one these elements. Communion, a sense of connection, intimacy, of being heard, reduces both isolation and the risk of suicide. Practitioners can reduce isolation by asking questions such as, "Who do you turn to when you are troubled?" or "In whose presence do you feel most calm?" (Siris, 2000). We also reduce isolation through our presence, the act of hearing our patients, and recognizing their suffering.

Despair is countered by identifying hope and desire. The open-ended question, "On difficult days, what keeps you from giving up?" allows patients to uncover sources of perseverance. Patients may also discover purpose by asking what makes their life meaningful, impactful, and inherently good. Purpose may take the shape in their connection with others. For instance, one might inquire, "For whom, or for what, does it matter that you continue to live?" Purpose can also be found in spirituality or religious beliefs. We can ask, "What does God hope you will do in the days to come?" The objective of these questions is to begin a dialogue with patients. The questions remind both the patient and ourselves of the patient's strengths and reasons for living. Bringing resilience and strength to the mind, can help tip the scale toward life rather than death.

TREATMENT

Treatment Setting

Patients and providers intersect at various levels of care. Treatment settings range from outpatient-clinic visits to day-treatment programs, to locked inpatient psychiatric hospitals. The goal is to meet our patients at the level of care they need. When individuals are at significant risk of harming themselves or others, psychiatric hospitalization is often warranted and necessary. Admitting individuals with psychosis to the hospital may be a voluntary process but can also be a forced hospitalization. Once patients are stabilized, our task is to successfully transition them to a less restrictive level of care. For instance, patients may participate in a day-treatment program or be seen more frequently by outpatient providers following hospitalization. Other options include enhancing outpatient supports by adding case managers, home-care nursing, involving family members, or referring for psychotherapy.

Clozapine

Clinicians should strongly consider using clozapine when treating individuals with schizophrenia who are at high risk of suicide or who have a history of suicide attempts. There is robust support in the literature documenting that clozapine reduces the risk of suicide, suicide attempts, and suicidal ideation in individuals with schizophrenia (Kasckow et al., 2011). This risk reduction appears unique to clozapine and does not generalize to other second- or first-generation antipsychotic medications.

Researchers have demonstrated clozapine reduces rates of suicide upward of 80–90 percent in both controlled studies and large retrospective clozapine database reviews. Meltzer initially described the antisuicidal property of clozapine in a study of treatment refractory schizophrenia patients. The authors followed patients for two years and identified that the rate of suicide attempts decreased by 86.4 percent following treatment with clozapine (Meltzer & Okayli, 1995). Most recently, in a randomized, two-year prospective study of schizophrenic and schizoaffective patients at high risk for suicide, clozapine was shown to decrease the relative risk of suicidal behavior suicide by 24 percent compared with olanzapine (Meltzer et al., 2003). In response to this broad evidence base, the U.S. Food and Drug Administration (FDA) now includes clozapine as indicated treatment for suicidal behavior in individuals with schizophrenia.

Antidepressants

The American Psychiatric Association also recommends using antidepressant medications for patients with schizophrenia or schizoaffective disorder who experience comorbid major depression (Lehman et al., 2004). A number of double-blind randomized control trials have evaluated the efficacy of SSRIs for treating depression in individuals with schizophrenia or schizoaffective disorder. Although results have been mixed across studies, the largest study found augmentation with citalopram significantly reduced symptoms of depression and thoughts of suicide (Zisook et al., 2010). As discussed earlier, scales like the CDSS are specifically tailored to uncover signs and symptoms of depression among individuals with schizophrenia. In general, antidepressants should be used in conjunction with antipsychotic medications (AP) when individuals with schizophrenia experience unipolar depression (Lehman et al., 2004).

Psychotherapy

Antipsychotic medications are not cures for schizophrenia and many individuals (30–40 percent) suffer from symptoms that are refractory to antipsychotic medications. Even when clozapine is used, patients may continue to experience symptoms. And even when medications are effective, poor medication adherence due to side effects may lead to re-emergence of psychotic symptoms. Additionally, it is known that antipsychotics have limited effect on the negative symptoms.

Psychotherapy for individuals with schizophrenia has significantly changed since the nineteenth century. During the 1800s, countries in Europe and North America institutionalized many individuals in asylums. Patients did improve in the structured social milieu. Improvement manifested in daily interactions with compassionate staff and patients, in assigned work roles, and even pursuit of creative interests (Shorter, 1997). In some settings, physicians also used psychoanalysis to treat institutionalized patients. By the twentieth century, overcrowding of mental health facilities resulted in poor living conditions and inadequate patient care. A combination of poor conditions and emergence of pharmacotherapies precipitated the deinstitutionalization of mentally ill individuals.

In present times, research has shown cognitive behavioral therapy, family therapy, and cognitive remediation are helpful for individuals with schizophrenia. Psychotherapy is helpful for individuals with psychosis for a number of reasons. In psychotherapy, a trusting relationship is created between the provider and patients. Once an alliance is secured, the therapist helps patients explore other explanations for the inaccurate thoughts and inaccurate sensations.

Family therapy is particularly effective for decreasing high interpersonal stress. This type of stress, "High E," makes patients and their families less resilient and adaptive. It is critical to teach family members techniques to decrease stress, accept the patient's limitations, improve self-esteem, and reduce isolation (Pilling et al., 2002). Family therapy is helpful in objective measures as well. Specifically, family therapy reduces symptom relapse, decreases rehospitalization rates, and improves medication adherence. There

TABLE 17.4 Therapy Benefits for Patient with Schizophrenia

Improvement Area	Family	CBT	Cognitive Remediation
Depression		X	
Suicidal Ideation	?	X	
Hallucinations		X	X
Fewer Relapses	X		
Fewer Readmissions	X		
Med Compliance	X		
Psychosocial Functioning			X
Cognitive Performance			X

is also some evidence that family therapy is helpful in reducing suicide rates, however, sample sizes are too low to verify this hypothesis (Table 17.4).

In the same meta-analysis of trials, CBT was shown effective in reducing Brief Psychiatric Rating Scale (BPRS) scores. Meaningful reductions were observed in positive psychotic symptoms, dysphoria, and improvements in insight (Table 17.4). More recently, Bateman and colleagues evaluated whether CBT could reduce suicidal ideation in a group of 90 patients with chronic schizophrenia (Bateman, Hansen, Turkington, & Kingdon, 2007). Patients were randomized to CBT or a control group involving a befriending intervention. The CBT intervention focused on maximizing coping skills and reevaluating psychotic symptoms. Although both groups demonstrated a mean decrease in sucidality, the decrease was only statistically significant for the CBT group.

Most recently, mental health practitioners developed a new behavioral intervention, termed cognitive remediation, for the treatment of schizophrenia. The objective of this therapy is to treat the cognitive and negative symptoms. Specific goals include improving attention, memory, social cognition, and psychosocial functioning more broadly (Wykes, Huddy, Cellard, McGurk, & Czobor, 2011). A meta-analysis of 40 cognitive remediation trials found cognitive remediation improved both cognition and psychosocial functioning (Table 17.4).

NONSUICIDAL SELF-INJURY

Mental health practitioners frequently treat individuals who engage in deliberate self-harm (DSH). Self-injury or self-harm are defined as the intentional destruction or injury of the body without suicidal intent. Diagnoses including borderline personality disorder, factitious disorder, malingering, and eating disorders often first come to mind when thinking of individuals at risk for DSH. However, individuals suffering from psychotic disorders are also at great risk (Haw, Hawton, Sutton, Sinclair, & Deeks, 2005). In fact, 38 percent of individuals with chronic schizophrenia have a history of DSH (Breier, Schreiber, Dyer, & Pickar, 1991).

Patients with schizophrenia engage in deliberate self-injury for a number of reasons. For instance, patients suffering from delusions of sin may self-harm to atone for perceived trespasses. In other instances, command hallucinations may demand patients to harm themselves. Self-injury may also manifest as a maladaptive behavior to manage general distress from the illness.

Occasionally the degree of self-injury is particularly severe among psychotic individuals. In a case review of patients with biblical delusions who engaged in DSH, all patients cited excerpts from the Biblical Book of Matthew as reasons for self-injury (Schwerkoske, Caplan, & Benford, 2012). The patients engaged in severe self-mutilation that included enucleation of the eye and amputations of limbs and genitals. A number of individuals who engaged in ocular enucleation cited Matthew 5:29, "But if thy right eye offend thee, pluck it out and cast it from thee: for it is profitable for thee that one of thy members should perish, and not that thy whole body should be cast into hell." These patients frequently perceived guilt about sexual acts as the motivation for self-mutilation. The ensuing castration or enucleation was viewed as atonement for sin. Patients felt relief after completing the act. Even long after the act of self-mutilation, these patients did not regret the loss of limbs, eyes, or genitals. Although these acts are infrequent, individuals with psychotic disorders appear at unique risk of severe self-mutilation. For example, research has shown 87 percent of males who engaged in genital self-mutilation suffered from a psychotic illness (Greilsheimer & Groves, 1979).

Though these severe acts are infrequent, mental health practitioners must be vigilant for at-risk individuals and foster interdisciplinary communication. It is notable that many psychotic individuals complete surgical consultation requesting the removal of a body part prior to completing the act themselves (Waugh, 1986). Thus, the medical community should view the surgical consultation as a critical opportunity. Specifically it is an opportunity to teach surgical providers skills to detect high-risk individuals and immediately refer patients to mental health providers. The overarching objective is to prevent potentially catastrophic tissue damage.

The severity of self-injury in these cases is pronounced. However, other forms of self-injury are practiced among individuals with psychosis. In fact, research has shown that more moderate or superficial self-injury is seen with much greater frequency (Harvey et al., 2008). Specifically, Harvey et al. evaluated the incidence and type of self-harm behavior among individuals presenting in their first psychotic episode. The most frequent types of self-harm behaviors included cutting (30 percent), overdoses (29 percent), hitting (9 percent), or jumping from heights (9 percent). Thus, the vast majority of self-harm behavior resulted in less severe tissue injury in this much larger prospective study cohort. The authors also documented the overall frequency of self-harm behavior during the first episode of psychosis was 11.3 percent. Although lower than the rate observed among individuals with chronic schizophrenia (38 percent), this lower frequency is impacted by the shorter duration of illness in this first episode cohort.

This evaluation of patients with first episode psychosis also highlights that self-harm behavior manifests for a variety of reasons. In this cohort, only 19 percent of individuals noted hallucinations or delusions directing them to injure themselves. Rather, the vast majority of patients (71.4 percent) reported distress from their symptoms as the reason for DSH. These findings have been replicated in a meta-analysis of risk factors for self-harm among people with schizophrenia (Bateman et al., 2007). The study found that distress and severity of negative symptoms was predictive of self-harm behavior. However, command hallucinations and delusions were not correlated with DSH.

Researchers have uncovered additional risk factors for DSH among individuals with psychosis. There is significant overlap between risk factors for suicide (Table 17.2) and risk factors for self-harm behavior (Table 17.5). Overlapping risk factors include depression, histories of self-harm, or psychiatric hospitalization. Enhanced insight to the illness is also correlated with self-harm behavior. It is believed that insight highlights how the illness derailed one's life. Common losses include endings of intimate relationships, employment terminations, and academic suspensions. Loss can manifest as hopelessness, despair, and even self-loathing to the point of self-injury. In some instances, self-harm may be perceived as revenge on a body that has failed oneself.

TABLE 17.5 Risk Factors for Non-Suicidal Self Injury

Present	Risk Factor
☐	Male gender (for first episode patients)
☐	Insight to illness
☐	Longer duration of untreated illness
☐	Depression
☐	Substance use
☐	History of self-harm behavior
☐	History of psychiatric hospitalizations

Substance Use, Psychosis and Self-Harm Behavior

Complex relationships exist between psychosis, substance use, self-harm behavior, and suicide. First, it is widely known that many illicit substances induce psychotic symptoms including amphetamine compounds (stimulants, methamphetamine, cocaine, PCP), hallucinogens such as LSD, and cannabinoids. Within the last decade, a new class of synthetic drugs commonly called bath salts, has emerged and precipitates psychotic symptoms. The psychosis manifests via the amphetamine-like properties of bath salts (Ross, Reisfield, Watson, Chronister, & Goldberger, 2012). Bath salts are produced synthetically and thus, have made regulatory enforcement difficult. These substances are easily purchased over the Internet or at community head shops.

Similar to other amphetamine-like compounds, adverse physical effects from bath salts include tachycardia, hypertension, arrhythmias, diaphoresis, and myocardial infarction. Care in the emergency department is largely supportive, but also focused on reducing the risk of seizures. Users of bath salts may also experience anxiety, extreme agitation, paranoia, hallucinations, and self-mutilation or even suicide. In emergency departments, drug induced psychoses are often acutely managed with neuroleptic medications (Harvey et al., 2008). However, due to the risk of seizures associated with bath-salt use, practitioners have recommended using benzodiazepines as opposed to antipsychotics for symptom control.

It is clear that illicit substances can induce psychotic symptoms. However, this relationship is further complicated because individuals with schizophrenia use illicit substances at a much higher rates (40–50 percent) than the population as a whole (16 percent). Hadock and colleagues(2013) characterized the frequency and risk factors for DSH among 327 patients with schizophrenia and illicit drug or alcohol use disorders. Of these individuals, 28 percent engaged in DSH or a suicide attempt during the two-year study. The severity of positive psychotic symptoms, both hallucinations and delusions, increased the risk of self-harm up to three times the baseline rate. This finding is notable because hallucinations and delusions do not consistently increase risk for self-harm among other populations with schizophrenia. Overall, 30 percent of the enrolled patients experienced command hallucination to harm oneself. Similar to studies in other psychotic populations, distress from psychotic symptoms was associated with self-harm behavior (Haddock, Eisner, Davies, Coupe, & Barrowclough, 2013)

CONCLUSION

Individuals with schizophrenia and related psychoses commonly engage in deliberate self-harm. The character of self-harm can vary widely in presentation. A minority of incidents may be gruesome, even catastrophic self-injury in response to command hallucinations or delusional content. Evidence exists that individuals with comorbid substance use and schizophrenia are at greater risk of DSH secondary to positive psychotic symptoms. However a more frequent self-injury presentation is moderate or superficial self-injury. Most self-injury occurrences are attributed to attempts to manage distress from psychotic symptoms. The overarching objective for mental health practitioners is to create a space for open dialogue with patients. Then, one must ask meaningful questions to understand and prevent further self-harm.

REFERENCES

Addington, D., Addington, J., & Schissel, B. (1990). A depression rating scale for schizophrenics. *Schizophrenia Research, 3*(4), 247–251.

Bateman, K., Hansen, L., Turkington, D., & Kingdon, D. (2007). Cognitive behavioral therapy reduces suicidal ideation in schizophrenia: results from a randomized controlled trial. *Suicide and Life Threatening Behavior, 37*(3), 284–290.

Breier, A., Schreiber, J. L., Dyer, J., & Pickar, D. (1991). National Institute of Mental Health longitudinal study of chronic schizophrenia. Prognosis and predictors of outcome. *Archives of General Psychiatry, 48*(3), 239–246.

Drake, R. E., & Cotton, P. G. (1986). Depression, hopelessness and suicide in chronic schizophrenia. *British Journal of Psychiatry, 148*, 554–559.

Falcone, T., & Timmons-Mitchell, J. (Dec 11, 2013). Psychosis and suicidality in adolescents. *Psychiatric Times* (20–22).

Greilsheimer, H., & Groves, J. E. (1979). Male genital self-mutilation. *Archives of General Psychiatry, 36*(4), 441–446.

Griffith, J. L., & Gaby, L. (2005). Brief psychotherapy at the bedside: countering demoralization from medical illness. *Psychosomatics, 46*(2), 109–116.

Haddock, G., Eisner, E., Davies, G., Coupe, N., & Barrowclough, C. (2013). Psychotic symptoms, self-harm and violence in individuals with schizophrenia and substance misuse problems. *Schizophrenia Research, 151*(1–3), 215–220.

Harvey, S. B., Dean, K., Morgan, C., Walsh, E., Demjaha, A., Dazzan, P., ... Murray, R. M. (2008). Self-harm in first-episode psychosis. *Br J Psychiatry, 192*(3), 178–184.

Haw, C., Hawton, K., Sutton, L., Sinclair, J., & Deeks, J. (2005). Schizophrenia and deliberate self-harm: a systematic review of risk factors. *Suicide and Life Threatening Behavior, 35*(1), 50–62.

Healy, D., Le Noury, J., Harris, M., Butt, M., Linden, S., Whitaker, C., . . . Roberts, A. P. (2012). Mortality in schizophrenia and related psychoses: data from two cohorts, 1875–1924 and 1994–2010. *BMJ Open, 2*(5), 1–10

Kasckow, J., Felmet, K., & Zidook, S. (2011). Managing suicide risks in patients with schizophrenia. *CNS Drugs, 25*, 129–143.

Kelleher, I., Corcoran, P., Keeley, H., Wigman, J. T., Devlin, N., Ramsay, H., . . . Cannon, M. (2013). Psychotic symptoms and population risk for suicide attempt: a prospective cohort study. *JAMA Psychiatry, 70*(9), 940–948.

Lehman, A. F., Lieberman, J. A., Dixon, L. B., McGlashan, T. H., Miller, A. L., Perkins, D. O., . . . Kreyenbuhl, J. (2004). Practice guideline for the treatment of patients with schizophrenia, second edition. *American Journal of Psychiatry, 161*(2 Suppl), 1–56.

Lindenmayer, J. P., Czobor, P., Alphs, L., Nathan, A. M., Anand, R., Islam, Z., . . . Chou, J. C. (2003). The InterSePT scale for suicidal thinking reliability and validity. *Schizophrenia Research, 63*(1-2), 161–170.

McGlashan, T. H. (1999). Duration of untreated psychosis in first-episode schizophrenia: marker or determinant of course? *Biological Psychiatry, 46*(7), 899–907.

Meltzer, H. Y., Alphs, L., Green, A. I., Altamura, A. C., Anand, R., Bertoldi, A., . . . Potkin, S. (2003). Clozapine treatment for suicidality in schizophrenia: International Suicide Prevention Trial (InterSePT). *Archives of General Psychiatry, 60*(1), 82–91.

Meltzer, H. Y., & Okayli, G. (1995). Reduction of suicidality during clozapine treatment of neuroleptic-resistant schizophrenia: impact on risk-benefit assessment. *American Journal of Psychiatry, 152*(2), 183–190.

Nordentoft, M., Jeppesen, P., Petersen, L., Bertelsen, M., & Thorup, A. (2009). The rationale for early intervention in schizophrenia and related disorders. *Early Intervention Psychiatry, 3*(Suppl 1), S3–S7.

Pilling, S., Bebbington, P., Kuipers, E., Garety, P., Geddes, J., Orbach, G., & Morgan, C. (2002). Psychological treatments in schizophrenia: I. Meta-analysis of family intervention and cognitive behaviour therapy. *Psychological Medicine, 32*(5), 763–782.

Potkin, S. G., Alphs, L., Hsu, C., Krishnan, K. R., Anand, R., Young, F. K., . . . Green, A. (2003). Predicting suicidal risk in schizophrenic and schizoaffective patients in a prospective two-year trial. *Biological Psychiatry, 54*(4), 444–452.

Preston, E., & Hansen, L. (2005). A systematic review of suicide rating scales in schizophrenia. *Crisis, 26*(4), 170–180.

Ross, E. A., Reisfield, G. M., Watson, M. C., Chronister, C. W., & Goldberger, B. A. (2012). Psychoactive "bath salts" intoxication with methylenedioxypyrovalerone. *American Journal of Medicine, 125*(9), 854–858.

Rudd, M. D., Berman, A. L., Joiner, T. E., Jr., Nock, M. K., Silverman, M. M., Mandrusiak, M., . . . Witte, T. (2006). Warning signs for suicide: theory, research, and clinical applications. *Suicide and Life Threatening Behavior, 36*(3), 255–262.

Sadock, B. J., Sadock, V. A., & Ruiz, P. (Eds.). (2009). *Kaplan and Sadock's comprehensive textbook of psychiatry* (9th ed.). Philadelphia, PA: Lippincott Williams & Wilkins.

Schwerkoske, J. P., Caplan, J. P., & Benford, D. M. (2012). Self-mutilation and biblical delusions: a review. *Psychosomatics, 53*(4), 327–333.

Shorter, E. S. (1997). *A history of psychiatry from the era of the asylum to the age of Prozac*. New York, NY: John Wiley & Sons.

Siris, S. G. (2000). Depression in schizophrenia: perspective in the era of "atypical" antipsychotic agents. *American Journal of Psychiatry, 157*(9), 1379–1389.

Siris, S. G., Addington, D., Azorin, J. M., Falloon, I. R., Gerlach, J., & Hirsch, S. R. (2001). Depression in schizophrenia: recognition and management in the USA. *Schizophrenia Research, 47*(2-3), 185–197.

Tandon, R., & Jibson, M. D. (2003). Suicidal behavior in schizophrenia: diagnosis, neurobiology, and treatment implications. *Current Opinions in Psychiatry, 16*, 193–197.

Waugh, A. C. (1986). Autocastration and biblical delusions in schizophrenia. *British Journal of Psychiatry, 149*, 656–658.

Wykes, T., Huddy, V., Cellard, C., McGurk, S. R., & Czobor, P. (2011). A meta-analysis of cognitive remediation for schizophrenia: methodology and effect sizes. *American Journal of Psychiatry, 168*(5), 472–485.

Zisook, S., Kasckow, J. W., Lanouette, N. M., Golshan, S., Fellows, I., Vahia, I., . . . Rao, S. (2010). Augmentation with citalopram for suicidal ideation in middle-aged and older outpatients with schizophrenia and schizoaffective disorder who have subthreshold depressive symptoms: a randomized controlled trial. *Journal of Clinical Psychiatry, 71*(7), 915–922.

/// 18 /// EMERGENCY MANAGEMENT OF THE AGGRESSIVE AND VIOLENT PATIENT

STEPHEN MILLER, MATTHEW KRUSE, and ROBERT HAIGHT

INTRODUCTION

Psychotic illness has been associated with an increased risk of violence in both community and institutional settings (Douglas, Guy, & Hart, 2009). When a person with psychosis is seen in an emergency department or inpatient unit, there may be additional risks associated with the person's belief that treatment or hospitalization is unwarranted. For a person with psychosis, the process of hospitalization and treatment may feel like an assault on his or her rights and person, increasing the likelihood of conflict with staff. Like other decisions in medicine, choosing an intervention requires consideration of the diagnosis, potential risks and benefits of a given intervention, alternative interventions that are available, and the consequences of not intervening. Each element of this decision-making process will be discussed in this chapter. It should be noted that due to the challenges inherent in performing controlled trials involving emergency interventions, guidance for physicians who encounter these clinical decisions comes mainly in the form of expert consensus guidelines (Allen, Currier, Carpenter, Ross, & Docherty, 2005; Wilson, Pepper, Currier, Holloman, & Feifel, 2012).

DEFINING AGITATION

Aside from actual physical aggression (e.g., hitting, kicking, pushing, spitting, charging at staff) clinically meaningful behaviors that may warrant emergency intervention include:

Intimidating behavior.
Restlessness, pacing, or excessive movement.
Explosive and/or unpredictable anger.
Physical self-harm.
Demeaning or hostile verbal behavior.
Uncooperative or demanding behavior.
Resistance to care.
Impulsive behavior.
Low frustration tolerance.

There are several rating scales available to quantify agitation, though their specific metrics and intended use in clinical settings vary (Swift, Harrigan, Cappelleri, Kramer & Chandler, 2002; Palmstierna & Wistedt, 1987; Yudofsky, Silver, Jackson, Endicott, & Williams, 1986). Nevertheless, use of an objective instrument may help identify the need to intervene earlier (Richmond et al., 2012).

GOALS OF INTERVENTION

Although it is possible to use medications to induce sleep, this is not considered to be the goal of emergency management of aggression. Expert consensus guidelines in the United States and the United Kingdom (National Institute for Health and Clinical Excellence, 2009; Wilson et al., 2012) agree the most appropriate goal of emergency medication intervention is calming the patient without sedation. This allows care providers to continue assessing the patient and tailor further interventions accordingly.

INITIAL ASSESSMENT

Time is often limited when assessing an agitated patient, but prompt, efficient evaluation may yield critical clinical information to help guide treatment. Assessment should begin with vital signs, a medical history, and a focused physical exam to identify any medical cause for agitation or aggression. Special attention should be paid to signs of head trauma, respiration, heart rhythm, smell of alcohol, diameter/reactivity of pupils, lacerations, nuchal rigidity, and fractures. Initial laboratory exams should include blood glucose measurement and urine toxicology (drug screen). If a medical etiology is identified, treatment should focus on correcting the underlying condition. In terms of psychiatric assessment, the interview should be sensitive to broad categories of illness, including psychosis, mania, intoxication, and withdrawal (Allen et al., 2005).

During evaluation, striking a tone of kind-hearted curiosity may reduce the risk of aggression toward the examiner. Interview questions might include the following:

1. "Hello Mr. X, my name is Dr. Y. How are you feeling today?"
2. "In order to keep you and others here safe, there are some questions I'd like to ask you. First, what brought you into the emergency room today?"
3. "Have you used any substances recently that might still be in your system?"
4. "Do you think you might be in withdrawal from any substance?"
5. "Are you having any thoughts that are bothering you? Are your thoughts going so fast, you can't keep up with them?"
6. "Do you ever hear strange things, such as voices when nobody else is around? Do you ever see things that disturb you?"
7. "Do you feel like people are out to get you or trying to harm you? Do you have any special abilities?"
8. "Have you been having any thoughts of wanting to hurt yourself or others?"
9. "Have you ever been on a medicine for psychiatric symptoms in the past? What was it called? Was it helpful? Can we offer you a medicine now to help you calm down?"
10. "Is there anything I can do to help you?"

NONMEDICATION INTERVENTIONS

For agitated or aggressive patients who refuse to take an oral medication for the purpose of calming, a few interventions should be tried before a medication is forced by injection. Verbal de-escalation is a well-established intervention and will be described in detail in the next section. The patient may be asked to walk to his or her room and stay there for a set period of time (e.g., 30 minutes). If the patient complies and is able to calm down on his or her own, more restrictive interventions such as seclusion or restraints may be avoided. If these initial methods are unsuccessful, a "show of force," in which extra staff members are called to the area, may discourage the patient from being aggressive and allow for redirection. If restraints are needed, it is recommended medications be given concurrently rather than using restraints alone (Allen et al., 2005).

Verbal De-escalation

The goal of verbal de-escalation is to help the patient calm him- or herself and develop an internal locus of control. Richmond et al., 2012 outline a three-step process for de-escalation: (1) verbally engage the patient, (2) establish a collaborative relationship, and (3) employ a de-escalation technique suitable to the particular patient and situation. To accomplish these steps, several of the following strategies may be employed.

Establish clear goals and reassurance. Regardless of your role on the treatment team, it is important to explain to patients you are there to keep them safe and make sure no harm comes to them or anyone else. Reassure patients you want to help them regain control of their behavior. Do your best to identify what patients want. If it isn't clear, ask them to tell you and listen actively. Clarifying statements such as "tell me if I have this right. . ." can be very helpful. (Richmond et al., 2012)

Use Miller's Law, which states, "to understand what another person is saying, you must assume that it is true and try to imagine what it could be true of." The patient will sense you are truly trying to understand. If the patient has a delusion that someone intends to cause him harm, imagine how this is true from the patient's standpoint. Engage the patient in a conversation about why this is happening and ask who would want to harm him. The patient will begin to see that you care. (Richmond et al., 2012)

Another technique is to find something about the patient's position with which you can agree. There are three ways to do this:

1. **Agree with the truth**. For example, if a patient is agitated after being informed of an involuntary hospitalization, you might say "Yes, you've been hospitalized against your will and you're angry about that."
2. **Agree in principle**. For example, if a patient is complaining he was disrespected by the police, you don't have to agree with his opinion but you can say "I believe everyone should be treated with respect."
3. **Agree with the odds**. For example, if a patient is agitated about having to wait to see the doctor and states anyone would be upset in that situation, you might say, "many people would be upset by that."

In finding a way to agree, you might feel as though you are stating very obvious truths. However, it should never be assumed that the patient *knows* or *believes* that you are intending to be helpful, and making explicit statements to foster that belief is very important. If pressed to agree with a delusion, one might respond "Although it sounds unlikely to me, I have no way of proving right now that you're wrong." (Richmond et al., 2012)

If you've listened empathically and attempted to find some areas of agreement, you will now be in a better position to set clear limits. Tell the patient any injury to him or others is unacceptable. If the patient's behavior is making you feel unsafe, it's often helpful to verbalize this. Sometimes a patient will be unaware their behavior is making others feel uncomfortable and will react with appropriate regret. Verbalizing your feelings can sometimes help the patient consider another perspective, even if only for a moment. You can combine an expression of your feelings with a directive statement, such as "I'd like you to sit down; when you pace like that, I feel frightened and I can't pay attention to what you are saying." (Richmond et al., 2012)

Finally, offer choices. If the situation is escalating, be assertive and quickly propose alternatives to violence. These might include food, water, blankets, magazines, or access to a phone. Offers should be realistic and promptly provided if chosen. You might also ask "What helps you at times like this?" This invites the patient to consider options, and may be a good segue into a discussion of medication. Current guidelines recommend patients should be involved in the selection and route of administration of any medication. (Allen et al., 2005; Richmond et al., 2012; Wilson et al., 2012) State "I think you would benefit from a medication." Ask what medications have been helpful for the patient in the past. If this doesn't produce an acceptable option, a short list of viable alternatives can be given (see the following section for specific recommendations based on provisional diagnosis). If the agitation is severe enough to warrant forced intramuscular (IM) medication, giving the patient a choice between an oral medication or receiving a shot allows the patient some element of control. You can say "I can't let any harm come to you or anyone else. I would like to offeryou some medication now to help you stay in control. Would you like to take it by mouth or by injection?" (Richmond et al., 2012)

Following any type of involuntary intervention (e.g., forced medication, restraints, or seclusion), it is important to debrief the patient in order to restore the therapeutic alliance. Explain why the intervention was necessary. Let the patient express his perspective. Help him explore alternatives for managing similar feelings in the future. Teach the patient how to request a time out and how to express anger in an acceptable way. Discuss how medications may be used earlier to avoid further aggression if agitation is escalating.

Any statements that can foster optimism about the situation are a good way to conclude. State your belief that things are going to improve for the patient, and your hope that he or she will have a safe and healthy life outside the hospital. Often, the patient's desire is to "get out of here." State that you want that as well. You can say "I don't want you to be here any longer than necessary; how can we work together to help you get out of here?"

SELECTION OF A MEDICATION BASED ON PROVISIONAL DIAGNOSIS

When initial, nonpharmacologic interventions are unsuccessful, medications to calm a patient may be necessary. In these situations it is important to first identify a provisional diagnosis to guide the selection of an appropriate medication. Unfortunately, many patients who become aggressive or violent are new to the treatment setting (emergency department or psychiatric unit). Patient symptom and medication histories may be limited, if available at all.

The administration of a medication should also be timed appropriately. If a patient is given a medication too early or too aggressively, any attempts to engage them in a psychiatric evaluation may be disrupted. If medications are delayed, the patient, staff, and others may be at risk for harm. Patients with worsening agitation or who were not calmed by the initial dose may require repeat administration and/or escalating doses.

There is no class or specific medication considered to be the "best" in all cases of agitation. Available classes that have the most clinical experience and research include

1. First-generation antipsychotics.
2. Second-generation antipsychotics.
3. Benzodiazepines.

The route of administration should also be considered, and if possible, discussed with the patient. Although not available for all medication options, routes may include the following:

1. Oral tablets.
2. Orally dissolving tablets.
3. Intramuscular injections.

No Provisional Diagnosis

The patient may not be able to meaningfully participate in an interview because of thought disturbances or agitation. In cases in which the only observed sign or symptom is agitation, the recommended treatment is oral or IM lorazepam. Oral risperidone, IM ziprasidone, IM olanzapine, and IM haloperidol are also considered first-line options. Second-line options include oral olanzapine, haloperidol, or quetiapine . The aforementioned medications should generally be avoided if the agitation appears to be caused by a general medical condition, delirium, or dementia, and instead, treatment should focused on treating the underlying cause. (Allen et al., 2005).

Provisional Diagnosis: Psychosis

When a patient presents with agitation and some indication of perceptual disturbance (appears to be responding or attending to unseen others verbally or physically, indicating auditory and/or visual hallucinations) or difficulty with reality testing (e.g., delusions such as a belief that he or she is being poisoned, monitored, or targeted for attack), then a provisional diagnosis of psychosis is reasonable. Even without a more definitive diagnosis (schizophrenia, bipolar mania with psychosis, etc.), the recommended treatment for agitation is an antipsychotic medication, since it would likely help to alleviate the underlying cause of the agitation while also providing time-limited sedation. (Allen et al., 2005; Wilson et al., 2012)

Selecting an antipsychotic medication the patient has benefited from in the past is preferred, particularly if the medication is a reasonable choice for providing an immediate calming effect (i.e., it is not an extended release formulation).

Olanzapine (oral or IM) or haloperidol plus lorazepam (oral or IM) are recommended as first-line options. Ziprasidone IM, either alone or combined with lorazepam IM is also a first-line option. Oral ziprasidone is not generally used as a PRN for agitation. (Allen et al., 2005)

In a retrospective chart review of 146 consecutive, agitated patients, those who received 10 mg IM olanzapine had similar outcomes and lower rates of additional medication intervention (AMI) compared to 5 mg IM haloperidol combined with 2 mg IM lorazepam. The rate of AMI observed in patients who received IM olanzapine alone was 9 percent, compared to 22 percent of patients who received combined IM haloperidol/lorazepam, and 45 percent for patients who received IM haloperidol alone. (MacDonald et al., 2012).

In this study, adding IM lorazepam to IM olanzapine did not significantly reduce AMI compared to IM olanzapine alone (MacDonald et al., 2012). The manufacturer does not recommend concurrent IM olanzapine with benzodiazepines due to the potential risks of excessive sedation, orthostatic hypotension, or cardiorespiratory depression. (Zyprexa (olanzapine) product information, Eli Lilly—December 2014). A separate study that evaluated outcomes of patients receiving IM haloperidol or olanzapine, with or without benzodiazepines found the combination of IM olanzapine + benzodiazepines was not associated with hypotension. However, the combination was found to have a risk of decreased oxygen saturation, particularly in patients who were alcohol-positive. The authors of both studies felt the combination of IM olanzapine + benzodiazepines did not have an increased risk of hypotension, but declined to recommend the combination due to lack of evidence for improved efficacy compared to IM olanzapine alone and the need for additional research. (Wilson, MacDonald, Vilke, & Feifel, 2011; MacDonald et al., 2012)

If a patient with a presumed psychotic disorder has received the usual maximum dose of an antipsychotic, and the patient has calmed down somewhat but is still moderately agitated, addition of oral lorazepam is recommended. Giving another dose of the same antipsychotic is a second-line option. Adding divalproex or a different antipsychotic are third-line options. (Allen et al., 2005).

Provisional Diagnosis: Mania

When a patient presents with agitation along with typical symptoms of mania (e.g. pressured speech, grandiose ideas, flight of ideas, decrease in sleep), use of an antipsychotic is again recommended, either alone or in combination with lorazepam or divalproex. If oral administration is possible, olanzapine and risperidone are considered first-line. Quetiapine, ziprasidone, and haloperidol are reasonable choices as well. If divalproex is added, a loading dose of 30 mg/kg/day may be used for two days followed by 20 mg/kg/day thereafter. Although lithium is an evidence-based first-line treatment for bipolar mania, it may not be as helpful as divalproex in managing agitation. If IM administration is needed, olanzapine alone or haloperidol plus lorazepam are recommended. (Allen et al., 2005).

DOSAGE AND FREQUENCY

Medication doses should always be tailored to the individual patient and circumstance, with consideration given to age, body size, any knowledge of renal or liver function, and past experience with similar medications. The following dose ranges were considered appropriate for use in a behavioral emergency by 90 percent or more of an expert panel (Allen et al., 2005):

Oral lorazepam: 1–3 mg.
IM lorazepam: 0.5–3 mg.
Oral or IM haloperidol: 2.5–10 mg
Oral risperidone: 1–3 mg.
Oral olanzapine: 5–20 mg.
IM olanzapine: 5–10 mg.
IM ziprasidone: 10–20 mg

NEW THERAPEUTIC OPTIONS

A new, inhaled version of loxapine is indicated for the acute treatment of agitation associated with schizophrenia or bipolar I disorder in adults. Due to concerns about respiratory distress and arrest, all patients should be screened for a history of asthma, COPD, or other pulmonary disease. Use of the delivery device also requires patient cooperation. Loxapine inhalation powder is only available through a restricted program under a Risk Evaluation and Mitigation Strategy (REMS). To register for this program, sites must have access to on-site equipment and personnel trained to manage acute bronchospasm, including intubation and mechanical ventilation. Inhaled loxapine is not mentioned in any available guidelines for the treatment of acute agitation.

CONSEQUENCES OF NOT INTERVENING

In the case of less severe agitation or aggression verbal de-escalation, behavioral interventions, and voluntary medication administration are preferable, as these approaches better maintain the provider-patient alliance and may shorten hospitalization length of stay. When necessary, the risks of harm to the patient and staff with forced medication interventions, restraints, or seclusion is still tolerated in some cases as the risks of not intervening may be more serious. In the case of an acutely violent or aggressive patient, the risk of not intervening includes the risk of serious injury to self, staff, or fellow patients. In light of this, there is a higher tolerance for risk associated with the intervention than in situations in which the risk of not intervening is less serious, for example, during the phase of long-term maintenance treatment. For this reason, medications that are used commonly for management of acute agitation may not be the best choice for long-term treatment. Often, a switch from an acute treatment to a long-term treatment is warranted as the patient's behavior stabilizes.

REFERENCES

Allen, M. H., Currier, G. W., Carpenter, D., Ross, R. W., & Docherty, J. P. (2005). The expert consensus guideline series. Treatment of behavioral emergencies 2005. *Journal of Psychiatric Practice, 11*(Suppl 1), 5–108.

Douglas, K. S., Guy, L. S., & Hart, S. D. (2009). Psychosis as a risk factor for violence to others: A meta-analysis. *Psychological Bulletin, 135*(5), 679–706.

MacDonald, K., Wilson, M., Minassian, A., Vilke, G., Becker, O., Tallian, K., . . . Feifel, D. (2012). A naturalistic study of intramuscular haloperidol versus intramuscular olanzapine for the management of acute agitation. *Journal of Clinical Psychopharmacology, 32*(3), 317–322.

National Institute for Health and Clinical Excellence. (2009). *Schizophrenia: Core Interventions in the treatment and management of schizophrenia in adults in primary and secondary care (Clinical Guideline CG82).*

Palmstierna, T., & Wistedt, B. (1987). Staff observation aggression scale, SOAS: presentation and evaluation. *Acta Psychiatr Scand, 76*(6), 657–663.

Richmond, J., Berlin, J., Avrim, F., Ng, A., Bregman, B., & Andwrson, E. (2012). Medical Evaluation and Triage of the Agitated Patient: Consensus Statement of the American Association for Emergency Psychiatry Project BETA Medical Evaluation Workgroup. *Western Journal of Emergency Medicine, 13*(1), 3–10.

Richmond, J., Berlin, J., Holloman, G., Zeller, S., Wilson, M., Rifai, M., & Ng, A. (2012). Verbal De-escalation of the Agitated Patient: Consensus Statement of the American Association for Emergency Psychiatry Project BETA De-escalation Workgroup. *Western Journal of Emergency Medicine, 13*(1), 17–25.

Swift, R. H., Harrigan, E. P., Cappelleri, J. C., Kramer, D., & Chandler, L. P. (2002). Validation of the behavioural activity rating scale (BARS): A novel measure of activity in agitated patients. *Journal of Psychiatric Research, 36*(2), 87–95.

Wilson, M.P., MacDonald, K., Vilke, G., & Feifel, D. (2011). A comparison of the safety of olanzapine and haloperidol in combination with benzodiazepines in emergency department patients with acute agitation. *Journal of Emergency Medicine, 43*(5), 790–797.

Wilson, M.P., Pepper, D., Currier, G.W., Holloman, Jr. G.H., & Feifel, D. (2012).The psychopharmacology of agitation: Consensus statement of the American Association for Emergency Psychiatry Project BETA Psychopharmacology Workgroup. *West Journal of Emergency Medicine 13*(1), 26-34.

Yudofsky, S. C., Silver, J. M., Jackson, W., Endicott, J., & Williams, D. (1986). The overt aggression scale for the objective rating of verbal and physical aggression. *American Journal of Psychiatry, 143*(1): 35–39.

Zyprexa® (olanzapine) [package insert]. Eli Lilly and Company, Inc., Indianapolis, IN; December 2014.

/// 19 /// VOCATIONAL REHABILITATION AND RECOVERY

MORRIS D. BELL

INTRODUCTION

This chapter reviews the history of work programs in the treatment of psychiatric illness and how today's recovery movement has rediscovered and promoted the value of vocational rehabilitation as a therapeutic and empowering intervention for people with schizophrenia spectrum disorders. It describes the contemporary spectrum of work services and recent innovations that enhance vocational rehabilitation by addressing illness-specific work-related impairments.

BACKGROUND AND HISTORICAL PERSPECTIVE

Work activity was at one time viewed as a central component of comprehensive psychiatric treatment. In the mid-nineteenth century, the moral treatment of insanity regarded work as an essential therapeutic agent that could distract patients from their psychotic preoccupations, improve self-esteem through realistic accomplishment, and allow for the discharge of tension through physical activity. E Todd, MD, the superintendent of the Institute of Living, conveyed his conviction about the healing power of paid employment when he wrote in 1830 to the parents of a patient: "I cannot too strongly urge the advantage and even the necessity of his being engaged in some regular employment which shall hold out the promise of some moderate but fair compensation to his industry and prudence." (Brigham, 1847/1994).

At the beginning of the twentieth century, most asylums continued to provide patients with work activity—usually farming, cooking, maintenance, laundry, and cottage industries—because of its putative therapeutic benefit and because it reduced operational costs. Writing in the *Annual Report of the State Board of Charities and Corrections* to the governor of Virginia for the year ending September 30, 1911, superintendents at two state hospitals wrote:

> It has been said that occupation is a counterirritant to the brain, just as a mustard plaster is to a pain, and I hold this to be true, that suitable labor, recreation in the fresh air, and diversion will do the insane much more good than medicine out of a bottle. . . Therefore, a hospital for the insane should be a great workshop for the hands, with abundance of diversion and recreation (Dr. J. C. King, Southwest State Hospital).
>
> It is generally conceded by all practical and experienced alienists [public psychiatrists] that work therapy takes first rank as a remedial measure in all cases of chronic insanity (Dr. W. F. Drewry, Central State Hospital).

Recognizing that work activity to be effective must involve the interests of the patient and the encouragement of the staff, Dr. Drewry further wrote,

> Upon the hospital staff there rests a grave responsibility. Unless they take an active interest in devising ways and means of employment of the patients, and encourage them in their work, little or nothing can be accomplished.

In 1917, in the eighth volume of *Modern Hospital*, Dr. Fred Clark, Medical Superintendent at State Hospital, Stockton, CA, wrote an essay entitled, "Some Common Mistakes in Applying Occupational Therapy." It included a plea for what we now call individualized placement: "Work chosen must be adapted to the individual;" a recommendation that staff be specifically trained to high fidelity: "Work must be directed by trained teachers"; and an earnest warning that the patient's work activity should be in line with the patient's goals and interests: "Patient must not be allowed to become a drudge." A century later, versions of these principles will become central to contemporary vocational rehabilitation.

Dr. Clark had good reason to be worried about the quality of the work experience for residents in state hospitals for the insane. As America absorbed large waves of immigration, these institutions became overcrowded with displaced and desperate individuals, and chronic underfunding often led to the exploitation of patients as cheap labor. Many lived out their entire adult lives in these state hospitals where they had meaningful work in agriculture, cooking, cleaning or small shops, providing the bare necessities for themselves and sometimes servicing their doctors. In one shop, women took old sheets to sew dressing gowns for newly arrived patients; in another, donated scraps of leather from the town tannery would be used to repair worn out boots and shoes. Patients would care for the children of the doctors who lived on the grounds, cooked their meals and cleaned their houses. Some privileged patients would join their attendants in skating parties on the lake in winter, and generations of patients were buried in the cemetery on the hospital grounds. Although these institutions were a refuge for some, they were often a place of torment for others. Warehoused in back wards, patients were often stripped of their dignity, treated harshly, or neglected.

In the late 1950s and 1960s work activity at many of these institutions was reconceptualized as preparation for deinstitutionalization and community reintegration. One compelling reason for this change was the growing public recognition that patients were being abused and exploited. Concerns were raised about patient rights at a time when civil rights issues were at the forefront of public discourse in America. New legislation such as the Social Security Act amendments of 1965 and the Rehabilitation Act of 1973 began to address these concerns, and the deinstitutionalization movement got fully underway.

One inadvertent consequence of rapid deinstitutionalization was that many patients were deprived of the meaningful jobs they had performed while institutionalized. Since work programs in the community had not been created for these patients, hospital discharge usually meant unemployment and inactivity. Formerly institutionalized patients turned to community mental health centers for psychiatric treatment. Clinicians in these agencies seldom regarded work as their responsibility. Typically, they referred these patients to the vocational rehabilitation division of their state department of education.

This referral trend created a new set of problems and further reduced the emphasis on work as a necessary part of recovery from mental illness. Vocational rehabilitation counselors in state agencies were accustomed to assessing and training their clients with the goal of full-time competitive employment. They would make referrals to training programs that were not accustomed to the needs of mental health populations. Although appropriate for some, this procedure was not designed for the varied abilities, motivation, and level of psychosocial services needed to support someone in recovery. Moreover, since the aim of these vocational programs was to restore clients to full-time employment, these referrals had the ironic result of placing them into a system whose primary interest was economic rather than therapeutic. Instead of social reintegration and economic self-sufficiency, most people with mental illness failed to complete training or to find full-time competitive employment.

During this period in the early 1970s, some mental health programs continued to recognize the need for work activity as a therapeutic tool and attempted to provide work programs within a therapeutic context. Notably, psychosocial clubhouse programs included work components in their comprehensive services. The Boston University Center for

Psychiatric Rehabilitation was established to improve rehabilitation practice and promoted a "Choose-Get-Keep" vocational counseling approach (Determine what job is right for you, obtain the job, and get the supports you need to keep the job). In Europe, "Social Firms" began providing work opportunities in supportive environments; and as the recovery movement in the United States really got underway, Individual Placement and Support, an evidence-based supported employment program, was developed and promulgated.

It is now generally recognized that with medical, psychological, social, and community supports, people with mental illness can and do participate in meaningful social roles. Their recovery is enhanced when they participate in the world of work, earn an income, and join their communities as productive individuals. Their sense of identity, self-efficacy and self-esteem are enhanced. They become active citizens who contribute to the communities in which they live.

WHY WORK MATTERS

Until the recovery movement got underway, the prevailing clinical attitude was that people were so disabled by psychotic disorders that seeking employment and facing the demands of work would prove too stressful to them and might result in exacerbations of symptoms and relapse. This type of paternal and protective attitude, however well-intentioned, further discouraged patients who were already disheartened about trying to work. Moreover, there was no research evidence that workplace stress increased symptoms or led to relapse (Marrone & Galowaka, 1999), and this clinical attitude ignored the stress that unemployment causes—poverty, isolation, and social disenfranchisement.

Studies have shown that unemployment itself can lead to deterioration in mental and physical health among previously healthy individuals (Warr, 1987), and these consequences are all the more serious for those with severe mental disorders. Historically, the state of the political economy has been related to public health indicators of psychiatric illness, with increases in psychiatric hospitalizations during times of economic hardship (Warner, 1985). The modest income that federal and state disability programs provide is insufficient for independent living. Even with entitlements such as federal housing supplements, there is very little discretionary income left each month. In these circumstances, even a modest increase in income through part-time work can make a big difference in quality of life. More money means better food choices, participation in social activities, bus fare or gas to visit family or friends, and the opportunity to give to others. Supported education and employment interventions early in the course of illness can help many people experiencing prodromal symptoms or recovering from a first episode pursue their career plans by returning to college or employment. For them, vocational and educational supports may allow them to achieve full economic independence.

Having a work life expands opportunities to meet people and develop a social network that goes beyond family, therapists, and others with mental illness. In the course of a work day, there are common goals and activities that allow people to get to know one another and discover commonalities that may lead to friendships. The worksite is a place where social skills can be practiced, and as people with mental illness become more comfortable in their social interactions at work, they may begin to have more confidence in social relationships outside of work. Since most adults are workers, they can relate more easily to the experiences of others. When asked by new acquaintances, "What do you do?" they no longer need to feel embarrassed. There is the possibility of developing trusting and reciprocal relationships in which the person with mental illness feels that she or he has as much to give as she or he receives.

Instead of isolation and retreat into a private world of thoughts and fears, work life demands a reality orientation with focused goals and realistic problems to solve. Work is physically activating and gets people out of a sedentary life-style that may be deleterious to their health. Work is also cognitively stimulating and demands self-monitoring, impulse inhibition, planning, sequencing, and self-organization. These executive functions and other neurocognitive and social cognitive functions are often compromised by mental illness, and are related to difficulties on the job (Bell, Tsang, Greig, & Bryson, 2009). The work place may provide opportunities to practice those abilities or to learn compensatory strategies to cope with impairments in those abilities. Motivated by the desire to do their job well, people with mental illness can improve in these ways, and such improvements can generalize to other situations. For example, getting to work on time is an important requirement of most jobs; so learning to prepare for work by laying out clothes the night before; checking a calendar to determine the date and time; setting the alarm clock properly; having medications ready by the sink; having a grooming list taped to the full length mirror; preparing a fanny pack or purse with correct change for the bus fare, the house keys, work keys and identification card; and having the proper coat, hat, and shoes by the door makes it more likely that the person will get to work on time. Moreover, the person learns that the same strategies can be used to get to a doctor's appointment or a date on time. Mastery of competencies of daily living increases self-worth, confidence, and independence.

In addition to neurocognitive and social cognitive impairments, some with schizophrenia experience a loss of volition and other negative symptoms that affect work performance and employment (Lysaker & Bell, 1995a). These symptoms are fundamentally related to a sense of self and identity, which are necessary for the self-experience of purpose and will. The loss of a cohesive sense of self in schizophrenia leaves a person with no basis for setting goals or taking action to meet those goals (Lysaker & Bell, 1995b) and part of vocational rehabilitation becomes helping the person to create a narrative of their life that makes meaning of their experiences. Working may not only reactivate neurobiological reward system through doing, it may also help people begin to consolidate an identity. Through working, they discover or rediscover worthwhile features of themselves and begin to create a more integrated narrative of their recovery and their life. With that narrative can come specific and achievable goals that are meaningful to the person. Achieving those goals reinforces identity and generates new goals and directions.

Importantly, having employment in our society conveys status and promotes citizenship. People in their recovery from mental illness have learned to be empowered as consumers, making clear that there should be "nothing about me, without me." But although consumer power is important, greater empowerment occurs when people can give back to their communities as contributing members of society. One example of this has been employment of peer counselors by public mental health systems (sometimes called "prosumers" as a blend of caring professional and consumer). These trained counselors can use their lived experience of mental illness to enhance their understanding of their clients, and the clients in turn can identify with their counselor's successful recovery. Employment, whether part time or full time, reintegrates people into their communities and gives them a greater stake in civic affairs, making it more likely that they will relate to public concerns (e.g., buses need to run on time), be involved in community organizations, and vote in public elections. This reintegration is a key objective of the Americans With Disabilities Act (ADA) as well as the President's New Freedom Commission on Mental Health Report, *Achieving the Promise,* which reinforced the point that the goal of the mental health system is to help people with mental illnesses in "living, working, learning, and participating fully in the community" (President's NewCommission on Mental Health, 2003). In doing so, working may reduce the stigma of mental illness by decreasing its association with unemployment.

SPECTRUM OF VOCATIONAL REHABILITATION PROGRAMS

Vocational rehabilitation services have developed and progressed along with the recovery movement. Prevocational programs that were designed to prepare people for work but did not offer payment for work activities proved ineffective. These programs taught basic skills such as grooming and hygiene, regular attendance, building stamina, and getting along with others. However, being unpaid, many people would be unmotivated, and when they didn't show up to the program, staff would conclude that they were not "work ready." As a board member of the National Alliance on Mental Illness once described it, "Pre-voc is No Voc." Prevocational programs are still used by occupational therapists in inpatient settings where patients may do art projects, crafts, and gardening to help them be more active and attentive, but as psychiatric inpatient stays have become much shorter, these services are less likely to be used.

Much preferred are approaches to vocational training and employment that allow clients to quickly enter into paying jobs, even if only for a short period or for less than minimum wage. These programs include sheltered workshops, enclaves, transitional employment, social firms, supported employment, and job clubs.

Sheltered workshops were much more common in the mid-twentieth century than they are today. Charitable organizations or rehabilitation centers received contracts from businesses for piecework such as simple assembly, packaging, sorting, and labeling. Clients were paid by the piece and worked together, often at long tables carefully monitored by staff. These workshops were set up in environments segregated from other workers. They offered security, accommodations for a range of disabilities, and companionship. For some clients, the low expectations, the safety of only interacting with other clients and staff, and the daily routine seemed sufficient. However, these workshops had significant limitations: their work was repetitive and boring; there was no advancement; they reinforced an identity of disability; relationships were limited to other disabled people and staff; and the amount of pay was small. Although these workshops offered some of the psychological and social benefits of working, their limitations led to their discontinuation in most national programs serving psychiatric patients.

Work Enclaves are an advance over sheltered workshops because work is performed in a natural workplace often in work crews. The work has been especially set aside for workers with disabilities and is carefully monitored by staff. The work may be landscaping, housekeeping (often in public buildings at night), cleaning public parks, or assembling parts in a factory, and it may teach valuable work habits, social skills, and work skills. However, there is very little individual choice in the type of work, pay is modest, there is no advancement, jobs belong to the program and not to the workers, and workers remain segregated. Working in such jobs over time lowers self-expectations and becomes a comfortable "parking space" with no further vocational progress.

Transitional employment places clients with community employers, medical centers, psychosocial clubhouses, or rehabilitation centers. Clients work alongside and are supervised by regular staff. These experiences have direct relevance to community employment. What makes these programs "transitional" is that the job belongs to the program and not to the individual. They are time limited and their goal is usually to prepare clients to seek competitive employment. Usually these programs include counseling to prepare clients for transitioning into their own employment. These programs usually pay at least minimum wage and sometimes require that the person work full-time. There is considerable variation from program to program in the amount of vocational counseling, work expectations, accommodations for disability, and pay. What they have in common is that they are in conventional work environments, offer variety, have expectations for performance, and are integrated with nondisabled workers.

The Department of Veterans Affairs is the largest single provider of transitional work services in the United States, and it offers two levels of such service. One is called Incentive Therapy (IT) and provides work activity for up to 20 hours a week, usually in work sites around the VA Medical Center. It can pay no more than half minimum wage, and the payment is regarded as a therapeutic incentive rather than as employment earnings. Participation in IT cannot be considered in VA disability determination. IT is often used with veterans who may not plan to return to competitive employment but recognize the therapeutic benefit of work activity in a normal work setting, or it may serve veterans who will want to return to competitive employment but are so early in their recovery that stability and continuation in intensive treatments are more immediate concerns. Often these are patients with multiple comorbidities including medical conditions with chronic pain. IT provides accommodating work settings, schedules that do not interfere with treatment appointments, and counseling support as needed. Work placements are based on the client's interests, and new sites may be developed for that purpose. For example, a recovering veteran with a musical performance background worked with the occupational therapist in the VA nursing home, playing the piano while lunch was served; another wanting to help other veterans worked at the information desk; and a veteran with a technical background worked with the Medical Center engineers running blueprints and organizing files. IT has been shown to provide many of the mental health benefits that working can bring and can do so for veterans with significant limitations (Bell, Lysaker, & Milstein, 1996; Bell & Lysaker, 1997), but its goal is not necessarily to transition to competitive employment.

VA Compensated Work Therapy (CWT) is also regarded as a therapeutic program, so earnings do not affect disability determinations; but CWT is based on contracts for services either with the VA Medical Center or with area businesses. Pay is at least minimum wage, often requires a full-time commitment, and is usually fully integrated with the work of employees without disabilities. For example, the VA Medical Center may contract with CWT to provide housekeeping, inventory, or supply staff; or an area business may contract with CWT for landscape or maintenance work. CWT is usually combined with job counseling with the goal of transitioning to competitive employment. The demands of CWT may exceed what is possible for some veterans, and there remain questions about whether it succeeds in its primary aim of promoting competitive employment even for those without psychotic illness (Penk et al., 2010).

Affirmative Business and Social Firms are businesses that are created to employ people with disabilities and produce goods or services for the community at a profit. They provide stable employment opportunities while offering accommodations, security, and support for their workers. This model of employment for people with psychiatric disabilities first gained prominence in Trieste, Italy in the 1970s during a period of political activism when psychiatric institutions were rapidly closed and a sense of collective responsibility was at a high. A workers' cooperative was created that started out by providing cleaning services to public buildings, but by 1994 it had become a consortium of businesses that included a café, hotel, restaurant, transportation, and building renovation business. Several more social firms were later developed that provided shopping for the homebound, landscaping, bookbinding, and street cleaning (Warner & Mandilberg, 2006). The success of the Trieste experience influenced the development of social firms in Europe and eventually in North America, Australia, and elsewhere. According to the European Confederation of Social Firms and Cooperatives (CEFEC; www.socialfirmseurope.org), A Social Firm is a business created for the employment of people with a disability or other disadvantages in the labor market. It produces goods and services to pursue its social mission, mixes disabled and nondisabled workers, and all employees receive a fair-market wage for their efforts. Accommodations are made for disabilities and all employees share the same rights and obligations. It must also be a viable business that brings in an income, even if there are subsidies from private donors or government grants. For example, La Fageda is a for-profit dairy farm in Girona, Spain near Barcelona that employs 280 people, over half of whom have a mental illness. La Fageda produces a very popular yogurt that trails only Dannon and Nestle in yogurt sales. It also has vegetable gardens for jam production, a landscaping service, and a cattle-care facility (www.fageda.com). Workers are paid a fair wage, become shareholders in the cooperative, and have the option of living on the farm or on their own.

Supported Employment (SE) was promoted first for people with developmental disabilities but was adapted to psychiatric populations most successfully by Robert Drake and Deborah Becker at the Dartmouth Psychiatric Research Center. Named Individual Placement and Support (IPS), the Becker and Drake model has been accepted as an evidence-based practice since 2002 (Bond et al., 2002). Research has repeatedly demonstrated that it is more effective at improving competitive work outcomes than any other model of vocational rehabilitation for seriously mentally ill (SMI), with over 15 randomized controlled trials of "high fidelity" SE programs (Bond, Drake, & Becker, 2008). It continues to gain empirical support (Drake, Bond, & Becker, 2012) and is disseminated widely with the aid of a SAMHSA Toolkit (http://store.samhsa.gov/list/series?name=Evidence-Based-Practices-KITs). IPS aims to put anyone to work who wants to work regardless of the severity of their disability, and to do so by finding competitive employment in the community. Repeated studies indicate that employment rates for IPS of over 50 percent far exceed those of conventional vocational services (20 percent), with more than 30 percent sustaining work over long- term follow-up. One reason for their success is that IPS vocational specialists will develop jobs with community employers that suit the interests and limitations of their workers, and they provide wrap-around services and supports. Often these supports can be phased out as the worker becomes accustomed to the work environment, develops natural supports from co-workers and supervisors, and masters the skills necessary for independence. The main tenets of IPS are maximum inclusion, consumer choice, rapid job finding, competitive employment, and continuous support and follow-along services. A particularly important feature of IPS is that it specifies that SE services be integrated within mental health treatment teams, a principle believed to enhance job retention. Employment specialists focus exclusively on providing vocational services, facilitate integration of vocational and clinical services, avoid lengthy prevocational assessment and training, conduct rapid job searches for work in integrated community settings, strive to match consumers to jobs based on their preferences, and provide ongoing supports. IPS is particularly in tune with the recovery movement because of its principle that the only eligibility requirement is that the person wants to work. Although not all people with psychiatric disabilities may want to work, surveys suggest that more than 70 percent of people would like to have some kind of work in the community (Becker, Drake, & Naughton, 2005). As the mental health community becomes better at early detection of and intervention in psychotic illnesses, having the treatment team adopt IPS can be critical in helping individuals accomplish what they want in their lives (Drake, Xie, Bond, Mchugo, & Caton, 2013). When functional goals, rather than merely symptom reduction, become a treatment focus, the treatment team can work together to ensure that medication dosing is adapted to the work schedule (e.g., taking doses at night, so that the individual isn't drowsy on the job), that family is engaged in supporting their family member's work activities, and that, when a mental health crisis occurs, urgent attention is provided with minimal disruption to the person's work schedule (Ciardiello & Bell, 1988).

Although IPS has demonstrated its superiority to conventional vocational services, results are still limited. Despite employment rates of over 50 percent, in any one month, rates of employment are around 25 percent to 35 percent, and job complexity is generally low. It often takes about six months for a person to obtain a job, about half the people who get employed are not working at that job after six months (Cook et al.,

2005), and rates of employment are significantly worse for those with schizophrenia diagnoses (Razzano et al., 2005). Moreover, most of the jobs that people obtain are less than half time, and their earnings are insufficient for economic independence. Since most people enrolled in SE are receiving Social Security benefits, there are powerful disincentives that limit the number of hours and total earnings that they may feel they can earn without losing disability payments. Despite the Ticket to Work program (www.chooseworkttw.net) and other efforts to reduce disincentives, few people are willing to risk it. For this reason, benefits counseling has become a part of the IPS approach.

Job Clubs are for people with psychiatric disabilities who wish to look for work on their own (Azrin & Phillip, 1979). They are often people with established work histories, with additional resources such as transportation, and with a willingness to go on job interviews. Vocational staff provides structure to the job search, usually offering help in developing a resume or in completing job applications, often online. Vocational staff may have access to Department of Labor information about new job postings and are generally familiar with community employers that may be receptive to applications from their clients. Job Clubs are often centers where clients can use phones, computers, fax machines, and filing cabinets and get practical support from staff. They learn job-seeking skills, interview skills, and they are expected to set goals and meet them. Classes may be offered that address questions about whether to disclose their disability, what their rights are as workers with a disability, if they choose to disclose, what are reasonable accommodations once hired, how to negotiate their schedule, and how to handle the stress and frustration that is often a part of job searching. Much of the work of the vocational specialist is to encourage persistence. They also may encourage group support, and sometimes clients will buddy up, going on job interviews together. Daily goal setting that includes breaking down their goals into small steps and reviewing these goals provides a valuable structure for overcoming anxiety and following through on tasks.

PSYCHOLOGICAL INTERVENTIONS TO IMPROVE VOCATIONAL OUTCOMES

Supported employment may provide work opportunities; but modest vocational outcomes for those with schizophrenia spectrum disorders suggests the need for interventions to augment SE that target illness-specific work impairments (Bell, Choi, & Lysaker, 2007). Several psychological interventions to enhance work services include work behavior feedback groups with goal setting, work focused cognitive behavioral therapy, job-interview and work-related social-skills training, and neurocognitive and social cognitive training.

Work behavior assessments, feedback, self-appraisal, and goal setting have been strongly endorsed by management research as powerful methods to improve productivity. One review concluded: "With goal-setting theory, specific difficult goals have been shown to increase performance on well over 100 different tasks involving more than 40,000 participants in at least eight countries. . .In short, goal-setting theory is among the most valid and practical theories of employment motivation in organizational psychology" (Locke & Latham, 2002).

One systematic application of goal-setting theory to vocational rehabilitation has been the use of the Work Behavior Inventory (WBI; Bryson, Bell, Kaplan, & Greig, 1999; Bryson, Bell, Lysaker, & Zito, 1997) and the Vocational Cognitive Rating Scale (VCRS; Greig, Bryson, & Bell, 2004) to assess performance in the workplace, and the use of weekly worker meetings to provide systematic feedback from the WBI and VCRS to help workers set goals. The WBI scales include measures of work habits (e.g., punctuality); work quality (e.g., accuracy); social skills (e.g., relationships with co-workers); cooperativeness (e.g., willingly accepting direction); and personal presentation (e.g. hygiene). The VCRS measures attention, memory, and executive function in performing work assignments. In an hour-long workers' meeting, members receive feedback and participate in problem solving and goal setting. The vocational specialist leading the group encourages a process of accurate empathy in which true achievement is acknowledged and praised, and problems are realistically addressed. Self-appraisal is encouraged, and motivation is increased by setting realistic but attainable goals and by the group process of support and shared experience. Each week members report their progress and set new goals often based on their WBI and VCRS feedback. Goals might include increasing hours of work, taking on new responsibilities, taking fewer breaks, using self-talk to follow sequenced tasks, or approaching a co-worker about having lunch together. In programs of transitional employment (where direct observations for assessments are much easier than in competitive employment), feedback, self-appraisal, problem solving and goal setting can be done frequently (e.g., biweekly), which provides the individual with reassuring and reliable information that encourages progress.

There are several reasons this procedure is important for people with schizophrenia. First, this is a disorder with neurocognitive and social cognitive impairments that make it difficult to accurately understand what is going on in the complex social environment at work. Feedback provides information to workers about their work habits and quality, and importantly, about their social skills, cooperativeness, and personal presentation. These interpersonal behaviors are crucial for vocational success, but are usually not addressed. Work supervisors are comfortable giving feedback about work habits and quality (e.g., "You're late." Or, "Do this again; it's not right."), but they usually feel reluctant to talk with workers about social withdrawal, odd appearance, or difficulty taking criticism. Left alone, these problems can build up until there is a critical incident leading to job loss. Regular and systematic feedback can provide workers with schizophrenia a social prosthesis for their impairment in reading their social environment.

Second, motivation, sense of purpose, and self-confidence can be profoundly affected by psychiatric disorders. Regular feedback provides workers continual reassurance about what they are doing right and what they need to work on. Since feelings of worthlessness often lead these workers to think that others regard them as inadequate, getting accurate feedback about how they are viewed can reduce mistrust and increase confidence. As goals are set and attained, workers feel less hopeless and have a growing sense of mastery and self-efficacy.

Third, identification of vocationally related problems in attention, memory, and executive function can inform a plan for compensatory strategies in the workplace. These may include having a special color-coded work notebook with a section devoted to lists that breaks down work tasks into their specific steps and sequence. It may include calendars with specific daily instructions. It may have names of co-workers and supervisors that the worker has trouble remembering, and contact information for the vocational specialist or other support staff. It may include a section to write down problems or questions to bring to a supervisor, vocational specialist, or group. Accommodations in the workplace (e.g., shorter schedules, more breaks, quiet work space) can also be developed based on the WBI and VCRS; their effectiveness can be determined, and strategies can be refined as needed.

Finally, work feedback and goal setting can be combined with the other psychological interventions described in the following paragraphs. It is a procedure that is suitable to transitional and supported employment programs, directly addressing some of the illness-specific problems of workers with schizophrenia spectrum disorders.

Cognitive Behavior Therapy has been most specifically adapted to vocational rehabilitation in the Indianapolis Vocation Intervention Program (IVIP; Lysaker, Bond, Davis, & Bryson, 2005). IVIP targets beliefs and behaviors that interfere in sustaining work. These include beliefs like having the expectation of being rejected no matter what the worker does or having a behavioral tendency to be verbally aggressive when criticized. Groups are used to teach didactic material, and individual sessions are used to apply those to weekly work experience. The curriculum covers thinking errors (e.g., self-defeating beliefs), problem-solving methods, coping with emotions, learning from feedback, effective self-expression, self-appraisal of strengths and weaknesses, and managing success. Individual counseling focuses on reviewing and applying these lessons within a therapeutic alliance that motivates change. Initially, four self-defeating beliefs are identified collaboratively.

At each session, workers report on how well they accomplished their between-session assignments related to changing these beliefs and give a brief update of the past work week including any mental health concerns. Written practice assignments from the lessons are also reviewed. Using these methods, workers with schizophrenia spectrum disorders learn to identify and monitor their own thoughts and behaviors regarding work. They learn to recognize the links between their thoughts, feelings, and behaviors and to explore and change how they see themselves and work. They can use the individual sessions to create a narrative of their illness and recovery in relation to work that enables them to persist at work and to sustain their hope and enthusiasm over time.

Neurocognitive and Social Cognitive Training: A growing body of evidence has identified cognitive impairments as one of the main sources of functional loss and disability in schizophrenia and related disorders (Green, 1996). Cognitive impairments are common and often precede onset of illness, and these impairments may be linked to core neurobiological substrates of the disorder. The relationship between cognition and work outcomes has also been amply demonstrated (McGurk & Mueser, 2006). Recently, research has begun to focus on social cognition as an important area for investigation, particularly in understanding social dysfunction related to mental illness. Social cognition includes such abilities as emotion recognition, theory of mind, cognitive and emotional empathy, and social attribution bias. Although these aspects of mental life may be dependent on neurocognition, they appear to have explanatory power of their own (Couture, Penn, & Roberts, 2006). For example, in one study, social cognition measures explained vocational outcomes independent of neurocognition (Bell et al., 2009), and there is evidence that social cognition plays an important role in social-skills deficits (Bell, Fiszdon, Greig, & Wexler, 2010; Mueser et al., 1996). Several small intervention studies to address social cognition have been reported, and more are underway (Fiszdon & Reddy, 2012).

Programs to remediate neurocognitive impairments (programs such as CogPak; Brain HQ; PSS Cog Rehab) have gained increased attention with several meta-analyses generally supporting their efficacy (e.g., Wykes, Huddy, Cellard, McGurk, & Czobor, 2011). These methods rely principally on computer-based drill and practice to increase performance.

Several approaches that integrate neurocognitive training with vocational rehabilitation include Thinking Skills for Work (TSW; McGurk & Mueser, 2005), Neurcognitive Enhancement Therapy (NET; Bell, Bryson, Greig, Corcoran, & Wexler, 2001), and Integrated Psychological Therapy (IPT; Roder, Muller, Brenner, & Spalding, 2010); and NET and IPT also have social cognitive training groups included. They have all demonstrated improved cognitive functioning and better functional and work outcomes during follow up (McGurk, Mueser, Feldman, Wolfe, & Pascaris, 2007; Bell, Zito, Greig, &

Wexler, 2008; Mueller, Schmidt, & Roder, 2015). At least one study suggests that this approach may be particularly important for people with poor community function and may be less necessary for others (Bell, Choi, Dyer, & Wexler, 2014).

Although these approaches differ in regard to which neurocognitive and social cognitive training approaches are used, how long they are used, and how they are integrated into vocational rehabilitation, they share the core elements of cognitive training and some type of group experience that relates their cognitive training to vocational goals. Preliminary evidence suggests that this type of approach may be particularly effective with people in their first episode (Ventura et al., 2011).

Work Related Social Skills Training takes advantage of behavioral learning methods such as errorless learning, shaping, and social modeling and can thereby change behavior despite cognitive limitations (Liberman, 2008). One example of skills training that takes full advantage of these methods is a recently developed computer-based virtual reality job-interview training program (www.jobinterviewtraining.net). It uses implicit learning through repetition of role plays to improve performance, shaping behavior through feedback and reward, and scaffolding difficulty to optimize challenge while reducing error and discouragement. But, as important as it is to practice job-interview skills, people must also learn to overcome their fear of going on job interviews if they are to ever use those skills. Almost everyone is anxious to some degree when they go on a job interview, but for people with schizophrenia spectrum disorders this fear can be a significant barrier to their vocational success. The computer-based simulations help people overcome this fear through repeated exposure, taking advantage of the basic principles of exposure therapy (Wolpe, 1969). Virtual reality role play allows repeated exposure to the feared stimulus in a safe environment in which the trainee can exercise maximum control and gradually gain an increasing sense of mastery. People with schizophrenia spectrum disorder readily accept this virtual reality training (Bell & Weinstein, 2011), and in one study, they were significantly more likely to receive job offers than those that were randomized to usual vocational services (Smith et al., 2015).

Social skills training more broadly is an evidence-based practice that is aimed at improving social competence across a range of different areas, such as the quality of social relationships, job performance, or interacting with healthcare professionals (Heinssen, Liberman, & Kopelowicz, 2000; Dilk & Bond, 1996). All such programs involve teaching complex social skills by breaking them down into smaller steps and practicing the skills in role plays and in community settings. Work Place Fundamentals is a video-assisted training curricula developed by the UCLA Social and Independent Living Skills Program that focuses on learning and practicing fundamental problem-solving skills in the workplace. Using easy to understand language, the program talks about the "Gives" (what is expected of you) and "Gets" (what you can expect to receive) of work and the "Sweats" (your challenges) and "No-Sweats" (your worker strengths) at work. Videos are shown of work situations to promote discussion and to illustrate teaching points. For example, an employee who does not know how to do a task approaches a supervisor for help, but he refuses, saying he's too busy. Group members are asked about what they would do and brainstorm alternatives, and then weigh their pros and cons (Liberman, 2008, p. 388). This training has been used with SE to help people get more out of their job experience and to enhance job tenure. The program teaches three broad skill sets: identifying key procedures in the workplace (Gives and Gets), becoming alert to problems (Sweats), and finding ways to solve problems (mental and physical health, substance abuse, interactions with supervisors and co-workers, work performance, and motivation). To promote using these skills in the workplace, Liberman and colleagues developed In Vivo Amplified Skills Training (IVAST). IVAST uses a specialist case manager who provides community-based instruction to help generalize the lessons learned in Work Place Fundamentals (Liberman, Glynn, Blair, Ross, & Marder, 2002). Evidence for this approach is still accumulating, but one study found that knowledge and skills were retained over 18 months, and there was less job turnover and greater job satisfaction for those in SE who received this training as compared to SE alone (Wallace & Tauber, 2004).

CONCLUSIONS

Since moral treatment in the nineteenth century, American psychiatry has recognized the healing potential of productive activity. Today, families, consumers, and professionals want paid employment of some kind to be a goal of integrated psychiatric care for most people with schizophrenia spectrum disorders because it promotes recovery and social reintegration. A spectrum of vocational services has developed that offers various opportunities for employment. These services differ in the amount of support they provide, the demands for performance, and their degree of integration into the world of competitive employment. For younger people experiencing their first episode of schizophrenia spectrum disorder, having SE integrated into their treatment team may make it more likely that they can continue in their career path and not suffer the painful and deteriorating effects of unemployment. Employment services may be enhanced with other interventions that address neurocognitive, social-cognitive, and social-skills deficits in order to help people get jobs, keep them and gain greater satisfaction from them.

Although many of the interventions described in this chapter have only been developed in the past two or three decades, and although there is much more to learn about them and how they may work together, there is enough empirical support to warrant wider dissemination. By doing so, many more people with schizophrenia spectrum disorder can get the help they need to lead a more productive life. Their recovery will be aided by reintegration into a meaningful social role that gives them personal satisfaction and greater economic and social independence.

REFERENCES

Azrin, N. H., & Philip, R. A. (1979). The job club method for the job handicapped: A comparative outcome study. *Rehabilitation Counseling Bulletin, 23*(2), 144–155.

Becker, D. R., Drake, R. E., & Naughton, W. (2005). Supported employment for people with co-occurring disorders. *Psychiatric Rehabilitation Journal., 28*, 332–338.

Bell, M. D., Bryson, G., Greig, T., Corcoran, C., & Wexler, B. E. (2001). Neurocognitive enhancement therapy with work therapy: effects on neuropsychological test performance. *Archives of General Psychiatry, 58*(8), 763–768.

Bell, M. D., Choi, J., & Lysaker, P. (2007). Psychological interventions to improve work outcomes for people with psychiatric disabilities. *Journal of the Norwegian Psychological Association, 44*, 606–617.

Bell, M.D., Choi, K., Dyer, C., & Wexler, B. (2014). Benefits of cognitive remediation and supported employment for schizophrenia patients with poor community functioning. *Psychiatric Services, 65*(4), 469–475.

Bell, M. D., Fiszdon, J. M., Greig, T. C., & Wexler, B. E. (2010). Social attribution test—multiple choice (SAT-MC) in schizophrenia: comparison with community sample and relationship to neurocognitive, social cognitive and symptom measure. *Schizophrenia Research, 122*(1–3): 164–171.

Bell, M. D, & Lysaker, P. H. (1997). Clinical benefits of paid work activity in schizophrenia: 1-year followup. *Schizophrenia Bulletin, 23*(2), 317–328.

Bell, M. D., Lysaker, P. H., & Milstein, R. M. (1996). Clinical benefits of paid work activity in schizophrenia. *Schizophrenia Bulletin, 22*(1), 51–67.

Bell, M. D., Tsang, H. W. H., Greig, T. C., & Bryson, G. J. (2009). Neurocognition, social cognition, perceived social discomfort, and vocational outcomes in schizophrenia. *Schizophrenia Bulletin, 35*(4), 738–747.

Bell, M. D., & Weinstein, A. (2011). Simulated job interview skill training for people with psychiatric disability: Feasibility and tolerability of virtual reality training. *Schizophrenia Bulletin*, 37 (Suppl 2) S91–S97.

Bell, M. D., Zito, W., Greig, T., & Wexler, B. E. (2008). Neurocognitive enhancement therapy with vocational services: Work outcomes at two-year follow-up. *Schizophrenia Research, 105*, 18–29.

Bond, G. R., Campbell, K., Evans, L. J., Gervey, R., Pascaris, A., Tice, S.,. . . Revell, G. (2002). A scale to measure quality of supported employment for persons with severe mental illness. *Journal of Vocational Rehabilitation, 17*, 239–250.

Bond, G. R., Drake, R. E., & Becker, D. R. (2008). An update on randomized controlled trials of evidence-based supported employment. *Psychiatric Rehabilitation Journal, 31*(4), 280–290.

Brigham, A. (1994). The moral treatment of insanity. 1847. *American Journal of Psychiatry, 151*, 10–15.

Bryson, G., Bell, M. D., Kaplan, E., & Greig, T. (1999). The Work Behavior Inventory: Prediction of future work success of people with schizophrenia. *Psychiatric Rehabilitation Journal*, 23 (2), 113–120.

Bryson, G., Bell, M.D., Lysaker, P.H., & Zito, W. (1997). The Work Behavior Inventory: A scale for the assessment of work behavior for clients with severe mental illness. *Psychiatric Rehabilitation Journal, 20*, 47–55.

Ciardiello, J. A., & Bell, M. D. (1988). *Vocational rehabilitation of persons with prolonged psychiatric disorders.* Baltimore, MD: Johns Hopkins University Press.

Cook, J. A., Leff, H. S., Blyler, C. R., Gold, P. B., Goldberg, R. W., Mueser, K. T.,. . .Burke-Miller, J. (2005). Results of a multisite randomized trial of supported employment interventions for individuals with severe mental illness. *Archives of General Psychiatry, 62*(5), 505–512.

Couture, S. M., Penn, D. L., & Roberts, D. L. (2006). The functional significance of social cognition in schizophrenia: a review. *Schizophrenia Bulletin*, 32(Suppl 1), S44–S63.

Dilk, M. N., & Bond, G. R. (1996). Meta-analytic evaluation of skills training research for individuals with severe mental illness. *Journal of Consulting and Clinical Psychology, 64*, 1337–1346.

Drake, R. E., Bond, G. R., & Becker, D. R. (2012). *Individual placement and support an evidence-based approach to supported employment*. New York, NY: Oxford University Press.

Drake, R. E., Xie, H., Bond, G. R., Mchugo, G .J., & Caton, C. L. (2013). Early psychosis and employment. *Schizophrenia Research, 146*, 111–117.

Fiszdon, J. M., & Reddy, L. F. (2012). Review of social cognitive treatments for psychosis. *Clinical Psychology Review, 32*(8), 724–740.

Green, M. F. (1996). What are the functional consequences of neurocognitive deficits in schizophrenia? *American Journal of Psychiatry, 153*(3), 321–330.

Greig, T. C., Bryson, G. J., & Bell, M. D. (2004). Theory of mind performance in schizophrenia: diagnostic, symptom, and neuropsychological correlates. *Journal of Nervous and Mental Disease, 192*(1), 12–18.

Heinssen, R. K., Liberman, R. P., & Kopelowicz, A. (2000). Psychosocial skills training for schizophrenia: Lessons from the laboratory. *Schizophrenia Bulletin, 26*(1), 21–46.

Locke, E. A., & Latham, G. P. (2002). Building a practically useful theory of goal setting and task motivation: A 35-year odyssey. *American Psychologist, 57*(9), 705–717.

Liberman, R. P. (2008). *Recovery from disability: manual of psychiatric rehabilitation*. Washington, DC: American Psychiatric Publishing.

Liberman, R. P., Glynn, S., Blair, K. E., Ross, D., & Marder, S. R. (2002). In vivo amplified skills training: Promoting generalization of independent living skills for clients with schizophrenia. *Psychiatry, 65*(2), 137–155.

Lysaker, P. H., & Bell, M. D. (1995a). Prominent negative symptoms and work impairment in schizophrenia. *Acta Psychiatrica Scandinavica, 91*, 205–208.

Lysaker, P. H., & Bell, M. D. (1995b). Work and meaning: Disturbance of volition and vocational dysfunction in schizophrenia. *Psychiatry, 58*(4), 392–400.

Lysaker, P. H., Bond, G., Davis, L.W., Bryson, G. J., & Bell, M. D. (2005). Enhanced cognitive behavioral therapy for vocational rehabilitation in schizophrenia: effects on hope and work. *Journal of Rehabilitation Research and Development, 42*(5), 673–682.

Marrone, J., & Golowka, E. (1999). If work makes people with mental illness sick, what do unemployment, poverty, and social isolation cause? *Psychiatric Rehabilitation Journal, 23*(2), 187–193.

McGurk, S. R., & Mueser, K. T. (2005). *Thinking skills for work: An integrated program for cognitive rehabilitation and supported employment*. Concord, NH: Dartmouth Psychiatric Research Center.

McGurk, S. R., & Mueser, K. T. (2006). Cognitive and clinical predictors of work outcomes in clients with schizophrenia receiving supported employment services: 4-year follow-up. *Administration and Policy in Mental Health and Mental Health Services Research, 33* (5) 598–606.

McGurk, S. R., Mueser, K. T., Feldman, K., Wolfe, R., & Pascaris, A. (2007). Cognitive training for supported employment: 2–3 Year outcomes of a randomized controlled trial. *American Journal of Psychiatry, 164*(3), 437–441.

Mueller, D. R., Schmidt, S. J., Roder, V. (2015). One-year randomized controlled trial and follow-up of integrated neurocognitive therapy for schizophrenia outpatients. *Schizophrenia Bulletin, 41(3)*, 604–616.

Mueser, K. T., Doonan, R., Penn, D. L., Blanchard, J. J., Bellack, A. S., Nishith, P., & DeLeon, J. (1996). Emotion recognition and social competence in chronic schizophrenia. *Journal of Abnormal Psychology, 105*(2), 271–275.

Penk, W., Drebing, C. E., Rosenheck, R. A., Krebs, C., Van Ormer, A., & Mueller, L. (2010). Veteran Health Administration transitional work experience vs. job placement in veterans with co-morbid substance use and non-psychotic psychiatric disorders. *Psychiatric Rehabilitation Journal, 33*(4), 297–307.

President's New Freedom Commission on Mental Health. (2003). *Achieving the promise: Transforming mental health care in America: Final report.* (DHHS Pub. No. SMA-03-3832). Rockville, MD: Substance Abuse and Mental Health Services Administration.

Razzano, L. A., Cook, J. A., Burke-Miller, J. K., Mueser, K. T., Pickett-Schenk, S. A., Grey, D. D.,. . .Ann Carey, M. (2005). Clinical factors associated with employment among people with severe mental illness: Findings from the employment intervention demonstration program. *Journal of Nervous & Mental Disease, 19* (11), 705–713.

Roder, V., Muller, D. R., Brenner, H. D., Spaulding, W. D. (2010). *Integrated Psychological Therapy (ITP) for the treatment of neurocognition, social cognition and social competency in schizophrenia patients*. Gottingen, Germany: The Hogrefe Group.

Smith, M. J., Fleming, M. F., Wright, M., Jordan, N., Humm, L. B., Olsen, D., Bell, M. D. (2015). Job offers among individuals with severe mental illness after virtual reality job interview training. *Psychiatric Services, 66*, 1173–1179. PMID: 26130002.

Ventura, J., Subotnik, K. L., Guzik, L. H., Hellemann, G. S., Gitlin, M. J., Wood, R. C., Nuechterlein, K. H. (2011). Remission and recovery during the first outpatient year of the early course of schizophrenia. *Schizophrenia Research, 132*(1), 18–23.

Wallace, C. J., Tauber, R. (2004). Supplementing supported employment with workplace skills training. *Psychiatric Services, 55*(5), 513–515.

Warner, R. (1985). *Recovery from schizophrenia: Psychiatry and the political economy*. New York, NY: Routledge and Kegan Paul.

Warner, R., & Mandiberg, J. (2006). An update on affirmative businesses or social firms for people with mental illness. *Psychiatric Service, 57*(10), 1488–1492.

Warr, P.B. (1987). *Work, unemployment and mental health*. Gloucestershire, England: Clarendon Press.

Wolpe, J. (1969). *The practice of behavior therapy*. Elmsford, NY: Pergamon Press.

Wykes, T., Huddy, V., Cellard, C., McGurk, S. R., & Czobor, P. (2011). A meta-analysis of cognitive remediation for schizophrenia: methodology and effect size. *American Journal of Psychiatry, 168*(5), 472–485.

/// 20 /// STIGMA AND ITS IMPACT ON SCHIZOPHRENIA AND RELATED DISORDERS

SUE ABDERHOLDEN, LAURA PIENTKA, and S. CHARLES SCHULZ

INTRODUCTION

The majority of this volume has focused on several important aspects of mental illnesses from research in cognition to psychosocial treatments to evidence of the application of medication. These aspects are all a part of a multifactorial approach to treating people diagnosed with mental illnesses. However, an essential part of the care of the person living with a mental illness requires the recognition and consideration of the stigma surrounding mental health diagnoses.

WHAT IS STIGMA?

Stigma has been described as

> . . .a cluster of negative attitudes and beliefs that motivate the general public to fear, reject, avoid, and discriminate against people with mental illness.
>
> New Freedom Commission on Mental Health, p. 4, 2003

Despite many advances in the understanding and treatment of serious mental illnesses, stigma continues to be a significant barrier that precludes many individuals from getting the effective treatments and support they need. "Responding to stigma, people with mental health problems internalize public attitudes and become so embarrassed or ashamed that they often conceal symptoms and fail to seek treatment (New Freedom Commission on Mental Health, p. 4, 2003).

Due to stigma:

- People live an average of 10 years with their symptoms before seeking help.
- Only 60 percent of people with a severe mental illness actually receive treatment.
- A person's life span is reduced by an average of 20 years.

Furthermore, a survey of people with mental illnesses and their families, "identified stigma as one of the major barriers that discourage adults with mental illnesses, and the families of children and adolescents with serious emotional disorders, from seeking treatment," (U.S. Dept of Health and Human Services, 1999) and without treatment there is no relief from symptoms and negative impact on people's lives.

This chapter will focus on the stigma associated with mental illnesses, examine the causes, the impacts, and ways to change misconceptions associated with mental illnesses.

PERCEPTION OF MENTAL ILLNESSES

Perception is one the major factors contributing to the stigma surrounding serious mental illnesses. Many non-mental health diagnoses are generally viewed as "physical" illnesses that are associated with a specific dysfunction within an organ system or a disease process.

For instance, people with other types of illnesses such as cancer are often described characteristically as, "brave," "courageous," or "inspirational." People diagnosed with serious mental illness, however, are often described with derogatory terms such as "crazy," "loony," "dangerous" and with characteristics of being "lazy," "incompetent," and the "cause of their own illness."

In contrast to the characteristics associated with non-mental health diagnoses, the attributes associated with mental health diagnoses may imply that the illness may not be due to a dysfunction of an organ system or a disease process but rather caused by an inherent character flaw. (Kendell, 2001).

A report on mental health authored by the Surgeon General (U.S. Department of Healh and Human Services, 1999) stated that, "... everyday language tends to encourage a misperception that 'mental health' or 'mental illness' is unrelated to 'physical health' or 'physical illness'... In fact, the two are inseparable."

A quote from the British Journal of Psychiatry stated that, "[some people] assume that developing a mental illness is evidence of certain lack of moral fiber and if they really tried, people with illnesses of this kind ought to be able to control their anxieties ... But there is no reason, justified either by logic or by medical standing, why people suffering from, say phobic anxiety or depression should be able to exert more control over their symptoms than those suffering from myxedema or migraine. There is a further and equally damaging assumption that the symptoms of mental disorders are in some sense less 'real' than those of physical disorders with a tangible local pathology."

Recently, however, Reavley and Jorm (2014) published a survey study conducted in Australia that found some improvements within the opinions and perceptions of people living with schizophrenia. When compared to earlier surveys, it was noted that mental illnesses were felt to be associated with problems in childhood and inherited or genetic causes. It was also noted that there was a decrease in beliefs that mental illnesses are related to weakness or character abnormalities (Reavley & Jorm, 2014).

These findings demonstrate that the general understanding of serious mental illnesses may be gradually evolving from previously being viewed as weaknesses in character to being seen now as actual medical conditions.

STIGMA AND THE MEDIA

In addition to better understanding of mental illnesses as a true medical condition, the media can play a significant role in reducing stigma. Television shows, newspapers, social media, and music may influence millions of people on a daily basis and affect the perceptions and attitudes toward mental illnesses. Even advertisements can promote products using descriptions such as "crazy," "loco" "schizo" or "psychotic" at the expense of those with mental illnesses.

The media has a major impact in perpetuating stereotypes of violence and may contribute to an overall fear of people with mental illnesses. From hysterical, disheveled people living with a mental illness, to prison-like psychiatric wards and institutions, straitjackets, barbaric ECT treatments, and mind-numbing medications, these are the frightening images often associated with mental illnesses.

In fact, often characters with mental illnesses on television shows are portrayed as:

- Highly correlated with violent crime.
- Ten times more violent than other TV characters.
- Ten to twenty times more violent than in reality.
- Have a negative impact on society and a negative quality of life.

In addition, sensationalized news headlines, newspaper articles, and press about people with mental illnesses lead to further stereotyping, fear, and prejudice.

Based on a study published by UC Berkley, however, after a review of 305 violent events in the United States, only 12 percent were preceded by psychosis. "High-profile mass shootings capture public attention and increase vigilance of people with mental illness. But our findings clearly show that psychosis rarely leads directly to violence," said study lead author Jennifer Skeem, associate dean of research at University of California, Berkeley's School of Social Welfare (Anwar, 2015; Skeem, Kennealy, Monahan, Peterson, & Appelbaum, 2015).

This demonstrates the need for replacement of stereotypes that insinuate violence and dangerousness associated with people with mental illnesses with more accurate representation in the media.

THE IMPACT OF STIGMA ON PEOPLE LIVING WITH MENTAL ILLNESSES

Thus far, this chapter has discussed how the perception and media can influence opinions about mental illnesses. It is essential to remember, however, above all else, how stigma can affect people themselves as well as their loved ones. In a recent survey of people with a psychiatric illness it was found that 89 percent had experienced some discrimination because of having a mental illness. (Sarkin et al., 2014).

Dr. Mary Gullekson a psychologist (in Fink & Tasman, 1992) discusses her experience with her brother's schizophrenia and stigma:

> For me stigma means fear, resulting in a lack of confidence. Stigma is loss, resulting in unresolved mourning issues. Stigma is not having access to resources resulting in lack of useful coping skills. Stigma is being invisible or being reviled, resulting in conflicts regarding been seen. Stigma is lowered family esteem and intense shame, resulting in decreased self-worth. Stigma is secrecy, resulting in lack of understanding. Stigma is divisive, resulting in distrust of others. Stigma is anger, resulting in distance. Most importantly, stigma is hopelessness, resulting in helplessness. This all adds up to decreased potential, of self and for others.

Furthermore, when people with mental illnesses want to participate in activities of everyday life, they are still often faced with significant barriers. "Stigma leads others to avoid living, socializing, or working with, renting to, or employing people with mental disorders—especially severe disorders, such as schizophrenia" (New Freedom Commission on Mental Health, 2003, p. 4).

For instance, people with mental illnesses may face discrimination when applying for jobs and, as a result, 75 percent of people with schizophrenia are not currently in the workforce. People may face barriers to obtaining safe, affordable housing due to limited income. Additionally, for those who need it, they may live in a state that does not provide the in-home supports that would make it possible for people to live independently in the community. People with serious mental illnesses also report that they may have difficulty making friends or discussing their mental illness with others leading to a feeling of being isolated and alone. Outside of family members, it may be challenging for them to find others that might relate to their experience.

Not only can stigma affect how others view people with mental illness, it may also affect how they view themselves. Discrimination and negative labels can lead to internalization and identification with these labels creating a self-stigmatization. One article (Corrigan, Larson, & Rusch, 2009) discusses the process of self-stigmatization, which requires an awareness of a stereotype, agreement with it, and application to one's self. This leads to low self-esteem and often avoidance of activities of everyday life. This can lead to thoughts of "Why even bother?" or "Why even try?" "If others think I'm irresponsible, why even bother trying to get a job or live or alone?" This shows how stereotypes and negative public opinion of mental illness can contribute to low self-esteem, self-stigmatization and avoidance of opportunities of daily life.

IMPACT OF STIGMA ON THE FAMILIES OF PEOPLE LIVING WITH MENTAL ILLNESSES

The effect of mental illnesses on the entire family cannot be underestimated. Family members are often an essential part of a person's support group. However, the stigma surrounding mental illnesses can be very painful for not only the person with the diagnosis but for their family members as well. It has been shown that stigma and discrimination can lead to fewer community supports for people living with mental illnesses and their families such as fewer get well cards, less help with child care or fewer meals being brought over.

One person noted a very different reaction when her husband was hospitalized for heart disease and when he was hospitalized for depression. When he was treated with depression no one came to visit or called, and no meals were delivered.

Families may even feel lack of support from their loved one's provider. In surveys done for Mona Wasow's book *The Skipping Stone—Ripple Effects of Mental Illness on the Family* (1995), spouses saw little help from professionals: "They see us as the enemy. We are never told anything. Hiding behind the confidentiality issue—they never tell me what is going on." She also found that families are put in a no-win situation. If they ask questions about the treatment, professionals see them encroaching on confidentiality laws. If they say nothing, they are seen as uncaring.

Providers can help families feel more supported by continuing to improve their communication and connection with families. Engaging families means listening to and answering their questions. Families have stated that their goal in asking questions and discussing their loved one's illness with the doctor is to:

- Reduce anxiety and confusion.
- Determine appropriate expectation for their loved one.
- Learn how to motivate their relative to do more.
- Find out about the nature of serious brain disorders.
- Assure accessibility to a professional during a crisis.
- Understand the diagnosis and prognosis.
- Understand symptoms, medications, and side effects.
- Get specific suggestions for coping with problem behaviors.
- Deal with practical issues.
- Make contact with peer support groups.

When families are not engaged, people with serious mental illnesses often end up alone, vulnerable, homeless, or in the criminal justice system without someone to support or advocate for them.

Families can be essential in successful treatment; they know what medications and levels were used in the past and what worked and what didn't work. They can provide a list of the person's strengths, talents, and preferences. They know the history of the illness, the relapses, and the hospitalizations. They are a dependable early-warning system to relapse. They can keep you up to date on your client's day-to-day moods, problems, and progress. They know how their loved one has acted in the past and what worked and what did not. They are a reliable source for information on drug or alcohol use. One woman stated that, after living with her husband who has bipolar disorder for over 10 years, she was able to detect problems very early compared to the doctor who only saw him once every several months. Families want to be respected for their expertise and want to develop collaborative relationships with their loved one's doctor and treatment team.

The nonstigmatizing engagement of family further helps in areas for people with schizophrenia by addressing:

- Advice and encouragement.
- Family's ability to recognize early reemergence of symptoms.
- Advocating for the person in clinics, schools, and workplace.

In order to enable the families to provide this unstigmatized support, engaged clinicians can truly help by:

- Encouraging interactions to maintain hope of the person's outcome.
- Validating their worries.
- Diminishing any stigmatizing issue of families.
- Offering caring communication as some families feel stigmatized.

MOVING AHEAD FROM STIGMA

After discussing the significant impact stigma has on individuals and their families, it is important to consider ways to reduce stigma. In order to reduce stigma, it is important to start by changing how mental illnesses are viewed, talked about, and thought about.

The report, *Mental Health: A Report of the Surgeon General,* stated that "Promoting mental health for all Americans will require scientific know-how but, even more importantly, a societal resolve that we will make the needed investment. The investment does not call for massive budgets; rather, it calls for the willingness of each of us to educate ourselves and others about mental health and mental illness, and thus to confront the attitudes, fear, and misunderstanding that remain as barriers before us."

One way to reduce stigmatization and the negative impact it has is through the use of people-first language. There are many offensive terms associated with serious mental illnesses—especially schizophrenia. Removing hurtful and judgmental words such as "crazy" or "nuts" from a person's everyday language is a simple but important step forward. Moreover, clinicians may focus on connecting people living with mental illnesses with their care by not using terms such as "compliance" but vocabulary such as "adherence." Others have noted that calling a person schizophrenic may cause a person to feel defined solely by their illness and not as an individual. The phrase "a person living with schizophrenia" can be much more thoughtful.

In addition, Corrigan and Penn (1999) suggested three strategies to reduce stigma: education, contact, and protest. Education focuses on better understanding of mental illness in order to dispel any misconceptions. Contact emphasizes, ". . .challenging public attitudes about mental illness through direct interactions with persons who have these disorders." Protest involves advocating for change in the way mental health is portrayed in the media and working to promote more positive and accurate representations of people with mental health.

PROMOTING RECOVERY

In addition to recognizing and reducing stigma, the promotion of recovery should always be the highest priority. Promoting recovery involves fully connecting with people with mental illnesses and their families. NAMI has recommended that the first steps in this area are empowerment and a holistic approach.

In regards to empowerment, the whole team focuses on what the individual wants, including what their goals are and making it person-centered by focusing on their unique strengths and needs, preferences, and culture. The individual needs to participate in the decision making rather than have decisions made by others. Peer support and having a sense of belonging may also be helpful for promoting recovery.

An example of a program's empowerment is illustrated in the following case:

> *A young man with the diagnosis of schizophrenia was not responding to front-line antipsychotic medications. Unfortunately this led to homelessness and no support. He was arrested for taking food in a grocery store—he could not afford to purchase food. The police department referred him to a comprehensive schizophrenia program, which updated his medication to clozapine, engaged him in individual and group therapies, and helped him meet his goals. This young man graduated from a junior college,with a computer major, and became full-time employed doing this work for a company.*

This story demonstrates how engaging an individual in their treatment, utilizing peer support, and focusing on the individual's strengths and goals can lead to a successful recovery.

CONCLUSION

Stigma remains a major issue that continues to significantly impact people with mental illnesses as well as their families. Even as the fields of psychiatry and psychology advance the understanding of serious mental illnesses, education, advocacy, and willingness to challenge misconceptions related to mental illnesses are needed to reduce the fear and discrimination caused by stigma. This can lead to better support and thus better outcomes for people with mental illnesses and their families.

REFERENCES

Anwar, Y. (2015). Psychotic hallucinations, delusions rarely precede violence. [Berkley News Center]. Retrieved from http://news.berkeley.edu/2015/05/11/psychosisandviolence/

Corrigan, P. W., Larson, J. E., & Rusch, N. (2009). Self-stigma and the "why try" effect: impact on life goals and evidence-based practices. *World Psychiatry*, *8*(2), 75–81.

Corrigan, P. W. & Penn, D. L. (1999). Lessons from social psychology on discrediting psychiatric stigma. *American Psychologist*, *54*, 765–776.

Fink, P. J. & Tasman, A. (1992). *Stigma and mental illness*. Arlington, VA: American Psychiatric.

Kendell, R.E. (2001). The distinction between mental and physical illness. *The British Journal of Psychiatry*, *178*(6) 490–493

New Freedom Commission on Mental Health, Achieving the Promise: Transforming Mental Health Care in America. (2003). Final Report. DHHS Pub. No. SMA-03-3832. Rockville, Md.

Reavley, N. J. & Jorm, A. F. (2014). The Au stralian public's beliefs about the causes of schizophrenia: Associated factors and change over 16 years. *Psychiatry Research*, *220*(1-2):609–614.

Sarkin, A., Lale, R., Sklar, M., Center, K. C., Gilmer, T., Fowler, C., ... & Ojeda, V. D. (2014). Stigma experienced by people using mental health services in San Diego County. *Social Psychiatry and Psychiatric Epidemiology*, *50*(5), 747–756.

Skeem, J., Kennealy, P., Monahan, J., Peterson, J., & Appelbaum, P. (2015). Psychosis uncommonly and inconsistently precedes violence among high-risk individuals. *Clinical Psychological Science*, DOI:10.1177/2167702615575879

U.S. Department of Health and Human Services. (1999). *Mental Health: A Report of the Surgeon General*. Rockville, MD: U.S. Department of Health and Human Services, Substance Abuse and Mental Health Services Administration, Center for Mental Health Services, National Institutes of Health, National Institute of Mental Health.

Wasow, M. (1995). *The skipping stone: Ripple effects of mental illness on the family*. Palo Alto, CA: Science & Behavior Books.

REFERENCES

INDEX

Page numbers followed by *b*, *f* or *t* indicate boxes, figures, or tables, respectively.